Blind in Early Modern Japan

Corporealities: Discourses of Disability

Series editors: David T. Mitchell and Sharon L. Snyder

Recent Titles

A complete list of titles in the series can be found at www.press.umich.edu

Blind in Early Modern Japan

Disability, Medicine, and Identity

WEI YU WAYNE TAN

University of Michigan Press
Ann Arbor

Copyright © 2022 by Wei Yu Wayne Tan
All rights reserved

For questions or permissions, please contact um.press.perms@umich.edu

Published in the United States of America by the
University of Michigan Press
Printed and bound by CPI Group (UK) Ltd, Croydon, CR0 4YY

First published September 2022

A CIP catalog record for this book is available from the British Library.

Library of Congress Cataloging-in-Publication Data

Names: Tan, Wei Yu Wayne, author. | University of Michigan. Press, publisher.
Title: Blind in early modern japan : disability, medicine, and identity / Wei Yu
    Wayne Tan.
Other titles: Corporealities.
Description: Ann Arbor : University of Michigan Press, [2022] | Series:
    Corporealities: discourses of disability | Includes bibliographical references
    and index.
Identifiers: LCCN 2022009825 (print) | LCCN 2022009826 (ebook) |
    ISBN 9780472075485 (hardcover) | ISBN 9780472055487
    (paperback) | ISBN 9780472220434 (ebook)
Subjects: LCSH: Blind—Japan—Social conditions—Edo period, 1600–
    1868. | Blind—Japan—Occupations—Edo period, 1600–1868. | Guilds—
    Japan—Edo period, 1600–1868. | Ophthalmology—Japan—History.
Classification: LCC HV2113 .T26 2022 (print) | LCC HV2113 (ebook) |
    DDC 362.4/10952—dc23/eng/20220525
LC record available at https://lccn.loc.gov/2022009825
LC ebook record available at https://lccn.loc.gov/2022009826

Publication of this volume has been partially funded by Hope College.

Cover illustration: *A Blind Musician Plays the Koto to a Gathering of Women Dressed
in Ornate Kimonos*, by Utagawa Kuniyoshi (1849/1852); from the Wellcome
Collection.

The image on this book's cover is a colorful illustration divided into three
panels that depicts a bearded, blind musician on the right playing the *koto*
(a Japanese stringed musical instrument) to entertain nine women, one
man, and a dog. The women's kimonos feature fine embroidery and other
embellishments. The dog (also in finery) rests upon a pillow at the center of
the image. The cover is red on the left side with the title displayed above the
illustration. The right side is a gray band where the subtitle appears opposite
the title. The author's name (Wei Yu Wayne Tan) appears in the red half below
the illustration.

Contents

Digital materials related to this title can be found on
the fulcrum platform via the following citable URL:
https://doi.org/10.3998/mpub.9769233

Illustrations

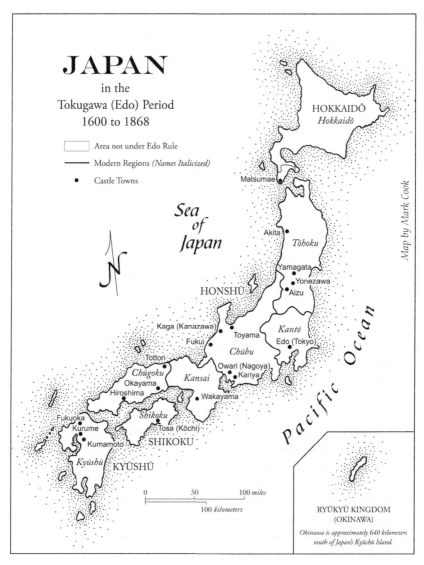

JAPAN

in the
Tokugawa (Edo) Period
1600 to 1868

Area not under Edo Rule

—— Modern Regions *(Names Italicized)*

• Castle Towns

Sea of Japan

HOKKAIDŌ
Hokkaidō

Matsumae

Akita

Tōhoku

Yamagata
Yonezawa
Aizu

HONSHŪ

Kaga (Kanazawa)
Fukui
Toyama
Kantō
Edo (Tokyo)
Chūbu
Tottori
Owari (Nagoya)
Kariya
Chūgoku
Kansai
Okayama
Hiroshima
Wakayama
Fukuoka
Shikoku
Kurume
Tosa (Kōchi)
Kumamoto
SHIKOKU
Kyūshū KYŪSHŪ

Pacific Ocean

0   50   100 *miles*

100 *kilometers*

RYŪKYŪ KINGDOM
(OKINAWA)

*Okinawa is approximately 640 kilometers
south of Japan's Kyūshū Island.*

Map by Mark Cook

Japan in the Tokugawa (Edo) Period, 1600–1868. Map created by Mark Cook.

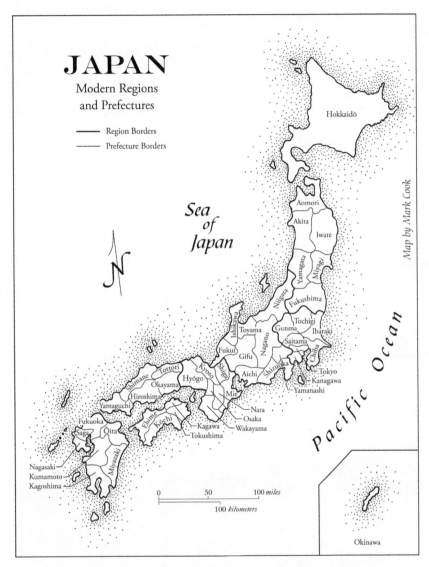

JAPAN
Modern Regions and Prefectures

—— Region Borders
— Prefecture Borders

Sea
of
Japan

N

Map by Mark Cook

Pacific Ocean

Hokkaidō

Aomori
Akita
Iwate
Yamagata
Miyagi
Niigata
Fukushima
Tochigi
Toyama
Gunma
Ibaraki
Ishikawa
Nagano
Saitama
Fukui
Gifu
Shizuoka
Chiba
Shiga
Aichi
Tokyo
Kyoto
Yamanashi
Kanagawa
Tottori
Hyōgo
Mie
Shimane
Okayama
Nara
Hiroshima
Osaka
Yamaguchi
Ehime
Kōchi
Kagawa
Wakayama
Fukuoka
Tokushima
Saga
Ōita
Nagasaki
Miyazaki
Kumamoto
Kagoshima

0   50   100 *miles*

100 *kilometers*

Okinawa

Regions and prefectures in modern Japan. Map created by Mark Cook.

Abbreviated List of Historical Periods

All years listed are in CE (common era) unless otherwise stated.

Timeline of Japan

Nara period (710–794)
Heian period (794–1185)
Kamakura period (1185–1333)
Muromachi period (1336–1573)
Tokugawa period (1600–1868)
Meiji period (1868–1912)

Note: While 1600 can be considered the beginning of the Tokugawa period, some scholars choose 1603 because that was the year Tokugawa Ieyasu officially became shogun.

Classical period: Nara and Heian periods
Early medieval period: 1100s–1300s
Late medieval period: 1400s–1500s
Early modern period: Tokugawa period
Modern period: from the Meiji period onward

Timeline of China

Han dynasty (206 BCE–220 CE)
Tang dynasty (618–906)
Song dynasty (960–1279)
Yuan dynasty (1279–1368)
Ming dynasty (1368–1644)
Qing dynasty (1644–1911)

Works consulted in this section: Jansen, *The Making of Modern Japan*, 1–31; Mass, *Yoritomo and the Founding of the First Bakufu*; Spafford, *A Sense of Place*, 1–29; Bulliet et al., *The Earth and Its Peoples: A Global History*, vols. 1 and 2.

A Note on Japanese Terminology and Names

In general, I follow the convention of listing a Japanese name with the family name preceding the personal name (or what we may call the first name). For example, the order of the name Ogino Chiichi tells us that Ogino is the person's family name and Chiichi is his personal name. In the secondary literature, scholars with Japanese names who write in English list their personal names before their family names; I respect that order in my references to them.

In the Tokugawa-period historical context, and in earlier historical contexts, I follow the convention of using a person's personal name instead of the family name. For example, I mention Ogino Chiichi by his full name the first time and subsequently refer to him as Chiichi. In later historical contexts, while it may be common to refer to a person by that person's family name after the first mention, I make some exceptions and use personal names to be specific, especially when a family name can refer to multiple people in those contexts.

Since this book is about blindness and about blind people, I anticipate that interested readers possess different degrees of vision. As far as possible, I use English translations of Japanese and Chinese book titles and terms in the main text. I do it mainly because this improves readability on a computer screen reader and also because this makes technical details that are originally in Japanese and Chinese accessible to a reader, especially one who is a nonspecialist reader. While I use standard English translations of some published Japanese and Chinese works, many of the translations are mine. I provide romanized transliterations of original Japanese titles and terms (and use pinyin for original Chinese titles and terms) in the notes for anyone interested in those references and sources. I place a macron over a vowel (such as ō or ū) to indicate a long vowel in the original Japanese—fully anglicized Japanese words such as Tokyo, Kyoto, Osaka, Shinto, and shogun, and others appear without macrons. Most tables and images in this book are accompanied by prose descriptions so that they are legible to readers using a computer screen reader.

In many references to Tokugawa domains, I indicate in the main text approximate correspondences with cities, prefectures, and regions in contemporary Japan. Maps that are specifically drawn for this book are included for reference.

Throughout the book, I tend to use disability-first language. For example, I say "blind people" because this phrasing foregrounds the experience and identity of blind people and also reflects the references in historical sources.

Many historical sources refer to guild members (blind men who were members of the Kyoto guild) by names associated with guild membership. Full names of blind individuals are not always available, so I use names as they appear in historical sources. Their personal names are often characterized by a "Jō-" prefix or an "-ichi" suffix. Sometimes, in a name, I add an apostrophe before the "-ichi" suffix to clarify how the name should be parsed. For example, I write Wa'ichi, instead of Waichi, so that it is clear that the name should be read as Wa-ichi, not Wai-chi.

Acknowledgments

Writing this book took a lot longer than I had expected, and now that I have completed it, there is no other book I would have wanted to write. The long journey of writing and rewriting drafts is now a memory I will cherish. Along the ups and downs of that journey, I benefited greatly from the kindness, wisdom, and generosity of the people around me.

At Harvard University, Shigehisa Kuriyama was the best mentor I could ever have—he is the kind of mentor I aspire to become. His insightful comments and critical questioning, coupled with his keen, affable demeanor, kept me deeply engaged with my research and also pushed me to find new, unexpected answers in everything I did. David Howell, Helen Hardacre, and Ian Jared Miller were simply models of scholarship, and their erudition shaped my thinking about Japanese history and Japanese religions. Edwin Cranston patiently taught me to read classical Japanese literature, as did Fumiko Cranston. Kuniko Yamada McVey expertly helped me to track down materials (often at short notice) through interlibrary loan. It was a great joy working alongside peers— Sean O'Reilly, Yan Liu, He Bian, and Bina Arch—whose scholarship set high standards for me.

At Kokugakuin University, Negishi Shigeo-sensei welcomed me into his Japanese history seminar, and the hospitality of the staff of the International Exchange Programs Office made my research stay in Japan delightful.

At Dartmouth College, where I was an undergraduate, and also where

I returned as a postdoctoral fellow, I found a great community of scholars: Pamela Crossley, Steven Ericson, Hua-Yuan Li Mowry, Sarah Allan, Soyoung Suh, Sachi Schmidt-Hori, Dennis Washburn, Mikhail Gronas (my first teacher of Russian), Lindsey Whaley, and others. Pamela Crossley, in particular, was the reason why, as an undergraduate, I dreamed of going to graduate school.

At Hope College, my colleagues in the History Department—Marc Baer, Albert Bell, Janis Gibbs, Lauren Janes, Fred Johnson, Alison Lechner, Jeanne Petit, and Gloria Tseng—make going to work a joy. They continue to inspire me. For giving me specific advice on writing, I especially thank Janis Gibbs and Natalie Dykstra. Michelle Yost's help with interlibrary loan eased the stress of the final phase of research.

Senior scholars—Harold Cook, Karen Nakamura, Kim Nielsen, Michael Rembis, and Sara Scalenghe—were gracious hosts. They offered me opportunities to present my research at various stages: at Brown University (2014), Yale University (2015), the University of Toledo (2017), the State University of New York—Buffalo (2017), and the National Endowment for the Humanities Summer Institute (2018). Their encouragement, as well as the questions and comments from audiences (among them, Daniel Botsman, Fabian Drixler, Daniel Trambaiolo, and Marta Hanson) at those events, helped me to rethink and reframe the big picture of my research for an interdisciplinary audience.

Over the years, I presented early ideas at annual meetings and conferences of several organizations, such as the American Association for the History of Medicine, the Association for Asian Studies, the American Historical Association, the Early Modern Japan Network, and the Midwest Japan Seminar. Panelists and audiences (Dennis Frost, Ethan Segal, Elizabeth Lublin, Susan Burch, Maren Ehlers, Amy Stanley, and too many others to name here) gave me much to think about as I was analyzing the materials for this book.

My research was supported by funding at different stages. Travel and research funding from Harvard University (Sinclair Kennedy Traveling Fellowship, Merit Term-Time Research Fellowship, grants from the Reischauer Institute for Japanese Studies), the Kokugakuin University Visiting Researcher Fellowship for research in Japan, the Andrew Mellon Postdoctoral Fellowship in the Humanities for a research year at Dartmouth College, and summer research grants from Hope College made my research and writing possible. I also thank the History Department and the office of the Dean for the Arts and Humanities at Hope College for providing a book subvention award.

At the University of Michigan Press, LeAnn Fields, Flannery Wise, Kevin Rennells, and the production and marketing teams have been incredible partners. Words are simply not enough to express my thanks to LeAnn for believing in this project from the very beginning and for giving me precise advice at moments when I was at the crossroads of lengthy revisions—she represents everything (and more) that any author could wish for in an editor. Kevin's timely advice helped me get the manuscript through the final stage. The anonymous reviewers engaged deeply with every aspect of this book, and their suggestions were what I needed to improve the book manuscript. For including my book in the *Corporealities: Discourses of Disability* series, I wholeheartedly thank the series editors, David Mitchell and Sharon Snyder. It means a lot to me to be part of the series.

An early version of chapter 5 was published in the *Journal of Japanese Studies* (45, no. 1, winter 2019), and parts of my early research for chapter 5 also appeared in the *Proceedings of the Association for Japanese Literary Studies* (vol. 15, summer 2014). I thank the journal editors for their permission to reproduce the works in this book.

Ann Sierks Smith read every line of a late draft of this book and offered prompt, perspicacious, meticulous comments that helped me to strengthen and clarify my writing. Anne Taylor provided insightful comments on making the final changes. Mark Cook offered his time to create the maps for this book.

Finally, I want to thank the people who made a tremendous impact on my life. Brian and Dorothy Finley supported me through good cheer and laughter. The Brouwer family (Tom and Mingwei), the Smith family (Stephen and Ann), and the Bast family (Peter and Sarah) warmly welcomed us into their homes. My parents, Larry and Lynette, made sacrifices so that I could pursue my passion. They have steadfastly stood by me, and their selfless, unconditional love is what sustains me. I honor my late grandparents, whom I dearly miss. I also honor my late parents-in-law, who were loving parents to my wife, Har Ye, and to her sister, Wai Ye.

To Har Ye: Thank you for all your love and patience. You give meaning to everything.

To Matthew, Emma, and Mitchell: You bring us much joy, brighten our universe, and make everything worthwhile. Someday, when you get to read this book, I hope that you know this.

Preface

A Personal Note

───◆───

I consider myself to be someone who is sighted, but mostly with the aid of corrective lenses. When I visited Japan for the first time in 2009, I was impressed with the blind-friendly culture in public urban spaces. Tactile pavement tiles along sidewalks and near the edges of train platforms caught my attention. These functional bright yellow tiles, some with tactile dots and others with tactile parallel lines, help people with visual impairment "read" their directions as they use canes to navigate their paths.[1] Also new to me were the engineered chirping sounds at crosswalks that give pedestrians an audio cue to cross the roads; I learned to wait to hear them every time I reached a crosswalk. Other first-time travelers to Japan may also have quite similar impressions of its blind-friendly culture.

After that visit to Japan, I knew that my research was going to be about blind people, but I certainly did not expect it to be about blind people in Tokugawa Japan, the early modern period from 1600 to 1868. As a historian of Japan, I wanted to find out how blind friendly (or disability friendly) Japan was in the twentieth century. Instead, my early research took me down a different path. Something greatly intrigued me: since the Tokugawa period, blind people have been employed as masseurs. Even today, there is a niche industry of blind masseurs in Japan and in other countries in East Asia.[2] It seemed logical to me that a person could perform massage without using much sight, but how did blind people in Japan become involved in massage in the first place? Were there social or cultural reasons to explain why blind people were suited to be masseurs? The more I focused on the Tokugawa period, the more I learned that blind people were active in medicine, music, and religion. Their contributions in all those contexts have had an enduring impact on Japanese society.

My fascination with the blind masseurs of the Tokugawa period led me to Zatōichi, arguably the most iconic blind fictional character familiar to modern Japanese audiences. In films and a television series set in that period, Zatōichi appears as a blind masseur and also as a musician.[3] But there is nothing ordinary about him at all: he embodies the kind of superhuman qualities that audiences, for better or worse, imagine blind people to possess. Armed with a sword that is as extraordinary as his prowess, he is remembered as a consummate swordsman dedicated to pursuing poetic justice. He fulminates against social injustices and stands up for the downtrodden masses. In tense moments of battle, he uses his extraordinary sense of hearing to detect the movements of his sighted adversaries, though he cannot see them. Darting with lightning speed, never faltering, he nonchalantly and deftly cuts them down with his sword with deadly precision. His lack of sight elevates the magnitude of his physical feats and exaggerates the melodrama of violence. With a larger-than-life personality, he towers over other blind characters in Japanese popular culture.

The realities of blind people's lives in Tokugawa Japan were much more ordinary than the drama of Zatōichi's adventures. But what the fiction about Zatōichi suggests is that he was special—and, by extension, that blind people were unique in the Tokugawa period.

There is truth to this latter interpretation. In that era in Japanese society, even in their ordinary lives, blind people were unlike other disabled people and unlike their sighted peers. We are compelled to reimagine our approach to disability because these blind people were different yet able. Difference and ability were integrated into blind people's experiences with disability.

Through many detours, my research kept taking me back to the starting point—the hyperreality where blind masseurs and Zatōichi loomed large. I could not help but ask myself time and again what it was really like to be blind in Tokugawa Japan. The sources from that period have a lot to say, and thus this book, organized by theme, presents a narrative that conveys some answers.

Introduction

———◁◦▷———

What Did It Mean to Be Blind in Early Modern Japan?

When I think about the broad topic of this book, three people come to mind—three notable men of Tokugawa Japan (or Tokugawa society), the early modern period in Japanese history from 1600 to 1868. Sugiyama Wa'ichi was an acupuncturist of the seventeenth century. He so excelled in his profession that he was honored by the shogunate (the central government helmed by and centered on the Tokugawa shogun in the capital Edo, which is Tokyo today). Wa'ichi positioned himself at the vanguard of Japanese acupuncture by promoting a new technique so effective that it continues to be applied in acupuncture clinics in contemporary Japan. No less accomplished was Ogino Chiichi, a musician of the eighteenth century. He was a master of the genre of the medieval epic *The Tale of the Heike*,[1] which contemporary audiences regard as a canon in Japanese literature. In Chiichi's time, his oeuvre, the culmination of a lifelong dedication, was studied and enjoyed by professional musicians, samurai connoisseurs, and amateur fans. The third notable person, Hanawa Hokiichi, lived from the mid-eighteenth century through the early nineteenth century. He was an influential scholar who earned his reputation by compiling and editing *The Collected Records of Various Subjects*.[2] This monumental encyclopedia still serves as an indispensable reference guide for scholars today.

These three men had one important thing in common: they all had become blind at a young age and achieved success later in life as blind people. The success stories of Wa'ichi, Chiichi, and Hokiichi, in their own ways, answer the main question that this book will explore: What did it mean to be blind in Tokugawa society?

The answer is complicated, because the historical records we have of medical, social, political, and cultural perspectives in Tokugawa society tell us that being blind was about being disabled but also about being enabled in particular ways. There were people who, because they were suffering from blindness, were visually impaired, as well as people who focused their work on curing blindness. The unusual feature of that culture and era is that there also were people who, because they were blind, acquired new professions, new alliances, and new identities as disabled people. Not all blind people lived precariously. In fact, many explored ways to leverage their identities in Tokugawa society.

Blindness was disabling because it was construed and experienced as impaired vision. Throughout the Tokugawa period, the medical literature warned of diseases such as smallpox and measles that attacked the eyes and caused blindness. Blind people were visually impaired people, and the social experience of suffering and getting cured was part of the experience of being blind. We do not know the details of the early lives of Wa'ichi, Chiichi, and Hokiichi, but it is reasonable to imagine that growing up with blindness in that time and place involved going through stressful ordeals to get treated. The options for treatment were limited during Wa'ichi's childhood in the early seventeenth century, compared with what had become available in the eighteenth century when Chiichi and Hokiichi were born.

At the same time, social and political conditions determined blind people's interactions with society. Through its top-down means of control, the shogunate emphasized that blind people were different from the rest of the population and systematically generalized their difference. In some ways, blind people were vulnerable to exploitation by institutions in society. In other ways, however, it was sometimes advantageous for blind people to assert their disabled identities. This may not seem intuitive to audiences today, who have grown accustomed to negative images and stereotypes of disability or who assume that early societies (societies before the modern period) were "backward" and rejected disability. But there were good reasons for blind people to thrive. Certain conditions in Tokugawa society enabled blind people to use their abilities to productively engage with society. Under the most opportune circumstances, blind people like Wa'ichi, Chiichi, and Hokiichi could secure important privileges stemming from their identities as blind individuals—privileges that enabled them to become exceptional.

Readers interested in Japanese history, particularly in a disability-focused approach to Japanese history, will find that the context of contemporary Japan is a good starting point for understanding the relationship between *impairment* and *disability*. The contemporary Japanese word for "disability" is *shōgai*, which can also mean "impairment" in many interchangeable contexts—for example, *shikaku shōgai* means "visual impairment" and also "disability due to visual impairment."[3] Japan's Basic Act on Persons with Disabilities, enacted in 1970 and revised over the years through 2016, defines disability as "physical, intellectual, and mental disabilities or impairments" and "other disabilities or impairments of the body or mind" and recognizes social barriers (*shakai teki shōheki*) that impede the daily lives and social activities of people with disabilities.[4] The contexts of impairment and disability generally overlap to denote impediment or deterioration of function, dysfunction, and disablement.

The word *shōgai* was not featured in texts from the Tokugawa period, and impairment was described through a range of medical, cultural, and historical terms. Although it is unlikely that *shōgai* in the Japanese language today had the same range of meanings in the Tokugawa period,[5] there are advantages in accepting the idea that disability encompasses impairment and also in adapting this approach to analyze blindness in Tokugawa society. First, the impairment-based approach to disability allows us to explain blindness as physical, physiological, and functional impairment. Second, in light of the literature on disability, which I will discuss in the next section, it will be helpful to expand on the impairment-based approach in order to contextualize and explain one important argument about disability: that disability exceeds medical definitions of impairment. Yes, disability is centered on impairment, but it is also an experience and an identity. It is a socially constructed experience of society's practices, thought, and attitudes surrounding impairment, and it reflects the forms and hierarchy of political authority in society. In the intersecting social and political contexts of disability in Tokugawa society, a blind person could benefit from having a disabled identity (this identity means an impairment-based social and political identity). In short, by also focusing on nonmedical contexts of disability, we can see how blind people lived with blindness.

In thinking about what it meant to be blind in the Tokugawa period, ophthalmology offers some clues for understanding medical studies of the impairments of the eyes and vision. A specialty discipline of medicine, ophthalmology was introduced from China to Japan many centuries before the Tokugawa period through medical exchanges between the two countries. Chinese medical thought, because it was highly regarded in Japan, greatly influenced the general course of the development of Japanese medicine—to such an extent that even today, Japanese medicine is also called Sino-Japanese medicine.[6] This would explain why in the context of Sino-Japanese medicine, Tokugawa Japanese ophthalmologists used analytical conventions from Chinese medical sources to expound their own interpretations and commentaries. Many Tokugawa-period medical texts of Japanese ophthalmologists have yet to be systematically analyzed and properly compared in historical studies of medicine; nevertheless, as chapter 1 will explain, those texts give us important insights into the analytical language used to describe eye conditions.

Medical specialists in Tokugawa Japan did not propose a consistent definition of blindness. The cultural vocabulary about blindness was pivoted upon various descriptions of visual impairment, linking discussions of visual impairment to those of disease, illness, and cure. The core analytical language remained stable over the centuries, even as new epistemologies from Europe were introduced into the context of Sino-Japanese medicine in the late eighteenth century and influenced the styles of medical inquiry through the nineteenth century.

Rich historical sources in Japanese ophthalmology give us more medical descriptions about a range of visual impairment than about functional sight for good reason: visual impairment was more remarkable, because it came with symptoms unassociated with and unnoticed in functional sight. Diagnostic and descriptive terms, however, were imposed upon the medical lexicon by sighted ophthalmologists and not by blind people themselves. Yet, because no uniform standard existed in Tokugawa society to evaluate vision or vision loss, it is significant that Japanese medical scholars, including ophthalmologists, systematized, protected, and propagated medical knowledge and texts. Their work ensured that the epistemologies and discourses were kept fairly consistent over time in the intellectual context and professional practices of ophthalmology.

Exploring perspectives on blindness using medical and nonmedical sources, as chapter 2 will argue, can also open a new window onto ideas and practices of cure in popular medical culture. As early as the late seventeenth century, professional medical knowledge was being translated into vernacular scripts and circulated in print for the reading public. Certainly, by the eighteenth century, the flourishing print culture had stimulated new curiosity and spurred the spread of consumer culture across urban and rural areas. In her book about the information culture in Tokugawa society, Mary Elizabeth Berry introduces us to "open audiences of consumers, who were implicitly entitled to information, familiar with its frames of reference, and invested in self-discovery."[7] New modes in the consumption of information in the public realm informed contemporary mindsets and stimulated a constantly growing appetite for knowledge.

Particularly during the eighteenth and nineteenth centuries, as the array of approaches to health and healing dramatically expanded, people suffering from blindness were enabled by choices: as patients, they enjoyed increased access to physicians and medicines; as consumers, they received useful information from health manuals, gazetteers, and travel books. As diaries and medical case histories reveal, from a patient-centered perspective, blindness was framed by the experience and understanding of disease, illness, and cure. People complained about eye afflictions, such as debilitated vision, blurred vision, and red and painful eyes. But there seemed to be a treatment, or a promise that one existed, for every troubling eye ailment, from a slight eye infection to a persistent visual impairment.

To explore what it meant to be blind in Tokugawa Japan, we should also understand what the limitations with historical sources mean for our perspectives on blind people in the period's social and political contexts, which will be discussed in chapters 3 through 6. We do not know whether people with disabling eye conditions who sought treatment were fully cured, unless the records tell us so. It is also difficult to know how many visually impaired individuals who failed to get treated or cured then went on to assume disabled identities as blind people. We must take several leaps of faith in attempting to bridge the distance between the medical context and the social and political contexts. We have to assume that a person who became visually impaired temporarily from an illness had fewer reasons than a person with chronic visual impairment to be permanently identified as a blind, disabled person. We also have to assume that not every person sought medical treatment and that even among those who were not cured, not all were persuaded to declare their disabled identities.

Claims of disabled identity were subjective, and also subjective were differences in the degrees of vision between sighted people and blind people. Being sighted could mean having sufficient sight to perform essential tasks that required sight and, for that sighted person, would

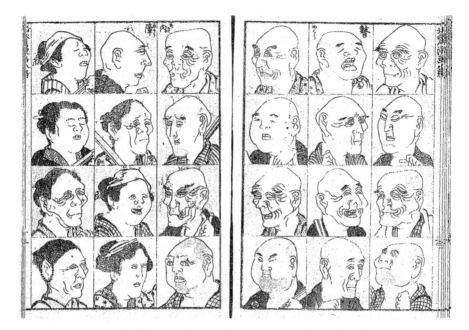

Fig. I.1. Sketches of the faces of blind men and women by prolific Japanese woodblock print artist Katsushika Hokusai. The faces appear to be those of elderly blind people. It was common for sighted people to form their impressions of blindness by observing the physical appearance of a blind person. Hokusai illustrates that blindness is etched onto each face as an identity marker of physical difference and as a brand of impairment. No two faces are alike; each face is imbued with its individuality. The variety suggests the appearances of various degrees of impairment affecting one or both eyes, including visible scars around the eyes, eyelids completely or partially sealed, blank stares, and deformed eyes. The Japanese scripts above include words referring to blindness: *ko* (blind or blindness), *mekura* (dark eyes), and *akimekura*. The *kanji* characters of *akimekura* say "internal obstruction"; the accompanying *kana* characters mean "blind but with clear and normal-looking eyes," a reference to the medical diagnosis of what are likely cataracts. From *Hokusai manga*, vol. 8 (Nagoya: Katano Tōshirō, 1878). National Diet Library Digital Collections.

mean not having to claim disabled identity. It is also impossible for us to say how "blind" one person was compared with another, so I rely on context to determine who blind people were. In the historical sources that discuss the social and political contexts of disabled identity, common references to blind people used a number of words: *mōjin* and *kosha* (a blind person or blind people), *zatō* (blind man or men), *mōjo* and *goze* (blind woman or women), *mekura* (dark eyes), *meshii* (blind), and *katameshii* (blind in one eye). Hence, when I refer to blind people, I think of these references to "blind people" and "blind man/woman/person"—that is, I refer to visually impaired people who were identified (or self-identified) and named as blind people in the sources.

The political administration of Tokugawa society provides the context for further discussion of blind people's disabled identities. The Tokugawa regime was largely stable through the centuries, peaking in the early eighteenth century and crumbling in the mid-nineteenth century. Tokugawa Ieyasu, the first shogun, inaugurated the Tokugawa polity at the dawn of the seventeenth century. Its capital, Edo, was founded in 1603, and its polity was politically and geographically organized into territorial units called domains.[8] The shogunate appointed a samurai lord[9] to govern a domain with the support of his clan, samurai vassals, and a wide base of government officials. As domain rulers, samurai lords commanded autonomous power to govern domain matters but submitted to the overarching authority of the shogunate. In each domain, government officials mediated contact between ordinary subjects and the domain lord.

The Tokugawa shogunate was largely successful in governing Japan's population because it employed the system of *status-based rule*[10] (or the status system), which it enforced in every domain at every level of government starting in the early seventeenth century. Status rule broadly represented the hierarchy of society and manifested the will of the shogunate. David Howell's study of status notes that the system created status groups as a means of formalizing military obligations to the shogun; over time, as the urgency of military rule was eclipsed by the need to maintain long-term administration, the divisions were solidified.[11] Status groups were defined by occupations, and by this I think of Howell's analysis of occupation as economic work related to one's status (and such work may be seen as a political obligation to the status system).[12] People across society belonged to status groups, such as samurais, commoners, temple and shrine clergy, outcasts, and others,[13] and in addition to their occupations were identified by the ties to where they lived.[14] Commoners made up the most prevalent group. The occupations that they were involved in were diverse, encompassing peasants and townspeople. Samurais, who commanded exclusive privileges, were in the minority.

Local government was organized according to status group membership, with status groups placed in charge of their status communities in administrative areas, such as villages, towns, and cities. As Howell also reminds us, "by ceding a measure of autonomy to status groups, including the domains, the shogunate abstained from intruding into those aspects of daily life deemed external to national concerns."[15] This means that status groups were granted some autonomy in local government without the shogunate's direct intervention in every routine matter. The autonomy was, in most cases, still bound by and exercised within the frameworks of domain-based government and shogunate laws. This complex bureaucratic structure served the shogunate well.

In the status system, the shogunate created a unique collective status category for blind people (the blind status category) and oversaw it through the guild of blind men (*tōdō* or *tōdōza*,[16] which is commonly translated in contemporary English-language scholarship as "the guild"). The guild was founded in Kyoto in the medieval period as an elite academy to train blind male musicians to perform *The Tale of the Heike* (*Heike* music). Music was a profession in which blind people were also popular throughout the Tokugawa period. As will be explained in chapters 5 and 6, it became less lucrative for guild members in Tokugawa society to be musicians of *Heike*, and over time many blind people, including those without ties to the guild, branched into fashionable musical genres or ended up working as masseurs. The popular imagination that enlarged ideas of blind people's abilities, such as their extraordinary faculties of hearing and memory, their uncanny connection with otherworldly realms through music, and their intuitive knowledge of touch, could have facilitated blind people's entry into those professions. The original medieval Buddhist idea that linked a person's blindness to karma (deeds in previous lives) appeared to have lost its negative connotations in the Tokugawa period.

In view of the guild's medieval heritage, as chapter 3 will show, in the early Tokugawa period the shogunate transformed the guild into the main political institution with the mandate to govern the blind status category. While some people had the flexibility to assume different status identities through multiple occupations, embodying what Howell calls the "situational character of status identities,"[17] the guild made guild membership exclusive but was open to accepting members from across status groups—though, as chapter 3 will explain, the guild excluded outcasts (an autonomous status category, associated with certain occupations and discriminated against by society). Typically, a blind man gave up his original status identity in order to adopt the new blind status identity. However, what constituted blindness was not at all defined by the shogunate or the guild and hence was left open to interpretation.

In the analytical framework of disability that this book employs, I interpret the blind status identity as the disabled identity tied to membership in the Kyoto guild (or guild membership). The guild maintained a collective identity that cohered with its powerful ideology about the common descent of all blind people from legendary blind ancestors. As an institution, it was singular in Tokugawa society in giving an institutional framework and foundation to empower guild members' disabled identities. It was a dependable platform with branch offices and leaders across Japan to represent guild members. Over the centuries, with its sweeping authority over the blind status category upheld by the shogunate, the guild, in principle, had power over anyone who claimed to be blind.

From the vantage point of disability history (or the history of disability), it is clear that in Tokugawa society disabled identity overlapped with the status system, and disability, as it related to blind people, was organized around guild membership. In Japanese-language and English-language scholarship, Katō Yasuaki and Gerald Groemer have given us useful overviews of the history of the guild and the guild's important place in Tokugawa history.[18] This book reframes the discussion around the social and political meanings of disability to examine how guild membership confirmed both the enabling and disabling aspects of disabled identity. Guild membership was expensive and came with significant financial and ritual obligations, but it gave a blind man a chance to learn vocational skills, collect alms, and be represented by the guild in routine matters, and it perhaps even gave him a chance to earn prestigious political appointments and strategically accumulate power through connections. This was true until the end of the Tokugawa regime. Enablement through the guild's government was a privilege that the shogunate had intended and had tried to systematize for the blind status category. It is no coincidence, then, that in their rise to power, blind people like Wa'ichi, Chiichi, and Hokiichi began their careers as guild members.

This analytical approach to disability explains that factors like a blind person's social and political ties, financial capacity, and gender that were enabling for some guild members also contributed to the tensions and inequities of disabled identity among guild members and nonmembers who lacked those advantages. The politics of enablement was matched by the politics of disablement. For example, the guild rewarded well-to-do guild members but discriminated against poor blind men without influential social or political connections. Blind men of affluent families did not need the prestige of appointments from the guild, and those who had sufficient support from their families also did not need support from the guild. Thus, someone of relatively good circumstances could retain his status and still validate his disabled identity without guild membership and without paying any dues to the guild. His forgoing of guild membership undermined the guild's authority.

Gender discrimination excluded blind women from the guild, but though they could not be guild members, they were quite arbitrarily considered by the guild to be bound by its authority over the blind status category. Among blind women, blind female musicians were the most prominent professionals who organized their own groups with all-female membership. Groemer's book-length study of blind female musicians exposes the hardships that they encountered to procure "emancipatory interests" and discusses how these blind female musicians, because of their gender and disability, "began to search for ways to organize in order to counter some of the worst effects of the economic exploitation, political domination, social marginalization, ability-based discrimination, and cultural restrictions that Tokugawa rule brought on as well."[19] Regardless of guild or group membership or one's gender, a blind person could, as a last resort, beseech the home community to provide food and material relief in hard times—a basic right of all needy people that government authorities tried to honor.

No other disabled social group was represented by a shogunate-backed institution like the guild. Deaf people did not gain the recognition of the shogunate through special institutions or appointments. Perhaps one reason was that deaf people, though hearing impaired, were assumed to be physically able-bodied and sufficiently sighted, so they were expected to perform physical tasks and had less conspicuous identities than their blind peers. As the earlier woodblock print illustration of blind people by Hokusai suggests (see figure 1), visual impairment in Tokugawa society was associated with observable physical qualities and deformities; deafness was less marked than blindness in visual appearances, and deaf people could more easily pass as "ordinary" than blind people could. Deaf culture, which emerged after the Tokugawa period, is a largely coherent culture in Japan today; but, as Karen Nakamura demonstrates, it is formed around mixed cultural identities and communities in the deaf population.[20]

Some documents of the Tokugawa period mention physically impaired people. Perhaps because physically impaired people were involved in a wide variety of occupations, and also perhaps because they were not unified by one core impairment, they did not have a cohesive disabled identity in the status system. The situation was significantly different much later after World War II, when physical impairment became the main focus of Japan's first disability-based legislation. Under Japan's Law on the Welfare of People with Physical Disabilities, a national law introduced in 1949,[21] physically impaired people—many of whom were disabled war veterans—were collectively recognized as a legal category and accorded rights to healthcare and social services for physical therapy and rehabilitation. Physical disability was broadly defined to include blindness and deafness—even in Japan today, this is a broad category of disability.

For the sake of comparison, let us briefly compare the blind status category in Tokugawa Japan to people with leprosy,[22] who made up another disabled status group (the leprosy status category) in that society, perhaps the only other disabled status group with organized rights and autonomy that were quite similar to those of the blind status category. Members of these two status groups all shared impairment, broadly speaking, as the common denominator in their constructed and lived identities. But people of the leprosy status group linked their disabled identities to the physical condition of leprosy, and their association with leprosy distinguished their identities from the blind status identity. What is also an important difference between the two status groups is that Tokugawa society discriminated against people with leprosy to such an extent that sometimes they were forced to live apart from the main population. Medical attitudes toward leprosy, as Suzuki Noriko and Susan Burns highlight, condemned the "bad blood" of leprosy as contaminating family bloodlines, further ostracizing people with leprosy as well as people with family histories of leprosy.[23] Unless it was caused by leprosy, blindness was not framed as a disease of the bloodline or stigmatized as a hereditary condition, and blind people, in general, did not face the same kind of discrimination.

As their impairments were interpreted and valued differently, blind people and people with leprosy encountered dissimilar fates in Tokugawa society's social organization of status. An important study by Yokota Noriko focuses on leprosy-afflicted people who formed their community in one part of Kyoto.[24] Autonomy and physical segregation were characteristics of a "leper" village, which made up a social unit of the leprosy status category. Among the activities in which a "leper" village exercised its rights and autonomy, the collection of alms was perhaps the most important. This practice grew out of the Buddhist worldview in the medieval period of begging for salvation and was secularized as routine begging sometime in the seventeenth century. Yokota's study highlights that even though people with leprosy were not clearly identified as outcasts, it appears that the status system placed the leprosy status group under the rule of the outcast status group. This subjugation of status only deepened the discrimination against leprosy and its sufferers. Though outcast leaders claimed to have the same authority over blind beggars, the guild stubbornly refused outcast rule.[25] The result was that guild members who earned a living from collecting alms were protected by the guild.

Clearly, examples such as those about the guild's authority suggest that there is much more that needs to be said about how the guild operated in Tokugawa society. One goal of this book is to shed light on this area, and this is what I will do, especially in chapters 3 and 4. Recent scholarship is correct in emphasizing the guild's sweeping mandate and its influence on blind people's professions, but it is also a significant fact that there was no normal or normative profile of a blind person. Rather, there were exhortations about what a blind person could or should do. The reality was complex, though this point has been understated in current scholarship. Through decrees and commands, particularly in the time of social and political reforms of the late eighteenth century and thereafter, the shogunate went to great lengths to maintain the fiction that most blind people were beholden to the guild. However, it is clear that blind people had different circumstances and made choices based on their circumstances. Well-to-do or privileged blind people were not the only ones who avoided the guild. Even through the nineteenth century, many of those blind people who did not join the guild worked hard for a living but still lived as they wished, as they had done before the repeated government decrees.

My discussion of blind people's professions, on one level, focuses on how blind people were enabled by their disabled identities to find work. There are important historical explanations, and they will be discussed in chapters 3 through 6. In general, when I consider the contexts of blind people's professions, I acknowledge Howell's argument that livelihood was the kind of work that a person did for a living, which often could be work unrelated to the occupation tied to that person's status.[26] Because guild members were usually employed in niche professions in music, medicine, and religion, I do not make a distinction between engaging in a livelihood and performing that same work as an occupation to serve the guild. I think of guild members' livelihoods as their occupations, and also as their professions and careers, and discuss what it meant to be blind and a guild member, as well as what it meant to be blind and not have to be a guild member. The shogunate and the guild had broad interpretations of acceptable livelihoods of blind people to make it convenient for blind people to join the guild, but the goal of expanding the guild's authority did not always meet with success.

My discussion, on another level, reconsiders how for blind people, being employed in niche professions was also about exploring ways to engage with the traditions of those professions. But because current scholarship emphasizes the niche nature of blind people's professions, it is easy to overlook the fact that many blind professionals were innovators on their own terms. The perspectives that are emphasized in chapters 5 and 6 will illustrate that some blind people embraced past traditions while many more adapted to the evolving demands of sighted society.

In music, my discussion of blind musicians and the *Heike* genre goes beyond the existing scholarship about musical history by notable scholars of Japanese music, such as Hugh de Ferranti, Kinda'ichi Haruhiko, and Komoda Haruko.[27] Blind musicians in the seventeenth century inherited the musical and religious traditions of the medieval period. It is true that *Heike* music was past its prime in the seventeenth century and also true that many blind musicians from that time specialized in more fashionable musical genres to broaden their repertoire. However, what deserves greater emphasis is that some elite blind musicians continued to teach *Heike* music through the eighteenth and nineteenth centuries. They did so in ways that demonstrate the relevance of *Heike* to the guild and to some audiences beyond the guild. The process of composing *Heike* texts was not only a literary process but also a social process in which blind musicians organized and shared knowledge through their social and literary networks, drawing in sighted amateurs who interacted and collaborated with them.

In medicine, the scholarship on blind acupuncturists and masseurs needs greater contextualization as much as it needs specific discussion of the roles of the guild and medical thought and practices. In the seventeenth century, the guild's leaders promoted new roles for blind people in acupuncture, which had historically been a mainstream medical specialty of sighted people. Blind pioneers of acupuncture were elite members of the guild who wielded their political influence with the support of the shogunate to teach acupuncture to guild members. Massage, which was related to acupuncture in this medical context, emerged in the eighteenth century as a common profession among blind people. When popular medical culture accentuated the benefits of massage in cultivating health, in disproportionately large numbers many blind people became masseurs. Massage required less technical training than acupuncture, so it was easier for a blind person to be trained in massage than in acupuncture. By openly associating themselves with expertise through their professional roles, blind people became visible in the public eye in Tokugawa Japan.

The Challenge of Doing Disability History: An Interdisciplinary Approach

Readers interested in disability studies may want to know that I develop my analytical framework around some basic and common concerns of disability history and that I also use the focus on Tokugawa society to bring out the complex meanings and specific experiences of enablement, which were not typical of other societies in that same time period.[28]

Today, there is no universal, cross-cultural consensus about disability. A definition of disability with a scope and depth that would apply unambiguously to every society and culture is elusive, even impossible. It would be unreasonable to expect to find a ready or formulaic expression of disability in early societies. The present legal standard for disability laws in the United States comes from the landmark Americans with Disabilities Act (ADA), which was passed in 1990 and amended in 2008. According to the ADA of 1990, disability is, as it concerns an individual, "(A) a physical or mental impairment that substantially limits one or more of the major life activities of such an individual; (B) a record of such an impairment; or (C) being regarded as having such an impairment."[29] Among the amendments to the ADA in 2008, a list of "major life activities" was enumerated, and additional clauses were added to clarify point (C) of the 1990 ADA.[30]

Japan's laws today recognize different categories of disability (see table 1). Katharina Heyer's survey of recent Japanese legal history explains that two key external factors were instrumental to the changes in Japan's context of disability: the ADA and the United Nations International Decade of Disabled Persons (1983–92).[31] In an important step toward normalizing disability in society, Japan's laws affirmed the state's role to engage with people with disabilities through their "independence and participation in society, both fundamental aspects of the normalization principle."[32] On this note, Carolyn Stevens argues that neoliberalism and normalization continue to be major guiding principles in contemporary Japan's approach to disability: "Generally speaking, neoliberalism is a particular sensibility or imagining whereby problems and solutions are defined in economic terms, and behaviours are moulded in terms of

Table I.1. Categories of Disability in Contemporary Japan

Physical disabilities	Intellectual disabilities	Mental disabilities
Original source of disability certification		
Law on the Welfare of People with Physical Disabilities (1949)	System for certifying intellectual disabilities (1973)	Law on Mental Health and the Welfare of People with Mental Disabilities (1950)
Major health conditions		
• Visual impairment • Hearing impairment (and impairment affecting balance) • Vocal or linguistic impairment • Impairment affecting the limbs or torso (also mobility functions affected by impairment of the brain) • Impairment of the heart • Impairment of the kidneys • Impairment of respiratory functions • Impairment of the bladder, colorectum, or small intestine • Impairment of the liver • Impairment of the immunity due to HIV	• Intellectual disabilities (this is a broad category)	• Various kinds of psychosis • Epilepsy • Schizophrenia • Emotional and mood disorder • Organic mental disorder • Developmental disorder • Other mental illnesses
Number of certified/registered people (2018 data)		
5,087,275	1,115,962	1,062,700

Source: Created by translating, compiling, and editing data from "Section on Disability Identification Card," Ministry of Health, Labour, and Welfare, https://www.mhlw.go.jp/stf/seisakunitsuite/bunya/hukushi_kaigo/shougaishahukushi/techou.html

In Japan, people with disabilities seeking benefits are required to be evaluated for the nature and severity of their health conditions in order to receive identification cards issued by the government. Stevens cites the view that the law is vague about intellectual disability and does not define it (Stevens, *Disability in Japan*, 30–31).

business interests."[33] (The modern principles of neoliberalism and normalization were absent in the Tokugawa context of status rule.) With the announcement in 2013 of the new anti-discrimination law, which was later fully enacted in 2016, Japan completed the series of reforms to ratify the Convention on the Rights of Persons with Disabilities (a 2014 United Nations treaty).[34] Within Japan there is fairly broad agreement on legal principles, but Japanese society continues to debate the future of reforms and activism.

From a global historical perspective, modern legal and political discourses about disability started to come to life by the early nineteenth century. Kim Nielsen's historical survey of disability in the United States explains that although disability was codified through the Revolutionary War Pension Act of 1818, impairments were not considered to be disabilities if they did not impede the impaired person's capacity to work.[35] This narrow scope of disability that is focused on work instead of the broad range of activities subsumed under the ADA suggests one framework for thinking about the context of blindness in Tokugawa Japan: that a person's blindness, though disabling as most impairments were, did not translate into the inability to work.

The lack of a uniform assessment of blindness in Tokugawa Japan is a fact that we also note in historical studies of other societies. For example, Zina Weygand's analysis of modern French society tells us that in France at the turn of the nineteenth century, blindness was understood as vision that was so impaired as to impede a person's ability to self-navigate.[36] French medical encyclopedias expounded interpretations of blindness, but they were of little use to anyone then who was looking for a clear, objective, standard definition of vision loss.

In Tokugawa Japan, while it is true that there were blind people who were too physically disabled to perform labor or look for work (which chapter 3 will discuss), this was often not due to blindness alone. Disability would not have simply meant being too impaired, and hence too disabled, to work. This was only to be part of the contextual interpretation. A blind person's disabled identity had a significance in Tokugawa society that was not found in the contexts of other societies: on the one hand, because disability denoted and enabled different ability in the economic sense, disabled identity could be a positive factor in the social mobility of a blind person, but on the other hand, that same identity could impose on the blind person, particularly someone of the guild, certain social and political duties as a price for individual enablement.

While it is important to represent blind people's perspectives in disability history, one of the greatest challenges for any author writing about premodern periods—interpreted broadly here and henceforth to mean the medieval and early modern periods—is the scarcity of sources written by blind people themselves. The problem is, of course, not unique to Tokugawa society. Even modern French society in the early nineteenth century, though it had been transformed by Enlightenment thought in philosophy and literature and by revolutionary ideas of human rights in the French Revolution, did not seem to publish many works by disabled people. Sighted people took great interest in blindness to advance various agendas. Blindness fascinated eighteenth-century French philosopher Denis Diderot so much that he wrote about how a blind person, upon acquiring sight, would comprehend the world that he had previously only learned about without sight.[37] In education, philosophical inquiries imparted a new momentum to pedagogical thought and experiment. As Weygand explains, before Louis Braille's invention of the Braille system, Valentin Haüy was a pioneer in blind education who devoted his energies to devising tactile methods of reading.[38]

In the sea of works by sighted people in France, Weygand and a fellow historian of disability and medicine, Catherine Kudlick, came across the memoir of a blind French woman named Thérèse-Adèle Husson, who lived in the nineteenth century. The memoir was discovered by happenstance in the archives of the preeminent Quinze-Vingts, a hospice and facility for blind people founded by the French royal house in the thirteenth century.[39] Weygand suggests that it may be the first substantive work by a blind person about the plight, dreams, and ideals of blind people,[40] and it is all the more significant because it expresses the perspectives of a blind woman who was trying to reconcile her gender role with her own disability. Husson's authorial voice, otherwise authentic, is at times intentionally stifled by idealistic, didactic tones to downplay her inner conflict with French society's expectations of her as a blind, disabled woman. This profile is useful as a point of comparison with other educated blind women of the nineteenth and twentieth centuries in the United States, such as Laura Bridgman, a blind-deaf protégé and star student of American pedagogue Samuel Gridley Howe at the Perkins Institution, and Helen Keller, the most memorable blind-deaf activist of her generation.[41]

In Tokugawa Japan, the problem of scarce sources by blind people could be explained by sighted people's marginalization of blind people's perspectives. While the purpose of writing this book is not to compare different societies, it is important to acknowledge that had women like Husson, Bridgman, or Keller lived in Tokugawa Japan, their voices would not have been represented in the historical record. Blind men of the Tokugawa period, in the little writing that they left behind, did not produce anything with the expressiveness of the modern autobiographical genre. The rich worlds of blind people's thoughts, aspirations, and emotions from that era remain out of reach. Their perspectives on their lived experiences in their own words are also buried somewhere in the pages of history. The stark reality of absent sources and perspectives is an unavoidable limitation of current historical research on Tokugawa Japan. Blind people, because of poor or limited vision, were not expected to read and write. Modern, Western-style education for blind and deaf people was not introduced in Japan until the Meiji period, and even then, the curriculum placed a strong emphasis on vocational training. Acquiring literacy was not as practical as learning skills for jobs for most blind people even during the Meiji period. It would not be shocking, then, that sighted people in Tokugawa Japan assumed that they, not blind people, would dictate the historical narrative to include or exclude blind people.

Historians of disability are right to insist that disability-centered analysis can turn a dominant narrative told through ableist perspectives (views by able-bodied people that determine who is able and hence enforce what is normal) inside out and upside down by recasting the story of society around disabled people. Susan Burch and Michael Rembis have compellingly argued that "recognizing disability as an analytic or interpretive frame, as a category or label, and as a lived experience forces us not only to re-member the past but also to rethink it."[42] (I understand "re-member" to mean "re-populate," that is to re-populate the story with disabled people.) Disability, as Burch and Rembis also argue, is "conceptual, lived, and interpretive."[43] How we interpret disability conceptually depends on our frameworks for interpreting the society under scrutiny; and how we interpret lived experiences of disability depends on what we do with the existing sources—the majority written by sighted people and the occasional ones written by disabled people.

How, then, do we fill in the gaps in the narrative about the Tokugawa context? The dearth of historical materials does not mean that the lived experiences and voices of blind people are irrecoverable from history. To quote Nielsen's argument about historical research on disability, "Structures of power, as well as individual human beings, reside *together* in historical contexts—sometimes seamlessly, sometimes uneasily, and sometimes messily."[44] For historians of disability, it is necessary to find a flexible solution: by approaching sighted people's sources differently, with a keen eye to clues about blind people that are mediated by these sources. Profiles of blind people do not substitute lived experiences, but they can help us reconstruct the historical content of blind people's lives and reimagine them as a plethora of lives alongside and entangled with those of sighted people.

In the rare instances in Tokugawa society in which blind people left behind records, we snatch a few glimpses, through separate accounts, of their musical studies and pursuits. More indirect accounts suggest the pain and suffering blind people would have endured because of eye afflictions and, on a more positive note, also reflect blind people's relentless will to carve out their careers. A recomposed picture of one blind person's life story does not easily replicate that of another blind person. The blind population was heterogeneous, even though the shogunate conveniently assigned one umbrella status to that population. Yet, together, these fragments of myriad lives from various sources allow us to grasp, albeit in an incomplete sense, the repertoire of choices and trajectories of blind people who had once lived in Tokugawa society; the mosaic picture that emerges would be our closest approximation of their personal histories and lived experiences.

In exploring perspectives on disability, this book broadly reflects on disability as framed by the *social* and *medical* models of disability in current scholarship about European and North American societies. The *medical* model views disability through a medical lens and, by medicalizing disability, analyzes it as an objectifiable, treatable, and even curable biomedical dysfunction of the individual person. According to Sayantani DasGupta, "The medicalization of disability, then, refers to how individuals with disabilities have been categorized as 'sick' and placed under the jurisdiction of the medical establishment and medical professionals."[45] The medical model's idea of equating disability with illness has a long history in the Euro-American historical contexts of the medical profession. In those contexts, medical professionals had the authority in the nineteenth century, if not before, to set medical categories of disability.[46] Historians of disability such as Beth Linker[47] point out that the medical model continued to provide the authoritative interpretive framework through the twentieth century to determine dominant narratives about disability. Under the medical gaze, disabled people were thought to be greatly inhibited by disability; they were undervalued and had to live with prescriptive and discriminatory ideas that they were ill, dependent, and weak. In the most simplistic vision of outcomes, disability could be cured so that disabled people could become "normal."

The medical model's generalization of disability has limited use in understanding Tokugawa Japan, especially in our understanding of the contexts of blind people's active participation in society. Tokugawa society did not have the same kind of medical infrastructure that characterized European and North American societies. In Tokugawa society, medical diagnoses were not used to determine a blind person's physical fitness to work or to collect alms. Disabled identity did not have to include a medical component. Blind people did not have to be medically certified by ophthalmologists or physicians to be declared blind, and blind people's abilities were not measured against a metric of work or labor.

The *social* model of disability can be seen as the model that was developed to counter the prevalence of the medical model. With a history that can be traced back to Europe and North America in the 1960s and 1970s, the social model became popular through disability rights activism for social justice for disabled people. Its proponents redefined disability by criticizing ableist views for labeling disability and for oppressing disabled people. Perhaps the most important characteristic of the social model is the idea that impairment and disability are separate. According to the model, *impairment* refers to biological and physiological impairments in a biomedical sense; *disability* is constructed purely around social and political agendas that find fault with impairment so as to justify the exclusion of impaired people from mainstream society.

In its early iterations, the social model overemphasized disability as an artificial concept and tended to resist a meaningful interrogation of the medical model, foreclosing discussions of the overlapping social, political, and medical contexts of impairment. As Tom Shakespeare writes, the social model was effective in mobilizing disabled activists to take back control of their lives and in freeing disabled people from feeling guilty about suffering from impairment.[48] But Shakespeare is also right to argue that the social model ignores impairment, that "it risks implying that impairment is not a problem."[49] G. Thomas Couser[50] offers constructive ways to think beyond the social model. He argues that illness and disability can be interrelated personal experiences: being ill and being disabled can coexist as cognitive, psychological, emotional, and physical states. Often the state of being disabled or feeling ill overlaps with experiences with impaired bodily functions—experiences that will be discussed in chapter 2. Like Couser, I do not seek to discredit the social model. These criticisms reflect current thought about updating the social model to advance its utility in disability studies.

Historians of disability have found uses for the social model by adapting its analytical framework in premodern historical contexts in which the language of disability was not formulated. Klaus-Peter Horn and Bianca Frohne argue in their work on medieval and early modern European societies that the concept of disability, though not described as disability in these contexts, can be broadly interpreted to encompass ideas about physical and bodily differences.[51] Sara Scalenghe[52] and Irina Metzler, who have examined disability in early modern Ottoman

Arab society and disability in medieval Europe, respectively, reiterate the current understanding that it is productive to focus on the various conditions of impairment in historical contexts in which disability was nebulous as a unifying concept. According to Metzler, "Medieval terminology relating to what we would now call 'disability' was notoriously vague, unless mentioning very specific physical conditions such as, in medieval parlance, the crippled, contracted or paralyzed person, or the sensory impairments of blind, deaf, and dumb."[53] Norms of disability in Tokugawa Japan, likewise, were not defined; so, because of that, our discussions of disability in an early modern society like Tokugawa society can be productively framed by the same approach of discussing particular types of impairment—discussing blindness as visual impairment and, also, as difference from imagined standards of vision.

I suggest that in disability history and disability studies, the social model gains new relevance when we reanalyze the contrast between impairment and disability within the model: disability and impairment are separable as analytical categories, but they are also historically inseparable and experienced together in actual lives. They depend on each other for their contextual meanings and are inalienable from the conditions that define real human experiences. Scalenghe's discussion of early modern Ottoman Arab society emphasizes "the privileged place of blindness within hierarchies of impairment."[54] Blind people in that society could earn positions in law and in religion because of "the paramount role of orality in the transmission of knowledge."[55] Certainly, some parallels can be drawn between Ottoman and Tokugawa societies. Popular ideas associating blind people with good memory and with enhanced sensitivity to orality and musicality are not unique to non-Western societies. But the traditions of blind people in Tokugawa society, such as their musical traditions, had distinctive origins and were tied to the guild's history. Blind people found jobs in music even as oral traditions of the past were absorbed by print culture. Though the shogunate did not formally create a "hierarchy of impairments," the disproportionate strength and representation of the blind communities in Tokugawa Japan's population, as a whole, would speak to the broad argument that different impairments were subjected to different cultural interpretations and appropriations, with unequal consequences in the experiences of disabled identity.

In one important respect, by following the social model of disability, my book argues for the understanding of disability through its social and political meanings. At the same time, this understanding crucially emphasizes that for the blind people living in Tokugawa society, embracing their disabled identities was a strategy of enablement. This seemingly counterintuitive argument goes against the social model's focus on protesting and resisting the disabled status. In the chapters to come, various case studies of the blind people of Tokugawa society concretely exemplify what disability studies theorist Tobin Siebers proposes as a new direction for the social model: "complex embodiment."[56] This thought asserts a disabled individual's autonomy to act according to an internalized sense of being and with the acquired knowledge of external situations of disability and nondisability. As Siebers highlights, "Passing as nondisabled and masquerading as more disabled, in addition to actions and statements of social critique, are practices where disabled people consistently self-identify as disabled, where they use the knowledge of society unique to them."[57] Nowhere is this idea by Siebers of "disabled subjectivity" and the "disabled subject as knowledge producer"[58] more evident than in the social behaviors of the blind people in Tokugawa society, who did not openly rebel against society or take to the streets to protest the status system, as the social model's advocacy of social justice and disability activism would lead us to expect. Instead, they mostly chose to embrace and enhance their agency in living by the terms and rules of the Tokugawa social and political order. In fact, as will become clear, those blind people—as individuals and in organized groups—played a role in scripting and enabling their lives: individually and collectively, they reacted to the conditions of disability as actors who were conscious and cognizant of the circumstances, employing their disability-based identities to their advantage and also, quite often, to the detriment of less able peers.

Take, for example, charity and disability in premodern societies. It may seem surprising, and even paradoxical, to find examples of agency in charity, because we are used to modern narratives about disabled people receiving welfare benefits and food relief, as if disabled people passively and indiscriminately accept aid all the time. Writing about blindness in medieval France and England, Edward Wheatley follows Metzler's argument to explain that distinguishing impairment from disability allows us to see how medieval ideas turned impairment into disability.[59] Wheatley rightly cautions that the association of charity with disabled people in the premodern Christian context, arising from the religious idea that the Church dispensed aid out of benevolence, can be misleading when it denies agency to disabled people.[60] Charity was also an arena in which we see how blind people in Tokugawa society exercised their agency to the fullest extent. Religion in Tokugawa society was organized around

Buddhist and Shinto institutions and also around indigenous local and regional traditions. Though religious views influenced ideas of charity, the ideological context of status rule was clearly what determined how charity was practiced. Blind people did not have to be physically disabled or incapable of working to receive charity. As blind people, and with their disabled identities, they could insist on the right to charity; if they were guild members, they could rely on the guild to demand alms on their behalf.

While arguing for a modified approach to the social model of disability, I also frame my argument in such a way as to engage with medical perspectives—that being disabled as a result of being blind can be understood through medical perspectives. This modified approach takes heed of Kudlick's exhortation to explore the social history of medicine and avoid the pitfall of couching "disability history's raison d'être exclusively in terms of being medical history's righteous opponent."[61] Medical perspectives, as this book highlights, are integral components of a society's culture and its culture of disability. Disability studies scholars such as Anne Waldschmidt and Sharon Snyder and David Mitchell remind us that culture, broadly identified and defined, is the vast matrix of society in which disability is embedded. Writing about the big picture of disability and culture, Waldschmidt observes that culture encompasses "the totality of 'things' created and employed by a particular people or society, be they material or immaterial"; what this explanation, by accentuating culture, denotes for disability studies is that "in short, the cultural model considers disability not as a given entity or fact, but describes it as a discourse or as a process, experience, situation, or event."[62] In the cultural understanding of disability, Snyder and Mitchell argue that the experiences and environments of disability are permeable: "The definition of disability must incorporate both the inner and outer reaches of culture and experience as a combination of profoundly social and biological forces."[63] What is "biological" about disability, as I think of it, can be interpreted as what is physical and physiological about the impaired body. The interpretations of physiology, as I argue, revolve around medical discourses—or "biological forces"—that also are informed by cultural and historical contexts. Hence, medical history is a basis (but certainly not the sole basis) of disability history, but current disability studies scholarship sometimes eschews medical approaches to disability so as to resist, and even undo, the influence of the medical model of disability.

One goal of my present task is to rehabilitate the value of medical perspectives, not so much that of the medical model of understanding

disability that was previously introduced. The approach I take transcends
the limited understanding of impairment of the social model, which current scholarship criticizes for taking impairment to be a static fact of an
ahistorical body inured from the historical influences of medical views.[64]
Medical descriptions of visual impairment in Tokugawa society were
shaped by cultural valences (or multivalences).[65] Yes, these may be medical terms that were introduced by sighted ophthalmologists and medical
scholars in Tokugawa society, and for some disability studies scholars,
this practice of using diagnoses imposed by sighted people points toward
the persistent problem of what David Bolt dubs "ocularnormativism"
and "ocularcentrism" of ableist terminology, which tends to privilege
sight as the norm and discriminates against visual impairment.[66] Yet, as
I suggest, investigating medical terms from within "ocularnormative" or
"ocularcentric" traditions can still be useful. Though subjective terms,
they can be seen as evidence of the historical traditions, ideas, and terminology of medical and clinical studies in Tokugawa society. It is certainly not unimaginable that many blind people were familiar with the
medical language dealing with blindness (and internalized a lot of the
basic knowledge) through their contacts with medicine and with popular medical culture.

Part of the impasse in scholarly conversations about disability has to do
with how cure, which some disability studies scholars still associate with
the medical model of disability, is quite often viewed as a synonym for the
oppression of disabled people. In her recent scholarship on cure, and
in a critique of medical cures, Eunjung Kim takes contemporary South
Korea as her case study—her work is a welcome addition to the growing
list of works on disability in East Asia. She brilliantly explains that cure is
transformative for disabled people but not through easy transitions into
or seamless reassociations with nondisability.[67] She writes that "curative
violence constructs the normative body by inducing metamorphosis"[68]
and "the violence associated with cure exists at two levels: first, the violence of denying a place for disability and illness as different ways of living and, second, the physical and material violence against people with
disabilities that are justified in the name of cure."[69] My approach does
not evaluate the ideas of cure as a violent kind of systemic oppression
and as a means to transform a "cured," disabled person's subjecthood—
not because those ideas are unimportant but because I want to recon-
sider the significance of cure for our social and medical perspectives on
the disability history of Tokugawa Japan.

The narrative of cure in the Tokugawa context can be read and told through the twin perspectives of the history of medicine and the social history of medicine. Together these perspectives let us flesh out a social and historical narrative of the intellectual and popular mindsets about medicine, particularly about what cures were, how they worked, what people did to treat impairments, and also what choices people had in getting treatment. This approach demonstrates that while the question of cure can still be thought of as a medical one, it does not have to be framed in binary terms with cure as the polar opposite of disability or with the idea of cure as an end in itself. There is, literally, more to cure than meets the eye. The medical history and social history of cure are equally important constituents of disability history. Discussions that avoid the question of cure because of an ideological position against it hence miss the opportunity to engage with the textual and visual sources that suggest to us that people in Tokugawa society actually had recourse to cures and tried to find them.

By centering each chapter's discussions on representative examples, the book's overall analysis sheds light on the characteristics of Tokugawa society that are central to the contextual framing of our answers to what it meant to be blind. The examples aim to show why accounts of disability that portray blind people as bland, hapless marginalized subjects, and a social or political history of disability that is pursued to the exclusion of literary and medical histories, are inadequate in describing blindness and the richness of blind people's lives in Tokugawa society. Instead of uncritically transposing today's negative assumptions about disability onto Tokugawa society, it is more productive to critically and analytically approach disability through the concrete contexts of the politics, traditions, identities, and experiences of blind people in that era.

Tokugawa society developed its institutional bases and infrastructure in a different light than the Meiji society that succeeded it. Compared with Europe and the United States of the nineteenth and twentieth centuries, Tokugawa society seems to have been oddly different. It did not seem to have invested in scientifically informed pedagogical programs for educating blind people or other disabled people. It did not set up institutions that we would associate with modern hospitals, nor did it introduce social policies that we would instantly recognize as modern welfare policies. Yet Tokugawa society was uniquely functional in dealing with the blind population: it served blind people according to its own political ideology, encouraging and promoting as well as exploiting their roles in professional employment and in nonprofessional activities, and nurtured vibrant cultural discourses and practices in medicine and in popular medical culture. For those blind people to thrive, the complex logic of enablement had to first assume the form of subjugation to the social and political system—and once the Tokugawa regime and its institutions completely collapsed, the mechanism of empowerment that was specific to and dependent on that system was quickly invalidated.

To restate the general arc of the narrative more succinctly, and to use the grammar and vocabulary of disability studies in the context of early modern Japanese history, this book elaborates on how blindness was socialized, politicized, and medicalized in Tokugawa society. With insights into both disability history and early modern Japanese history, the book thus responds to the urgency of writing a disability-centered narrative of Japanese society to meet the demand for non-Western cultural and historical perspectives on disability in current scholarship.

Chapter Summary

This book is organized in six chapters to explore interdisciplinary perspectives on the developments of medicine, institutions, identities, traditions, communities, and professions that made blindness and blind people's lives in Tokugawa society distinctive. The narrative is tied to the historical analysis and reexamination of published primary sources and digitized copies of historical, literary, and medical manuscripts (handwritten and print manuscripts) from the Tokugawa period. Each chapter explores one key theme across the Tokugawa period, telling the overarching story and context of that theme, providing detailed analysis of significant shifts in historical continuities over time, and commenting on contingencies in context, thought, and culture.

While I make every attempt to cover all the centuries of the Tokugawa period in this book, and, where possible, link the developments to broad chronological trends, there is a greater emphasis on the eighteenth and nineteenth centuries. The years after the late seventeenth century witnessed the growth of popular culture, consumer culture, and print culture, among many important developments, and the variety of sources that survived from that time is more conducive to contextualizing discussions of themes than the sources we have from the early or mid-seventeenth century.

Chapter 1 focuses on the medical thought and practices of Japanese ophthalmology. The chapter analyzes Japanese ophthalmologists' medical investigations of eye conditions and illustrates the historical background that informed the organization of medical knowledge about blindness. Chapter 2 explores sources of medicine and methods of treatment in popular medical culture and reimagines the experience of cure with patient-centered and consumer-centered perspectives.

Chapters 3 through 6 consider the diverse ways blind people lived, analyzing case studies to provide perspectives on the significance of blind people's contributions to Tokugawa society. Chapters 3 and 4 examine blind people's disabled identities and their activities through the guild and outside the guild. The two chapters survey what blind people did in their lives—and also, based on evidence, explain what they would have done in certain situations. They discuss the guild's complex mandate and operations to document that the guild was relevant to the political goals of government authorities. Chapter 3 argues that guild members, from the elite to the bottom tiers, used the guild to seek benefits. Chapter 4 considers examples of those blind people excluded from the guild, such as blind women and blind lay priests, to further discuss how blind people without guild membership, and marginalized groups among them, formed communities and looked for support.

Chapters 5 and 6 elaborate on the contexts in which Chiichi, Hokiichi, and Wa'ichi, the three blind men featured at the start of this introduction, achieved success. Chapter 5 focuses on *Heike* texts, music, and performances, which were traditionally performed by blind male musicians of the guild. The chapter argues that Chiichi embodied in his life and work what was exceptional about blind musicians and also what was ordinary about them. It addresses the striking similarities between Chiichi and Hokiichi in their lives and professional activities. By exploring print culture, musical lineages, and textual and performance histories, it surveys the choices of blind musicians and explains the contexts of collaborative endeavors between sighted people and blind musicians.

Chapter 6 analyzes the social and medical factors that enabled blind people to enter the new professions of acupuncture and massage. It discusses the profiles of blind pioneers in acupuncture, the most notable of whom was Wa'ichi. It also examines the emergence of trends in the cultivation of health to explore the popularity of massage and blind masseurs.

The six chapters interweave perspectives in an interdisciplinary analysis that makes it clear why the contextual study of Tokugawa society is imperative for understanding how and why being blind meant being disabled yet also being particularly enabled.

CHAPTER 1

Japanese Ophthalmology

Medical Studies of Eye Conditions

⎯⎯⎯⎯ ༒ ⎯⎯⎯⎯

This book begins with a study of blindness in order to introduce the medical and historical contexts of Tokugawa Japan in which people with medical expertise developed perspectives on what it meant to be blind. Ophthalmologists were among those people with intimate, expert medical knowledge of eye conditions. From the late medieval period through the Tokugawa period, Japanese ophthalmologists of the Majima lineage were influential. They were erudite medical scholars (scholars who studied and practiced medicine) whose medical thought and clinical techniques of treatment represented mainstream Japanese ophthalmology. The analysis of medical texts such as those of the Majima ophthalmologists helps us to understand how Japanese ophthalmologists investigated eye conditions.

Focused on the Tokugawa period, and with insights into earlier periods and contexts, this chapter's discussion of Japanese ophthalmology is organized around Japanese medical perspectives on a range of visual impairments that would likely have constituted blindness. This broad approach is necessary because Japanese ophthalmology did not have a fixed definition of blindness, and there was no objective standard for evaluating either vision or vision loss. Japanese ophthalmologists generally thought of blindness as disabling vision loss and poor vision, attributing it to eye diseases, afflictions, and injuries. They described the causes and treatments of functional disorders and impairments of vision, but their sources do not always give us details about the degrees of vision loss.

It is also significant that medical thought in Tokugawa Japan was centered on a system of lineages and texts. The Majima lineage of ophthalmologists is one example of a medical lineage. Medical lineages developed their thought and practices based on their founders' teachings, and selectively passed down knowledge from master to disciple through textual and verbal methods. Hence, medical texts were regarded as important written records of a lineage. This system validated historical traditions of interpretation and definition; the vocabulary, categories, and medical discourses in Japanese ophthalmology attest to this fact.

At a broader level, this chapter sheds light on the intellectual foundations of Japanese ophthalmology and discusses the introduction of European medical thought to Japanese medical scholars in the eighteenth and nineteenth centuries. The new wave of European medical scholarship in those years inspired approaches that studied eye conditions using a different analytical language but did not fundamentally change the traditional framework for understanding blindness.

Japanese Ophthalmology:
The Historical Background of a Medical Lineage

Ophthalmology in Tokugawa Japan was rooted in classical Chinese medical thought. By around the second and third centuries CE of Han-dynasty China, Chinese medical scholars had schematically articulated the human anatomy through terminology that mirrored the bureaucratic organization of the feudal state and economy. They understood the human body to be composed of organs and viscera[1]—or, more literally, "depots" (organs) and "palaces" (viscera)[2]—linked with one another through an intricate network of *qi* (breath; Japanese: *ki*) and blood flowing through vessels and conduits. Classical Chinese medical thought was cemented in *The Yellow Emperor's Inner Classic*,[3] a foundational medical text that has been studied extensively by contemporary historians of medicine, such as Paul Unschuld. The core anatomical discourses of medicine in Japan, known as Sino-Japanese medicine[4] because it was strongly influenced by Chinese medicine, traditionally focused on five organs (heart, liver, lungs, kidneys, and spleen) and six viscera (gall bladder, small intestines, large intestines, bladder, stomach, and a unique part called the "triple burner"[5]).

Classical Chinese medical thought primarily associated the eyes and vision with the liver. For example, according to *The Yellow Emperor's Inner Classic*, "the liver rules the eyes"[6] and "the liver opens an orifice in the eyes."[7] Vision, or what the eyes could see, depended on the uninterrupted flow of *qi* from the liver to the eyes. "The qi of the liver pass through the eyes. When the [qi of the] liver are in harmony, then the eyes can distinguish the five colors."[8] Historian of medicine Shigehisa Kuriyama highlights that the five colors (green, red, yellow, white, and black) were fundamental to classical Chinese medical thought, and together with the five phases (wood, fire, earth, metal, and water), they expressed the elemental unity of the human body and reflected the exterior macrocosmic environment.[9]

In the same classical Chinese medical thought, the eyes were also understood to be crucial nodal points among other sites around the body: "All vessels are tied to the eyes. All marrow is tied to the brain. All sinews are tied to the joints. All blood is tied to the heart."[10] Like their relationship with the liver, as the text tells us, the eyes were also said to reflect the qualities of the heart. "The luster of the heart shows in the face. The eyes are the emissaries of the heart."[11] Yet, despite the appearances of a strict hegemony, there was a dynamic equilibrium. As Kuriyama explains, there was a circular, complementary order in which the five organs governed one another and, in turn, were governed by one another: the heart governed the lungs but was governed by the kidneys; the spleen governed the kidneys but was governed by the liver; and the lungs governed the liver.[12] The eyes were thought to be passive pools of deposit from the liver and therefore inferior to the five (spirit) depots.[13]

In Japan's classical and early medieval periods, classical Chinese medical thought spread to Japan through Buddhism and through the Japanese imperial court of Nara and Kyoto. Medical knowledge was considered to be elite knowledge. The imperial court and Buddhist institutions sponsored the study of medicine, which included ophthalmology. Early evidence of Japan's reception of ophthalmology from China appears in the late tenth-century Japanese encyclopedia *Prescriptions from the Heart of Medicine*,[14] compiled by the courtier Tanba Yasuyori. As a collection of passages from Chinese medical texts, the encyclopedia gave educated elites, such as court physicians of the Bureau of Medicine,[15] insights into the historical thought and practices of Chinese medicine, including ophthalmology.

Across Buddhist cultures from India to China, there was an intimate relationship between Buddhism and ophthalmology. In her study of

Buddhist medicine, Katja Triplett explains that Nāgārjuna, an ancient Indian Buddhist philosopher, also was a famed practitioner of ophthalmology.[16] In light of Nāgārjuna's healing powers, *Nāgārjuna*, his name itself, became synonymous with divine cure for eye diseases in East Asian Buddhist traditions. Buddhism also informed medical knowledge about ophthalmology in Japan; Japanese Buddhist monks who traveled to China studied medicine in the Buddhist context.

The Majima lineage was a succession of generations of sighted ophthalmologists whose medical understanding and practices, it seems, were rooted in medieval Buddhist-medical learning.[17] A travel guidebook of the Tokugawa period, the *Illustrated Gazetteer of the Famous Places of Owari*,[18] tells us that this medical lineage traced its origin to the ancestral village of Majima in Owari province (in Aichi prefecture today). Although illustrated gazetteers (a genre of guidebooks) did not supplant official histories, they were widely enjoyed as works of travel literature because they regaled readers with stories and pictures about landmarks and attractions in different regions. The Owari gazetteer introduces us to Seigan Sōzu, supposedly the founder of the original Majima lineage in the early medieval period, and recounts the genealogy of the temple Myōgen'in, which was erected to honor the Medicine Buddha.[19] In the area around Owari, the Medicine Buddha was worshipped by mountain ascetics and devotees for his boundless benevolence and miraculous healing powers.[20] The religious culture of the Medicine Buddha had also been supported by the imperial court and court elites of Nara in the early eighth century.[21] Building on its early, strong reputation in ophthalmology, the Majima lineage bolstered its credibility in the Tokugawa period by claiming to have long-standing connections with the imperial family in Kyoto and with the shogunate in Edo.[22]

The Majima lineage enjoyed legendary status in the popular culture of the Tokugawa period.[23] According to the Owari gazetteer, the temple Myōgen'in was reportedly constructed in the early ninth century during the reign of Emperor Tenmu.[24] In the devastating medieval civil wars of the 1330s, nearly everything was burned to the ground, but the statue of the Medicine Buddha was miraculously salvaged. In the wake of the conflagration, the Majima founder devoted his life and energies to the reconstruction of the temple, restoring it to its former glory in 1357. As the story goes, one night, in a dream, the Medicine Buddha transmitted the secrets of ophthalmology to him and instructed him to apply those teachings to alleviate the sufferings of the world. When he was roused from his dream, at the altar he discovered a manual on ophthalmology.

This sacred manual was touted as a record of the secret teachings of the lineage, imbued with the divine authority of the Medicine Buddha.

The Owari gazetteer also outlines the miracles that the Majima lineage was said to have performed. In 1632, Enkei, a leader of the lineage, attended to Emperor Go-Mizunō's third daughter, who was tormented by a stubborn eye condition. Physicians from all over Kyoto were summoned, but none of them could deliver a cure. Enkei, however, astutely diagnosed the disease. At her bedside, he stuck a needle into her eye. Following that, he prescribed medicines that worked wonders. The lineage renewed its relations with the imperial family in 1766 when Enkai, a successor of the lineage, treated Emperor Momozono's son. Enkai's success recalled and rivaled Enkei's feat of healing performed more than a hundred years earlier. Though the historicity of either episode is not clear, the accounts are consistent in emphasizing the ophthalmologists' consummate skills. As will be clear in the subsequent discussion, the Majima lineage was known to use clinical techniques that involved needles (which I generally call needling or needling techniques), especially in treating eye conditions that required needles to break down impediments.

The Majima lineage in the Tokugawa period was composed of sublineages claiming descent from the parent lineage. As the parent lineage expanded, so too did sub-lineages grow in strength and compete with one another for authority.[25] They were also intent on recreating the original contents of the parent lineage's teachings without breaking with traditional, orthodox wisdoms. A disciple could train under a master and practice medicine in ways that were identified with that lineage. With the right connections and under ideal circumstances, a disciple could gain the right to practice medicine in an official capacity by being appointed as a physician to a samurai lord or, even better, as a physician to the shogun (a shogunate physician). As chapter 2 will highlight, Majima ophthalmologists who had broad connections with samurai lords were hired for their medical services. However, because there were no strict regulations on who could practice medicine, traveling medical vendors, religious healers, and pharmacists could also handle, prescribe, and sell medicines to the lay population anywhere; popular literature inveighed against quacks and charlatans. Hence, while many medical scholars were involved in medicine through the study and practice of it, in the broadest sense, professional medical practitioners encompassed people who engaged with medicine for a living: by teaching medicine, performing treatments with a variety of healing therapies and regimens, or selling medicines.

Eye Medicines of Majima Myōgen'in,[26] a medical text dated 1788, offers some insights into a typical account by a sub-lineage about its genealogical history.[27] As that text tells it, some generations earlier (in an unknown era), a priest of a local temple in Miura (in Sagami province; in Kanagawa prefecture today)[28] traveled to the Majima founder's temple to train as an ophthalmologist. According to the account, he cured more than ten thousand people of their eye diseases. In his seventies, he returned to his original home temple, where he carried on his work as a venerated ophthalmologist, and founded a sub-lineage. As we are told, the local temple gained repute as a center of ophthalmological care and served communities in the area. However, little evidence, if any, confirms this account and the priest's or the author's background. Yet, through aggrandized and uncorroborated claims, the inclusion of this narrative in the medical text justified the authority the sub-lineage had to practice ophthalmology in the name of the parent lineage.

Collectively, the Majima medical texts documented lineage-based knowledge. The entire corpus provides a solid textual basis for our analysis of the intersecting streams of medical thought, approaches, and practices. Comparison of the texts makes it clear that they generally agreed upon medical terms and made significant references to one another. Also, many of the texts were handwritten and privately owned and so were not as broadly circulated as other printed and published documents. This observation supports Peter Kornicki's argument that many handwritten medical manuscripts of the Tokugawa period were not meant for commercial sale.[29] Some texts disclosed secret recipes of medicines and were written to be read and studied by selected audiences. Though the authorship of many secret texts[30] cannot be verified, and secrets cannot be traced to exact sources all the time, the authors were firm in asserting their fidelity to the Majima parent lineage's original teachings.

The undated treatise *Secret Records: The Dawn of Eye Treatments,*[31] which it seems likely was copied sometime in the Tokugawa period, is especially significant for our study. It recorded the ophthalmological techniques of a sub-lineage. Like some medieval texts of the medical genre, it encrypted secrets to achieve a balance between openness and secrecy. Portions of the text that were to be taught by secret transmission to only distinguished disciples were abbreviated and encoded by brief phrases like "oral transmission of acupuncture treatment," "oral transmission of using needles," and "there is an oral transmission."[32] Despite their importance, texts of this sort were not intended to be substitutes for the transmission of knowledge directly from master to disciple. Although a disciple was bound by oath to protect the secrets of a lineage, by the late Tokugawa period the actual regulation of knowledge by any lineage had become quite flexible and certainly also quite untenable.[33]

As the number of works on ophthalmology in China grew, new ideas were introduced to Japanese ophthalmologists. *Essential Subtleties on the Silver Sea,* a representative Chinese ophthalmological treatise, was printed and circulated in Tokugawa society.[34] Compiled and edited sometime in sixteenth-century China, or possibly earlier, it crystallized the historical scholarship of Chinese ophthalmology.[35] For example, the eye was identified with the "five spheres"[36] and "eight boundaries"[37]— terminology that Jürgen Kovacs and Unschuld have analyzed as Chinese interpretations of Indian theories about the eyes.[38] This representation expanded on the earlier classical Chinese medical thought to schematically explain the correspondences between the eyes and other elements of the human anatomy and also between the eyes and the supreme cosmic elements. The model was reproduced in the Majima text of *Secret Records* (see figures 1.1 and 1.2 and table 1.1).

The Majima ophthalmologists adopted the idea from Chinese ophthalmology that the "spheres" and "boundaries" mapped the eyes' relationships with the organs and viscera. The eyes were most closely linked to the liver, as highlighted earlier in the discussion of *The Yellow Emperor's Inner Classic,* but as the correspondences show, the health of the other organs and viscera was also reflected in the health of the eyes. Ophthalmologists traced eye ailments to other parts of the body that were understood to be their sources. The "water sphere" and the "wind sphere" in the black region of the eye, which we know to encompass the iris and pupil, were matched with the kidneys and liver, respectively; the "blood sphere" at the inner canthus and outer canthus was linked to the heart; the "breath sphere" in the white area of the eye (the sclera) was associated with the lungs; the "flesh sphere" above the eye was believed to be related to the stomach and, below the eye, to the spleen.[39] The "eight boundaries"—the "swamp," "thunder," "mountain," "wind," "water," "earth," "fire," and "heaven" boundaries—were regarded as overlapping with the "five spheres" and were primarily associated with vessels and conduits of the organs and viscera.[40] This representation used by the Majima ophthalmologists also seems to have been accepted by other leading medical lineages in Japan.[41]

The next section focuses on the Majima ophthalmologists' understanding of eye diseases. While we do not know from the sources what

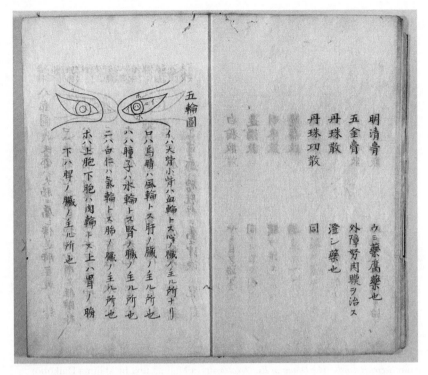

Fig. 1.1. Pages from a medical text including an image of the "five spheres" of the eyes. From *Secret Records: The Dawn of Eye Treatments* (a Majima text by Majima Daikōbō; Japanese title: *Ganryō tōun hiroku*). Main Library, Kyoto University Rare Materials Digital Archive.

degrees of vision loss made up blindness, we learn that Japanese ophthalmologists and, in general, Japanese medical scholars interpreted blindness as impaired vision. They all described the causes and mechanisms of visual impairment and the required treatments. There are significant technical details in the sources, and it is necessary to engage with those details in my analysis. Because many of the sources that I discuss were written by the Majima ophthalmologists, it is not clear how efficacious the clinical techniques and medical treatments were from their patients' perspectives or whether their patients were cured. What the technical discussions will tell us, however, is that there was consistency in the use of concepts and terms in medical lineages and that Japanese and Chinese ophthalmologists shared a common framework of interpretation.

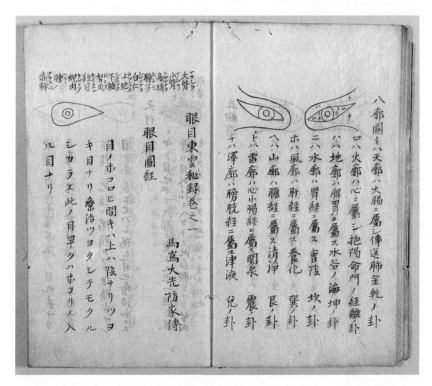

Fig. 1.2. Pages from a medical text depicting the "eight boundaries" of the eyes. From *Secret Records: The Dawn of Eye Treatments* (a Majima text by Majima Daikōbō; Japanese title: *Ganryō tōun hiroku*). Main Library, Kyoto University Rare Materials Digital Archive.

Table 1.1. Summary of the "Five Spheres" and "Eight Boundaries" and the Correspondences with the Organs/Viscera/Conduits of the Body

"Five spheres" and "eight boundaries"	Corresponding organs/viscera/ conduits in the body
"Blood sphere"	Heart
"Wind sphere"	Liver
"Water sphere"	Kidneys
"Breath sphere"	Lungs
"Flesh sphere"	Stomach and spleen
"Heaven boundary"	Large intestine and lungs
"Fire boundary"	Heart and the "Gate of Life" conduit
"Earth boundary"	Stomach and spleen
"Water boundary"	Conduit of the kidneys
"Wind boundary"	Conduit of the liver
"Mountain boundary"	Conduit of the gall bladder
"Thunder boundary"	Conduits of the heart and small intestine
"Swamp boundary"	Conduit of the bladder

Traditional Discourses of Vision: Finding the Causes of Impairment

REDNESS AND ATTACKS BY "WINDS"

According to classical Chinese medical thought, "winds"[42] were not merely air circulating in the outside environment; when they blew, they affected a person's health. Kuriyama writes that "winds (*feng*) cause chills and headaches, vomiting and cramps, dizziness and numbness, loss of speech. And that is but the beginning."[43] For example, *The Yellow Emperor's Inner Classic* discusses how the eyes and the connected body parts were susceptible to attacks by "winds." In life-threatening cases, the eyes were starved of nourishment; they appeared to be locked in a dead stare or to recede into the deep recesses of the sockets.[44] Which body part had to be treated depended on the source of the disease, and a physician could examine the condition of the eyes to find useful clues. When the head was besieged by "winds" (called "eye winds"), the eyes would turn cold or start to hurt and itch.[45] When the liver was assailed by "winds" (called "liver winds"), the person would succumb to periods of sadness and sweat profusely; green discoloration under the eyes was a symptom of this liver ailment.[46] Red eyes meant that the heart was affected by disease; white eyes were symptoms of diseased lungs; yellow and black eyes signified a diseased spleen and diseased kidneys, respectively.[47] This foundation of correspondences between the eyes and the connected body parts also prefigured relationships in the model of the "five spheres" and "eight boundaries" in later ophthalmological works.

"Winds" were thought to be linked to epidemics and contagion in the population. Daniel Trambaiolo's recent study tells us that seventeenth-century Chinese medical scholarship on epidemics revolved around discourses of unseasonal environmental conditions.[48] The condition of "epidemic red eyes"[49] discussed in Chinese and Japanese ophthalmological texts is one example of similarities between the medical categories of Chinese and Japanese ophthalmology. This condition was a disease of the eyes.

Comparing a Majima text such as *Secret Records* with *Essential Subtleties on the Silver Sea* allows us to examine intertextual references and to reimagine the intercultural significance of Chinese and Japanese medical diagnoses. The Chinese text *Essential Subtleties on the Silver Sea* explains that the cause of "epidemic red eyes" was the invasion of "winds." The text does not explain the routes of epidemic spread but warns of the danger of contagion. The infected eyes were not covered by a screen (or membrane)[50] and did not show signs of the invasion of fleshy matter.[51] Full recovery took about five days, but without treatment the eyes did not heal.

According to the Majima nosography (classification of diseases), "epidemic red eyes" were subsumed under the broader category of "diseased eyes,"[52] which were characterized by diseases of the eyes (conditions in which the eyes were affected by disease, or *yami*).[53] The redness associated with "epidemic red eyes" was a clear sign that the eyes had disease and that vision was impaired. Also related to "diseased eyes" were the "forty-eight eyes,"[54] a term that was probably based on a couple of things: the varieties of debilitating eye diseases with redness and impairment, or a reorganized classification of the seventy-two common eye diseases to which Chinese ophthalmological treatises refer.[55]

Contemporary historians of medicine may use historical descriptions as evidence to deduce the prevalence of certain diseases in the past, but this has to be done with the understanding that historical contexts of disease may be different from one another. In today's medical vocabulary, the Majima texts' "diseased eyes" category would have covered a good range of minor and severe eye inflammations. Redness of the eyes could have been caused by acute conjunctivitis or more serious infectious diseases. Despite the use of "epidemic" in certain categories in medical texts, eye diseases could be endemic, and impaired vision could have been experienced by anyone who contracted contagious diseases, such as measles and smallpox—diseases that Japanese medical scholars, including Japanese ophthalmologists, understood to affect the eyes (see this chapter's discussion of smallpox).

Using today's diagnostic definitions, symptoms like "ulcerations and granulations of the eyelids"[56] and "inward-growing eyelashes"[57] in *Essential Subtleties on the Silver Sea* and symptoms of "epidemic red eyes" and "diseased eyes" in *Secret Records* would correlate, among some possibilities, with classic clinical signs of trachoma infection. This infection, a bacterial disease caused by *chlamydia trachomatis*, is spread easily by human contact with contaminated fluids and secretions. The bacteria can also cause other kinds of infections that are linked to sexually transmitted diseases.

Trachoma, which still is regarded as a significant cause of visual impairment in places with poor sanitation and underdeveloped public health infrastructure, posed risks to public health through the Meiji period in Japan and was likely widespread earlier in Tokugawa society. In an effort to eradicate trachoma, public health officials of Meiji Japan intensified their campaigns to spread health awareness about hygiene and sanitation.[58] Some military servicemen returning to Japan from China after the Sino-Japanese War (1894–95) appeared to have contracted trachoma during their service stints abroad, which suggests that it was prevalent in parts of China through the nineteenth century as well.[59] From what we understand about trachoma today, depending on the duration of the disease and the degree of scarring, visual impairment can be partial or total, temporary or permanent.

BLURRED VISION

Poor vision was sometimes described in medical texts as blurred vision; more literally, blurred vision was like "cloudy" or "muddy" vision.[60] A possible cause was acute eye irritation. From a modern perspective, the conditions could have been linked to glaucoma, macular degeneration, astigmatism, myopia (nearsightedness), and hyperopia (farsightedness). As chapter 2 will discuss, patients who had blurred vision and "aging eyes" complained that they could not see things clearly, and in serious cases, those patients described that they completely lost their sight. It seems that the treatments discussed in the Majima texts focused on short-term relief. *Secret Records*, for instance, explains how to counteract hotness and coldness. Camphor, native to Southeast Asia and one of the foreign substances frequently mentioned in the text, was thought to possess a cooling nature with the power to dispel heat.[61] It was an ingredient of cinnabar powder for the treatment of "diseased eyes" and could also be used independently in its solid form to relieve poor vision.[62] Another substance was borax, which was prepared by being soaked in water and then dried before use. With similar cooling properties as camphor, it was used to clear up vision.[63] Cataracts, a possible cause of blurred vision, were assigned to the category of "obstructive" eye conditions in the Majima texts.

EYE CONDITIONS WITH "OBSTRUCTION"

Chinese ophthalmologists discussed an eye disease known as "clear blindness,"[64] which was quite likely a medical term for visual impairment due to cataracts. The descriptions also fit a related disabling eye condition mentioned in some Chinese texts as "green/blue blindness" or "glaucous blindness with a green/blue screen."[65] "Clear blindness" was understood to severely impair vision, and the timeline of the disease's progression depended on each individual. According to *Prescriptions from the Heart of Medicine*, a tenth-century Japanese compilation of Chinese sources mentioned in the previous section, when the eye was affected by "clear blindness," a greenish-whitish impediment formed over the center of the eye.[66] But the growth of cataracts did not seem to be accompanied by pain, itch, or structural deformities of the eyes' exterior parts—hence the eyes appeared to be "clear eyes" that looked normal. The text goes on to say that in the advanced stages of impairment, the affected person could barely tell apart people and things or suffered from significant vision loss but still had sufficient sensitivity to light to tell the difference between day and night. Akin to the ancient medical technique of cataract couching to remove cataracts, a surgical procedure performed with a golden needle on the "clear eyes" could help to restore sight—literally, by causing the impediment in the eyes to be dissipated. The procedure is thought to be ahead of its time and was probably introduced to China by way of Indian Buddhism and medicine.

Another disabling eye condition discussed in classical Chinese medical texts appears to be pterygium.[67] This condition, from what we know today, is associated with the growth of tissue over the eye. As Chinese ophthalmologists understood it, the impediment started at the inner corner of the eye and grew to encroach onto the area that we know to be the cornea. Chinese ophthalmologists explained that the disease resulted when *qi* was forced to rush into the eyes, causing a wing-shaped, skin-like film of matter to envelop them.[68] There were two types of film: white film and red film. Over time, the matter thickened and spread and had to be surgically removed, lifted and excised promptly and carefully with a surgical knife or with a hooked needle.[69] The steps were consistent with descriptions documented in Indian ophthalmological texts. Vijaya Deshpande's study of Chinese medical texts suggests that there were specific words in Chinese for the surgical actions of turning, cutting, needling, and scraping—yet another example of the influence of Indian ophthalmology and the syncretic nature of Chinese medical knowledge.[70]

The Majima ophthalmologists, like Chinese ophthalmologists, understood "clear blindness" and other related conditions of impeded vision to cause severe visual impairment and had names for "obstructive"[71] eye conditions. As the word "obstructive" suggests, these were eye conditions in which impairment was associated with obstruction of vision. The Majima ophthalmologists also followed the convention in Chinese and Japanese ophthalmology of differentiating "internal obstruction" from "external obstruction" (deformities around the eyes). "Obstructive" eye conditions were listed in *Explanations of Disease Names*, a seventeenth-century Japanese medical encyclopedia of the origins of disease names in major Chinese medical texts.[72] The Japanese terminology can be traced to Chinese translations of Indian Buddhist and medical texts. For example, various Chinese translations of "obstructions" linked "internal obstructions" to shades or screens that blocked the eyes.[73] It seems that the Majima ophthalmologists preferred to use external therapies, such as eye ointments, to treat "external obstructions,"[74] perhaps because these "obstructions" occurred on surfaces around the eyes.

Japanese ophthalmologists' complex understanding of "internal obstructions" is evident in their classification of white, green/blue, red, yellow, and black "internal obstructions." This classification was based on the five colors of classical Chinese medical thought. "Internal obstructions" had interrelated symptoms.[75] In almost all instances, the affected eyes had to be treated in time with needling techniques to save that person's vision. For example, according to *The Majima Lineage's Secret Text on the Eyes*[76] (1765), "yellow internal obstruction" began as a white substance in the area that we know as the iris.[77] As the disease spread around the eye, the affected white area turned yellow. The Majima ophthalmologists advised waiting for the pupil to shrink before treatment. As *Secret Records* indicates, "red internal obstruction" turned white over a year or two.[78] The Majima ophthalmologists recommended surgery after the redness had subsided and fully transitioned into whiteness. "Green/blue internal obstruction" was possibly a condition related to glaucoma, but as one text says, this condition showed symptoms that were quite similar to those of "white internal obstruction."[79] Though not explained as cataracts, the Majima ophthalmologists' descriptions of "white internal obstruction" would fit our modern understanding of cataracts: white matter blocks the lens and obstructs vision to the extent that it causes blindness. The choice of treatment, whether with medicines or with needling techniques, was influenced by an ophthalmologist's diagnosis of the severity, size, and depth of the "obstruction." Untreated visual impairment of any color classification could worsen and result in severe damage to vision.

The Takeuchi lineage, contemporary with the Majima lineage, claimed to have proprietary knowledge of medicinal substances to treat "obstructions." The ingredients of secret recipes were known to and prescribed by ophthalmologists of different lineages. For the Takeuchi lineage, the core knowledge was centered on the methods and proportions by which six important ingredients—camphor, musk, cinnabar, tiger meat, pearls, and "heaven's stone"—were mixed and combined into medicines.[80]

SMALLPOX

Smallpox is a highly infectious and virulent disease whose symptoms include skin lesions and scarring. It does not always inflict damage on the eyes, but when it does, a possible dreadful consequence is permanent vision loss. Though there are no longer active infections of smallpox in modern societies today, smallpox was widespread until public health measures were successfully enacted to contain and eradicate it.

Smallpox was endemic in the Japanese population during the Tokugawa period with periodic epidemic outbreaks, and the risk of infection was constantly present.[81] Historically, because of the population's prolonged exposure to smallpox, Japanese medical scholars were familiar with the pernicious nature of the disease and employed traditional methods of treatment even after the cowpox vaccine was introduced to Japan. As Ann Jannetta's study highlights, the cowpox vaccine was successfully brought over to Japan from abroad through the Dutch by around 1849; the vaccine was then transferred from Nagasaki to Edo, where advocates of the vaccine had been appointed to positions of political influence.[82] But even so, the shogunate did not coordinate a national plan to vaccinate the population against the disease.[83] The top-down efforts to spread the vaccine mostly depended on the goodwill of domain lords and their allies. Progress was slow and uneven. Statistics on vaccination are incomplete, but it should be emphasized that the vaccine had limited impact on the actual treatment of the disease.

Tokugawa Japanese medical scholars generally subscribed to the traditional idea that some diseases had "poison"[84]—understood specifically in the Sino-Japanese medical context as disease poison. Smallpox was one of those diseases. Japanese medical scholars were careful to specifically characterize diseases with sores such as smallpox, syphilis, and measles as diseases with "poison"—the latter two diseases are contagious, active diseases that even today can potentially cause serious complications with vision. Yoshimasu Tōdō, an influential eighteenth-century Japanese medical scholar who championed ancient Chinese formularies and espoused discourses of "poison," argued that "poison," in general, was the root of all diseases.[85] According to *The Break with Medicine*,[86] which outlines his teachings, the "poison" of smallpox was especially deadly: it choked the body and led to death.[87] Treatments of smallpox had to focus on expelling the "poison" from the body.

Japanese ophthalmologists were among those medical scholars who discussed "poison" and wrote about it in medical texts. Many of the texts distinguished the conditions of eyes affected by smallpox[88] from other conditions like "diseased eyes" and "epidemic red eyes" because the underlying causes were different. (Japanese ophthalmologists usually grouped visual impairment caused by diseases with sores in categories closely identified with those respective diseases.) Eye conditions of smallpox, measles, and syphilis were closely related to one another because of their common relationship with "poison," which was understood to be a significant cause of visual impairment.

Other Japanese medical scholars such as specialists of smallpox remarked that visual impairment that was caused by smallpox was notoriously difficult to treat. *A Sequel: Discerning the Essentials of Smallpox Medicine* (1827)[89] by Ikeda Mukei, a follower of the Ikeda lineage that specialized in treatments of smallpox, warns that the eyes were vulnerable to disorders in the course of an active smallpox illness.[90] Fevers from smallpox, unlike other fevers, developed from the depths of the body and radiated outward. As heat remained trapped in the body, blood flowed in a reverse direction away from the eyes, allowing "poison" to travel from the liver to the eyes. Together with heat, "poison" caused "winds" that damaged the eyes.

Another text of the same Ikeda lineage, *Verbal Formulas of Treating Smallpox by Master Ikeda*[91] (undated, but quite likely a late eighteenth-century manuscript), elaborates that even after surviving the illness of smallpox, that person was still not safe from "poison." Residual smallpox "poison" in the liver could still rise to the eyes, inducing pain and redness.[92] "Cooling-diaphragm"[93] powder—prepared from mint, gypsum, *Gardenia jasminoides*, rhubarb, goldthread, *Phellodrendon*, Chinese skullcap, and *Forsythia*—was a medicine that worked by purging "poison" and heat from the liver. Attacks by active or residual "poison," if not properly treated in time, could lead to devastating vision loss.

EXTERNAL INJURIES

Traumatic force to the eyes can cause severe vision loss. Workplace accidents, accidents at home, and brawls were likely scenarios in the Tokugawa period in which a person could sustain eye injuries. Handbooks and manuals that were published starting in the seventeenth century were useful sources of home remedies (see some examples in chapter 2). Their publication over the next centuries indicates that they continued to be helpful to the populace. Take, for example, *Emergency Prescriptions of Broad Virtue*[94] (1790), a late eighteenth-century work endorsed by the shogunate. It was published as a practical survival and medical guide. The authors were Taki Motonori, a shogunate physician who succeeded his father as the head of the shogunate medical school,[95] and his son Motoyasu.

The section on eye medicines in that text focuses on eye injuries. As the text recommends, a person could apply to a mildly injured eye generous amounts of breast milk and an aqueous solution of sugar.[96] The roots of bunch-flowered daffodils,[97] grown in home gardens, could be ground and mixed with sugar to make a kind of salve or lubricant. A suitable substitute was a mixture prepared with the heads of houseflies, which were crushed, mixed, and blended with sugar or breast milk. To treat a serious eye injury, the text recommends applying to the injured eye pulverized, ground deer velvet antlers[98] mixed with breast milk. The text says that to help a person who had been so badly beaten that the eye was protruding,[99] it was necessary to place a moist towel over the injury and, without disturbing the connective threads, delicately shift the displaced eye back into its original position.[100] That eye was then to be bandaged and protected from cold "winds" for three days. Applying *Rehmannia glutinosa*, pounded and ground, onto the eye under the bandage was thought to expedite the healing process.[101]

A New Moment in Japanese Ophthalmology: The Arrival of Rangaku (Dutch Learning)

Beginning in the early seventeenth century, and for centuries thereafter, because of the shogunate's strict ban on Christianity, the shogunate restricted Japan's contacts with the Europeans. Only permitted representatives of the Dutch East India Company (Vereenigde Oostindische Compagnie, or VOC) could trade with Japan, and only in the port city of Nagasaki. The Dutch acted as intermediaries between Japan and Europe and conducted their activities under the close surveillance of the Nagasaki magistrate,[102] an important office of the shogunate. The Dutch kept Japanese intellectuals informed about European developments in science, technology, and medicine. *Rangaku* (Dutch learning), a term in Japanese that acknowledged the intermediary role of the Dutch in spreading European knowledge to Japan, was an active field of scholarship among Japanese scholars who focused on European knowledge. Scholarship in Dutch learning gathered momentum in the eighteenth century as intellectual and social circles of scholars expanded. The methods and results of Dutch learning inspired *ranpō igaku* (Dutch-method medicine), an offshoot of Dutch learning centered on medical studies.[103] By the late eighteenth century, Dutch learning had become adapted and indigenized in Tokugawa Japan as a legitimate branch of scholarship.

Dutch learning developed under shogun Tokugawa Yoshimune, who ruled from 1716 through 1745. Policies previously enacted to protect the political and intellectual climate of Japan from subversive thought, especially Christian thought recorded in books from Europe, were selectively repealed in the name of "practical learning."[104] This reversal in official attitude toward scholarship stimulated a mainstream culture of learning for practical results. Yoshimune's political agenda gave an impetus to *honzōgaku* (natural history or nature studies). As Federico Marcon's study demonstrates, Yoshimune oversaw the grand project of compiling the names of all the varieties of plant and animal species across the land, which he regarded as "objects to be inventoried, accumulated, and consumed as material and intellectual commodities."[105] The task required exhaustive, time-consuming processes: collecting specimens, locating physical traits, and deducing relational and categorical links. In that process, scholars of nature studies reoriented their epistemic framework toward the direct observation of actual things.

The idea that observing things directly could lead to new discoveries generated interest in reexamining the human anatomy. Sugita Genpaku, a Japanese medical scholar who in the late eighteenth century was considered to be a pioneer in Dutch learning in Japan, argued that dissection opened a new window onto the firsthand experience of knowledge. His academic foray into human anatomical studies was seen by scholars as the start of Dutch-method medicine.[106] European anatomical studies were discordant with Japan's historical medical paradigm with its traditional approaches to the five organs and six viscera. Genpaku himself witnessed the dissection of a human corpse to compare and confirm the anatomical records. With the help of Maeno Ryōtaku, Nakagawa Jun'an, illustrator Odano Naotake, whose genre was *ranga* (Dutch-style art), and others, Genpaku translated into Japanese the Dutch anatomical text *Analytical Tables of the Anatomy* by Polish medical scholar Johann Adam Kulmus.[107] The collaborative efforts led to the publication in 1774

of *A New Treatise on Anatomy*[108] (considered to be a Dutch-method medical text). Despite Genpaku's professed goal of using dissection-based
knowledge, his treatise was a model of translation and not an original
work based on his personal observations of dissection. It was illustrated
by Naotake, who created the anatomical drawings in his own artistic style
but did not stray from the illustrations he had imitated.[109]

Regarded in its own right, the field of Dutch-method medicine was
not entirely a precursor to Meiji-period Western-based medicine and
medical studies, as teleological studies would sometimes suggest; nor
was its development polarized by tensions that are imagined to exist
between indigenous and imported types of medicine.[110] Benjamin Elman
explains that Dutch learning signaled a progressive turn toward "Westernization"[111] in the intellectual sense but also that Japanese intellectuals
were not fixated upon the "Westernization" of medicine in ideological
terms.[112] Instead, they were interested in experimenting with modes of
investigating and acquiring knowledge by translating Dutch sources and
comparing texts with literal objects under scrutiny.

Lineages of Tokugawa Japanese ophthalmology mostly remained
rooted in Sino-Japanese medicine. Scholars today who emphasize the
importance of Dutch learning sometimes state that Japanese ophthalmology, until the arrival of Dutch learning, suffered from stasis because
Japanese medical scholars did not break the mold of Chinese medical
thought.[113] This perspective, however, fails to consider the historical significance of the intellectual foundations and developments of Japanese
ophthalmology. It is true, as I have discussed, that Japanese ophthalmology was steeped in the medical traditions of lineage-based knowledge,
but this base of knowledge is essential to us for understanding the historical categories and interpretations of blindness.

At the same time, Japanese ophthalmology was not completely insu-
lated from Dutch-method medicine. Dutch-method medicine's influence may have been marginal in practical terms, insofar as it did not
paradigmatically or fundamentally transform how traditional ophthalmology was practiced by major lineages. But Dutch-method medicine
stimulated the birth of new inquiry in Japanese ophthalmology and,
more important, initiated perspectives and practices that enriched and
coexisted with the Sino-Japanese medical worldview.[114]

For example, in 1815, a new, specialized text on ophthalmology was
published in Japan that was inspired by Dutch-method medicine. It was
published by Genpaku's son, Japanese medical scholar Sugita Ryūkei,
with a title that had unmistakable overtones of Genpaku's treatise: *A New*

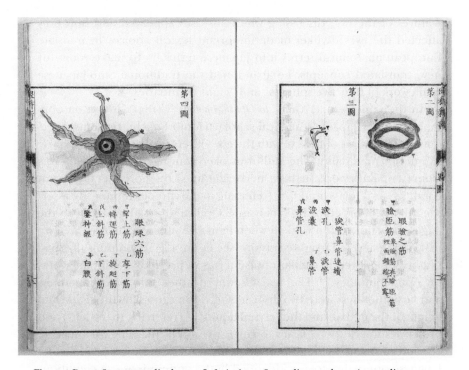

Fig. 1.3. Pages from a medical text. *Left:* A view of one dissected eye (according to the interpretations of Dutch-method medicine). *Right:* Views of eyelids and tear ducts. Compared with traditional Japanese renditions of the "five spheres" and "eight boundaries," the eye depicted here has a well-defined spherical shape and a solid form. For this reason, the eye is called an "eyeball." It is drawn with details organized around the emergent truths of dissection discussed in European texts (and oriented around the pivot of anatomical science), emphasizing a new materiality. The image shows six major tendons connecting the eye to the orbit. The seventh extension is described as a nerve conduit. The bluish matter of the eye is labeled as the "white membrane" (which appears to be the sclera). From Sugita Ryūkei, *A New Treatise on Ophthalmology* (Japanese title: *Ganka shinsho*), 1815. Main Library, Kyoto University Rare Materials Digital Archive.

Treatise on Ophthalmology.[115] It drew heavily from a Dutch translation of *The Instruction of Eye Diseases*[116] by Austrian physician and dermatologist Jacob von Plenck. *A New Treatise on Ophthalmology* features illustrations representing the eye with solid dimensions as a spherical mass. The illustrations methodically trace, through the eye's exfoliated surfaces, complex hidden structures that we may recognize as the sclera, optic nerve, and connected ligaments (see figure 1.3).[117] The juxtaposition of texts and illustrations visualizes and elaborates on the major morphological features of the eye, discussing where diseases appeared and how they affected the eyes. Ryūkei made important lexical choices to translate European anatomical terms into Japanese terms.[118] To make room for new, translated concepts, he abandoned the traditional Sino-Japanese framework of the "five spheres" and "eight boundaries."[119]

In the same vein, *A Guide to Ophthalmology*[120] (1831), a text on ophthalmology by Japanese medical scholar Honjō Fu'ichi, presents three-dimensional views of the eye with the eye's layers stripped away to expose its interior materiality. The author invoked translated anatomical terms from Genpaku's work, such as "nerve conduits" or, more literally, "spirit conduits" and "glass liquid"[121] (referring to the vitreous humor), to assert the validity of his empirical analysis.[122] Optical illustrations between the pages show how vision worked when light rays entered the eyes in "normal" vision and in farsighted vision (see figure 1.4), conditions that had not been explored in similar optical terms in previous traditional works on ophthalmology.[123] The text elsewhere notes that nearsightedness and farsightedness were two disorders of vision caused by the shape and height of the eyeball and the "crystal liquid"[124] (referring to the lens) and prescribes wearing eyeglasses to correct vision as the only treatment.[125] (Chapter 2 discusses eyeglasses and popular literature.) It is possible that Japanese ophthalmologists identified both conditions as eye conditions that could result in blindness because of their potential to cause severe disablement of vision.

Despite the empirical style of Dutch learning, which aimed to transcend past approaches by validating objective facts through the medical gaze of Dutch-method medical investigation, Dutch-method medical texts on ophthalmology provide important evidence of how Japanese ophthalmology still drew from the existing vocabulary of Sino-Japanese medicine to explain eye diseases. For example, a medical text on ophthalmology by shogunate physician Habu Genseki, who was trained in Dutch-method medicine, suggests that Dutch-method Japanese medical scholars still named eye diseases according to the conventional nomenclature, such as "epidemic red eyes," "wind-red eyes," "red eyes of fetal poison," and "inward-growing eyelashes."[126]

We can also find instances in the previously discussed Dutch-method medical texts, such as Ryūkei's *A New Treatise on Ophthalmology* and Fu'ichi's *A Guide to Ophthalmology*, that suggest that Dutch-method Japanese medical scholars adapted new perspectives from Dutch-method medicine but kept to the existing medical framework to explain blindness. Take, for example, the discussion in Ryūkei's text of *gankyū gan*

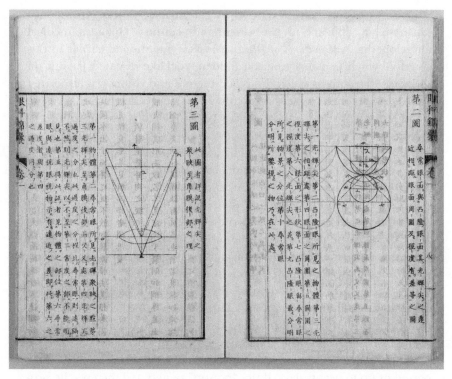

Fig. 1.4. Pages from a medical text. The drawing on the left depicts the optics of what we know to be farsighted vision. The text says that in farsighted vision, the light rays converge at a point behind the convergence point in "normal" vision. (In nearsighted vision, the opposite happens: the light rays converge at a point before the "normal" convergence point.) The key phrase in the text says that a person with this condition "cannot see clearly." The text suggests that vision can be corrected by adjusting the distance between the eye and the object. Though the actual science of vision is far more complex, the images and text in each frame indicate a new approach that translates vision and visual impairment into optical representation. These representations inspired by Dutch-method medicine mark a shift away from the traditional understanding that a person could see things when the eyes received blood from the liver. From Honjō Fu'ichi, *A Guide to Ophthalmology* (Japanese title: *Ganka kinnō*), 1831. Main Library, Kyoto University Rare Materials Digital Archive.

(disease of the eyeball).[127] The word *gan* means "cancer" in modern Japanese. It appears in the seventeenth-century Japanese medical encyclopedia *Explanations of Disease Names*,[128] mentioned earlier in this chapter, which explains *gan* as a hidden, rocklike diseased growth on the eye.[129] This mass, which destroyed the eye and vision, was associated with a debilitating disease[130] marked by sores, fevers, headaches, profuse sweating, and physical malaise. Ryūkei reintroduced *gan* in his context of Dutch-method medical translation to describe visual impairment as an alarming consequence of this specific eye disease.

Discussions of "poison" and visual impairment by Ryūkei and Fu'ichi show that traditional concepts for understanding blindness were still persuasive. Ryūkei discussed how the "poison" of smallpox could travel along the vessels and conduits to the eyes, causing the eyeball to swell and hurt.[131] As he described, in the most severe case, when disease had penetrated the eye orbit and thoroughly ravaged it, the entire eyeball had to be surgically removed. Fu'ichi explained that "fetal poison,"[132] which he thought to be latent in the body, could cause smallpox to develop with full-blown symptoms. The "poison" attacked by welling up from within the body and invading the eyes. (The symptoms were not distinguishable from those of measles.) Even after the scabs of smallpox sores had fallen off, the eyes were susceptible to residual "poison" for a period of up to twenty days. If the "poison" penetrated the eyes, he proposed applying white mustard plant parts (seeds or leaf tips)—ground and mixed—to the feet and placing leeches over the sores at the eyes to drain out the blood.[133]

Japanese scholarship on Dutch-method medicine was supported by forms of instruction that stimulated the sharing of knowledge. The European physician in Japan most visibly associated with Dutch-method medicine was Philipp Franz von Siebold, a physician employed by the VOC.[134] He arrived in Japan in 1823 and, in the following year, started the Narutaki academy, where he taught medicine and the natural sciences. Dutch learning academies set up by Japanese scholars—for example, Ōtsuki Gentaku's Shirandō in Edo (the first Dutch learning academy)[135] and Ogata Kōan's Tekitekisai academy in Osaka[136]—provided important platforms for teaching European medical subjects to aspiring Japanese intellectuals. Many of the academies' students paid fees to take lessons, but they did not always seek to practice medicine professionally. The academies' instructional methods preserved aspects of the traditional lineage system that confirmed the primacy of a master's authority.

Major cities were important nodes in intellectual networks. Japanese scholars read widely beyond their areas of interest and socialized freely with one another in their pursuits of learning and in well-connected communities.[137] In his survey of Dutch learning, Aoki Toshiyuki explains that enthusiasts from the Shinano area (in Nagano prefecture today) ventured into cities, such as Edo, Kyoto, Osaka, and Nagoya, to avail themselves of opportunities to study Dutch learning.[138] In less populated areas, academies were also important venues that promoted Dutch learning. Iinuma academy in Mino (in Gifu prefecture today), for example, opened its doors in 1781 as an academy of Sino-Japanese medicine but, in 1811, converted to teaching Dutch learning in response to popular interest.[139]

Ready access to VOC personnel and foreign texts played an important role in the development of Dutch learning at Nagasaki, where Japanese interpreters of Dutch were based. Siebold's academy, as Richard Rubinger highlights, was popular because Siebold himself taught his students.[140] One of his areas of instruction was ophthalmology, and at that time several well-known students who learned ophthalmology from him were shogunate physician Habu Genseki (whose scholarship, mentioned earlier, included a Dutch-method medical text on ophthalmology) and Kō Ryōsai. Siebold, however, ran afoul of shogunate laws and was summarily exiled from Japan in 1829.[141]

Siebold was reputed for his skills in performing eye surgeries, especially cataract couching. It is less clear how well Japanese ophthalmologists studied Siebold's techniques, but needling techniques had been practiced for a long time by the Majima ophthalmologists. What Japanese ophthalmologists like the Majima ophthalmologists probably wanted was greater precision in needling as they refined their clinical techniques. The pupil-dilating medicine that Siebold offered would have made the pupil of the eye significantly more visible during surgery and hence would have helped to reduce the margin of error. According to Siebold's original recipe, the medicine was mainly composed from *Atropa belladonna* (nightshade), which was not known to be a native plant species in Japan.[142] In 1826, at Nagoya, while on a tour to Edo, Siebold fortuitously convened with Mizutani Toyobumi, Itō Keisuke, and Ōkōchi Zonshin, who were Owari-based Japanese pharmacologists and natural history scholars. Through Siebold's expertise, they confirmed that the indigenous plant *Scopolia japonica* (Japanese belladonna)[143] had dilatory effects similar to those of nightshade. There were other eye medicines that Japanese medical scholars of Dutch-method medicine were thought to have produced, by learning the recipes either from Siebold or from other sources, to manipulate the dilation of the pupil. For example, *Records of Siebold's Prescriptions*,[144] written to describe the proven efficacies of Siebold's recipes, is a source that cites a prescription for the treatment of "black internal obstruction": calomel (a mineral form of mercury chloride), pulverized and mixed with aconite and sugar, was applied to the eye to treat an overly dilated pupil.

In one important respect, Japanese medical scholars learned to examine the inventories and formularies of Dutch-method medicine through different frames of analysis to find new utility for them. *Records of the Correspondences in Medicinal Products*,[145] a treatise by Siebold's student Ryōsai, gives us evidence of the comparative study to facilitate the understanding of Dutch-method medicine. Ryōsai's work compiled Sino-Japanese prescriptions, including information about common ingredients in Dutch-method medicine. Many ingredients, such as extracts of *Gentiana*[146] (a genus of herbaceous plants) and salix (or salicin),[147] and *Supurimāto*[148] (a Japanese gloss of the Dutch word "sublimaat"; a sublimate of mercury chloride), are mentioned by species or genus names and by chemical compositions alien to the traditional Sino-Japanese interpretive framework.

In another important respect, the significance of Dutch-method medicine in Japanese ophthalmology can be measured in terms of its contribution to studies of drugs. As Siebold's recipes tell us, Dutch-method treatments of eye diseases were centered on medicinal substances and their combinations. Dutch-method regimens complemented, and even affirmed, traditional methods of treating eye diseases. For example, mercury was an ingredient featured in various prescriptions for treating syphilis. Japanese medical scholars understood the "poison" of syphilis to act like the "poison" of smallpox: these "poisons" could cause blindness. In Japan, mercury in the form of red cinnabar and other mercury-based eye medicines of varying compositions and strengths were understood to be effective against the "poison" of syphilis. As Trambaiolo and Suzuki Noriko point out, Japanese medical scholars who studied Chinese treatises on syphilis would have learned much from reading about those medical recipes that listed mercury.[149] Japanese Dutch-method medical texts were also filled with formulas for eye medicines that included mercury, probably because European physicians had a long history of using mercury to treat syphilis-related eye ailments.

We find many examples of therapies with mercury in Dutch-method medical treatises. In *Essential Prescriptions for Expelling Syphilis*,[150] translated and published by Ryōsai in 1838, the text explains that a liquid mercury mixture relieved swelling and pain in the eyes (which we may understand as blindness) that was induced by the "poison" of syphilis.[151] The text recommends that opiates be used liberally with mercury in eye medicines. According to a mercury-based internal therapy documented in *Records of Siebold's Prescriptions*, calomel that was administered together with sulfur, antimony, and sugar was thought to act by expelling "poison" that had ravaged the eyes.[152] Another prescription mentions an analgesic opiate called Laudanum,[153] a tincture of European origin, as an ingredient of an eyewash.[154] The text says that the prescription could be modified by combining Laudanum and zinc flower (or zinc oxide).[155] Alternatively, eye lubricants could be made by mixing mercury and opium in water.[156] This combination of opium and mercury presumably had potent strength, because opium acted as a strong numbing agent and a good dose of mercury cleared vision.[157]

Overall, Dutch-method medicine enhanced Japanese medical scholars' knowledge about producing cures, but examples such as the references to "poison," mercury, and conventional disease names in discussions of blindness in the Dutch-method medical texts examined so far point to the dominance of traditional Sino-Japanese medical analysis.

Conclusion

From the Japanese medical perspectives presented in this chapter, being blind involved suffering from disabling eye conditions that caused visual impairment. The context of Tokugawa Japanese ophthalmology makes it clear that there was a range of those eye conditions and also highlights how the medical traditions that defined Japanese ophthalmology have a historical background.

Japanese ophthalmology adapted Chinese medical knowledge and developed in the context of Sino-Japanese medicine in Japan. By the early Tokugawa period, ophthalmology had become a specialty field recognized by the shogunate. Japanese ophthalmologists had organized lineages and formed their identities around core texts and teachings. This system of knowledge ensured that key terms in ophthalmology were properly interpreted, giving a solid historical basis for the medical vocabulary in use.

The vibrant intellectual heritage of lineages, as demonstrated by the Majima lineage, points to rich answers about blindness. Japanese ophthalmologists understood ideas of vision through Chinese medical traditions, including Chinese ophthalmology, and through lineage-based traditions in Japan. Blindness was analyzed in this medical context. Interpretations of disabling vision loss and poor vision were subjectively determined and described according to historical conventions. Though blindness was not clearly defined, texts clearly suggest that blindness was quite commonly disease-related visual impairment with numerous causes and recognizable symptoms that had to be treated. The axiom seems to have been that the sooner the underlying cause was determined, the sooner treatment could start—and delays in treatment or the inappropriate timing of treatment reduced the chances of saving vision. Blurred vision, attacks by "winds," "obstructive" impairments, and attacks by "poison" were some of the reasons why vision could be impaired. Treatments with needling techniques and recipes for pills, powders, ointments, and decoctions were standard topics in discussions and practices of cure.

In the late eighteenth century, Dutch-method medicine gained attention in Japan through the flourishing culture of Dutch learning, which had become an intellectual field of Japanese scholars. Through translated texts, Dutch learning, in general, introduced new epistemologies to ophthalmology. Japanese medical scholars, including ophthalmologists, were open to Dutch-method medicine, using analytical frameworks associated with it in their approaches to ophthalmology. Their intellectual output demonstrated a sophisticated understanding of new anatomical ideas and medical treatments of the eyes and vision.

CHAPTER 2

Eye Medicines

The Popular Culture of Cure

———— ❧ ————

This chapter examines sources in popular medical culture and other personal accounts to explore as well as reimagine what it was like for people in Tokugawa Japan to get treated for various eye conditions. It follows the previous chapter's approach of interpreting blindness in the context of conditions with disabling impairments of the eyes and vision. The sources that are discussed in this chapter do not explain blindness; rather, they focus on eye diseases and afflictions and suggest that visual impairment was a consequence. Complementing the previous chapter's discussion of the intellectual and medical views of Japanese ophthalmology, this chapter tells a different, yet related, side of the narrative through perspectives from the social history of medicine.

With a focus on the eighteenth and nineteenth centuries, this chapter argues that people in Tokugawa Japan who were disabled by blindness (or conditions of visual impairment) were enabled by options: they could decide what to do and where to go to find cures. This was true of other patients and consumers at that time, too. By the eighteenth century, developments in Japan's medical industry, print culture, and consumer culture had transformed consumers' habits and behaviors. General audiences, as patients and as consumers, engaged with medical services and with a popular medical culture of print and visual materials. While some medical knowledge—trade secrets and lineage secrets—mostly remained out of reach of general audiences because it was protected by commercial and noncommercial proprietors, as a rule even individuals who were not trained in medical and intellectual fields were sufficiently literate or informed to participate in the production, dissemination, and experience of medicine and medical knowledge.

Defining what is popular about any popular medical culture can be challenging because it presupposes that there is a clear division, in medicine and in culture, between what is elite and sophisticated and what is primitive and non-elite. This supposed dichotomy between elite medicine and non-elite medicine does not mesh smoothly with what we know about the vibrancy of discourses and practices in Tokugawa Japan's popular medical culture. For example, there was little to prevent an elite person like a samurai or a samurai lord from accessing various sources of information and buying medicines sold to the masses.

Tokugawa Japan's popular medical culture was enabled by consumer culture (mass consumer habits and commercial entrepreneurship) and also by the wide circulation of knowledge through print culture.[1] In the existing scholarship on popular culture in Tokugawa Japan, scholars such as Helen Hardacre, Nam-lin Hur, Laura Nenzi, and others have examined the ways people of a broad swath of social, political, and economic backgrounds engaged with popular religions, travels, and literature.[2] Along this line, I suggest that Tokugawa Japan's popular medical culture was inclined toward commonplace ways of thinking about medicine and cure, centered on accessible contexts of knowledge and prevalent treatments and cures.

There were diverse cures that were thought to perform their efficacies to treat eye conditions. In the culture of the eighteenth and nineteenth centuries, a full array of medical services was available to the populace. The physician-patient interface in the treatment of eye diseases, as seen in texts, conveyed anxieties about health, illness, and disease, as well as hopes of cure. In living vernacular traditions, many popular beliefs about cures for eye diseases and other diseases were infused with religious (and magical) beliefs that had complex histories of their own, while some elements of popular medical knowledge were also intertwined with intellectual medical traditions.[3] We may not know if people disabled by blindness were cured, or if they achieved their desired goals, but we can certainly imagine that there was no lack of choice in the social and cultural contexts of accepted practices.

Looking for Cures in Popular Texts

HOME RECIPES

Home recipes for cures were essential in the everyday experience of ill-ness. Medical services for the majority of the population were slow to develop in the early seventeenth century, and in the absence of physi-cians, people suffering from disabling eye conditions would have tried making remedies at home. Self-help health manuals were indispensable. Circulation of them to the public began sometime in the seventeenth century. These self-help books, characterized by their general instructive nature, were printed to be widely read. *Miraculous Medicines for Saving the Populace*[4] (1693) was a representative text of this genre.[5] The text by Hozumi Hoan, a physician of Mito domain (in Ibaraki prefecture today), honored the domain lord Tokugawa Mitsukuni, who had commissioned the work as a handy resource on health-related matters. The preface emphasizes in glowing language that the lord had extended a lifeline to the populace, especially during times of ill health when medical atten-tion was needed. According to the preface, ordinary subjects,[6] particu-larly those who lived in the wilderness or in the mountains, could not easily find medicines or access medical personnel in urgent situations. Households could prepare simple home remedies and save ailing family members from becoming physically impaired—or, literally, from becom-ing "handicapped" and "useless."[7] Ruling elites handed down medical knowledge through the political hierarchy to deploy privileged informa-tion about health as cultural capital and soft power.

The manuals were abbreviated so that readers could easily look up the main points for self-diagnosis and follow easy recipes for self-treatment. Those manuals mostly used the terminology found in medi-cal texts. Although it is hard to tell exactly how or where many of the customary formulas originated, the similarities with prescriptions of ophthalmological lineages, for instance, suggest that proprietary knowl-edge easily crossed over into popular medical knowledge. *Common Pre-scriptions*[8] (1729/30), like its predecessor *Miraculous Medicines for Saving the Populace*, was published in the early eighteenth century in the name of rescuing the populace. Written by shogunate physicians Niwa Seihaku and Hayashi Ryōteki, the work was endorsed by the shogunate under Tokugawa Yoshimune to dispense medical authority and project the image of benevolent rule.[9] It was a miscellany of recipes and remedies, and to increase their credibility the authors selectively ascribed some of them to Chinese texts, including the authoritative *Compendium of Materia Medica*[10] by Li Shizhen of Ming-dynasty China. (Because the venerable masters and the time-honored lore of Chinese medicine had said so, the advice had to be true.) Covering an expansive range of uncomplicated and intractable conditions, the work simplified for readers the vast knowledge of technical Chinese texts.

The two sources, *Common Prescriptions* and *Miraculous Medicines for Saving the Populace*, surveyed eye conditions that were mostly characterized by itch, pain, swelling, and redness, providing information about causes and giving concise directions for preparing drugs at home. Eye diseases of smallpox caused symptoms that could be difficult to treat. According to *Miraculous Medicines for Saving the Populace*, one treatment was to rub the resin of nutgall (a plant of the *Rhus* genus) with milk into the affected eye.[11] (Worms from a plant, possibly swallowwort,[12] of the *Cynanchum* genus also seemed to work.) Another treatment was to try using the blood of live eels as a medicine on the eye.[13] Children were particularly susceptible to smallpox, so the texts discussed in detail how someone (a lay person) could save children whose vision was threatened by the disease. *Common Prescriptions* instructed a person to drip the oil of gently seared bamboo shoots into a child's eyes,[14] pulverize goldthread, and apply it to the underside of the child's foot. To counter the invasion of smallpox "poison" (disease poison; see chapter 1) in the eyes, that text said to do this: mix yellow-red lead[15] powder with powdered mercury[16] and delicately blow the mixture into the ears—through the ears, the powder traveled to the eyes. If smallpox caused obstruction in the eye, it was good to give a decoction of these ingredients: equal proportions of hares' feces, sloughed husks of cicadas, *Akebia quinate*, and licorice (this formula was also listed in medical treatises).

There were other common eye ailments discussed by those texts. To treat night blindness[17] (an eye disease that Chinese and Japanese ophthalmologists recognized and categorized), *Miraculous Medicines for Saving the Populace* recommended the following: eat a dish of fermented sea bream paste[18] or the fat of red stingrays (the meat of Arctic lampreys appeared to work as well).[19] The same text recommended one easy way to treat "diseased eyes," a condition also discussed in specialized medical texts (see chapter 1): decoct goldthread (discarding the residue), mix that with water, and use the clear water of the mixture to wash the eyes.[20] Another eye condition, "wind eyes," could be treated with an eyewash made from a decoction of large leaves of tree ferns and a little cinnabar.[21]

POPULAR TRAVEL LITERATURE AND WONDER DRUGS

People's freedom to read popular travel literature and to travel was essential to how they were empowered as consumers. Peter Kornicki defines print culture in Tokugawa society as encompassing printed texts, handwritten manuscripts, and publishing culture.[22] Readers of books were consumers of knowledge circulated in print and hence were consumers of print culture. Richard Rubinger, whose recent scholarship has analyzed literacy in Tokugawa Japan, suggests that in the early eighteenth century, as commercial networks of urban, merchant centers expanded into rural areas, village administration and rural elites developed sophisticated literacy and reading habits; for example, the genre of agricultural manuals that circulated at that time indicates an educated readership in rural places.[23] While we do not have exact information on literacy rates across Tokugawa Japan, it is easy to imagine that the level of reading literacy only increased over time with more books in print and in circulation over the eighteenth century. This also provides the context for understanding printed and handwritten texts, which will be discussed in chapters 5 and 6.

Generally, in the context of popular travel literature, eye conditions were simply listed as medical conditions: they were all regarded, almost consistently, as diseases and ailments that caused visual impairment and as conditions treatable with the right kinds of cure. As print culture and consumer culture converged and burgeoned, and as travel networks percolated into distant corners of Japan, people traveled for pleasure and on business, especially from the eighteenth century onward. News about cures and where to find them quickly spread. To an imaginative reader who felt inspired to travel, a cure was worth traveling for and worth trying. We can imagine that blind people who could not read because of vision loss or poor vision could rely on their sighted families and friends to read travel books to them, as well as verbally relay to them information about cures.

Travelers would have known that big cities were important destinations on travel routes where choices of eye medicines abounded. For consumers looking for eye medicines in Kyoto, *A Convenient Guide on the Sale of Medicines in and around Kyoto*,[24] a travel guidebook of this genre of convenient guides, would have served a good purpose. The text even lists the market prices of drugs.[25] Similarly, *The Sands of Edo: A Sequel*,[26] written by poet and essayist Kikuoka Senryō in 1735, would have been useful for travelers to Edo.[27] The section on medicines rightly states that there was no lack of medicines and reputable physicians in Edo—court and sho-gunate physicians are included in the list of physicians.[28] Eye medicines[29] made up an important category of medicines. The text does not disclose secret ingredients (known only to producers, who guarded the knowl-edge) but advertises the locations in Edo where eye medicines could be purchased.[30] The Iōin eye medicine was sold on the compounds of Sensōji (a temple-shrine at Asakusa). "Five-spirit fragrance"[31] was sold by three families of former Masuda samurai vassals who had relocated to Edo sometime between 1624 and 1644. "Cloud-cutting"[32] eye powder, which was sold on the south side of Nihonbashi, continued to be sold through the Meiji period in places beyond Edo.[33]

The success of some proprietary and patented medicines depended on sellers' monopoly of markets and networks to reach consumers of those medicines. Some Buddhist temples had institutional networks to promote the commercialization of medicines. Duncan Ryūken Wil-liams's study of Sōtō Zen Buddhism in the Tokugawa period tells us that Dōshōan, a pharmacy in Kyoto with direct ties to the imperial house-hold, exploited its privileged status as an intermediary with Sōtō Zen head temples to sell its "poison-dispelling" pill[34] through the hierarchies of temples.[35] Another example of a famous wonder drug is the "soul-returning" pill[36] of Toyama (in Toyama prefecture today), which was one of the most iconic pills in the entire country at that time. A medicine for abdominal pains and myriad illnesses, the pill was apparently pro-duced from a secret mix of at least twenty-three ingredients.[37] While the original recipe is not known, it was linked to a physician named Mandai Jōkan of Bizen province (in Okayama prefecture today).[38] In one version of the narrative, Maeda Masatoshi, lord of Toyama in the early seven-teenth century, longed for the pill. After some years, a person named Kohē acquired the recipe and presented it to the lord. With the lord's approval, medical vendors obtained commercial licenses to sell the pill. Among the licensed sellers was the Matsui pharmacy. It was said that through the pharmacy the pill started to be sold widely across Japan. The factors of success were the traveling vendors' effective control of medical supplies, the top-down enforcement of commercial privileges by domain vassals, and, at the ground level, well-coordinated structures of monopoly through local and regional business groups.[39] The domain authorities—and especially medical vendors and pharmacies—were vigi-lant about methods of production and clamped down on the unlicensed sale of counterfeit medicines.[40]

Avid readers would have been familiar with illustrated gazetteers[41] (also known as illustrated travel guidebooks), a popular illustrated genre available from the late eighteenth century onward, as they searched for information about places to go to find cures. These texts appealed to the popular imagination by composing vivid pictures of local and regional cultures. Though they did not discriminate between the facts and fictions about cures, the books delighted readers with stories about the origins and histories of wonder drugs. For example, Myōgen'in, the ancestral site of the Majima lineage of ophthalmologists, is described in the *Illustrated Gazetteer of the Famous Places of Owari* as an attraction in Owari (in Aichi prefecture today) filled with hundreds of pilgrims at a time seeking cures for eye diseases.[42] Medicines with the Majima brand name, by association with the reputation of the site and lineage, were thought to have immense potential for healing ailing eyes. If blind people did not travel, or could not travel, they could entrust to their families and friends who traveled on their behalf the task of bringing home cures—many of which were light, portable things that could be carried around by travelers.

There are many examples of wonder drugs with broad curative powers. "Brocaded-pouch pill for ten thousand diseases"[43] was one of those drugs. The *Illustrated Gazetteer of the Famous Places of Edo*[44] tells us that the founder of the drug was a religious person who visited temples. At each temple, he cloistered himself to pray to the deities. During one visit, when he suffered from a swollen finger, he had a divine vision. In that vision, he received a pill from a brocaded pouch.[45] When he awoke, he realized that the pill had cured his affliction. Grateful for the miraculous healing, he opened a pharmacy in Edo and sold the pill to customers. "Rich-heart" pill,[46] described in the *Illustrated Gazetteer of the Famous Places of Yamato* (1791),[47] was a pill of Saidaiji,[48] the head temple in Nara of the Shingon Risshū Buddhist sect. "Ten-thousand-gold" pill[49] was sold at Noma teahouse near the Ise Inner shrine at Asama Pass (in Mie prefecture today), home to Asama village and many pharmacies.[50] As we are told by the *Illustrated Gazetteer of the Ise Pilgrimages*,[51] a long time ago the teahouse owners arrived from Owari using a secret prescription from Akita.

There was a practical solution, though not a cure, for people who were dealing with visual impairment. Those with mild to moderate visual impairment could get around with eyeglasses. In Edo, where splendid mechanical inventions and contraptions were sold, eyeglasses could be easily purchased. In his literary work *The Virtues of Eyeglasses for Flourishing Prosperity*[52] (1790), Koikawa Yukimachi, a popular author of the illustrated genre of *kibyōshi* (yellow-cover books, a satirical and comical illustrated genre), narrates a rags-to-riches fictional story about Gyōemon, an optician who makes huge profits by selling eyeglasses in Edo. Yukimachi's portrayal of Gyōemon encapsulates the spirit of individual entrepreneurship in the consumer culture of Edo. Timon Screech's study of Tokugawa Japanese popular culture highlights that this work amused readers in its time.[53] The social context of popular literature, such as that of this work, illuminates the importance of vision in everyday life. Because vision was essential for a person to read words, characters, and signs and to navigate the streets, visual impairment was at the very least an annoying inconvenience and also an impediment. People who were unable to read because of disabled vision had to rely on others to read things to them. Permanent visual impairment could have an impact on a person's identity and choice of livelihoods, as later chapters in this book will discuss.

POPULAR TRAVEL LITERATURE, RELIGION, AND MAGIC

The religious context of travel is important for understanding how people used pilgrimage as a reason to travel and to spend money on cures. Ise was one of many religious venues where pharmacies took advantage of the boom in popular religions to sell their medicines. Pilgrimages to the Ise shrines were part of the series of large-scale pilgrimages throughout Tokugawa Japan. The Ise pilgrimages were facilitated by organized networks of religious guides[54] of Ise. Starting in the eighteenth century, in some years, social factors spurred waves of pilgrims to flood travel routes.[55] People were willing to travel, and the sale of the famous "ten-thousand-gold" pill of Ise would have been impossible without the cooperation of religious guides as well as the marketing of the drug as a medicine and as a valuable pilgrimage keepsake.

In the popular consciousness, the populace did not purposely discriminate between the characteristics of Buddhism and Shinto. In discussing Japanese Buddhism, for example, Jason Ānanda Josephson highlights the term "prayer healing" (healing empowerment by praying). With an emphasis on worldly benefits, praying was a culturally specific act, tailored to the types of conditions for which treatment was being entreated; the purposes were diverse.[56] This logic of prayer for efficacy broadly applied to Tokugawa Japanese religions. Shinto was not a monolithic religion but rather had been absorbed by the Buddhist cultural and intellectual complex. It had coalesced, without a central identity, as an amorphous mass of local beliefs, deities, and localized religious customs centered on shrines and communities.[57]

While traveling on a pilgrimage, it was common for people with ailments to stop to worship at religious sites that specialized in treatments of those ailments. *A Convenient Guide on Prayers to Deities of Edo*[58] (1810s) of the genre of convenient guides would have been popular among audiences looking for solace through some kind of divine intervention that exceeded the possibilities of popular medicines. To cure an eye disease, the text suggests paying a visit to Cha no Ki (Tea Tree) Inari shrine, which was located midway up the slope of Ichigaya Hachimangū (a Hachiman shrine).[59] The small Inari shrine enshrined the Tea Tree Inari Daimyōjin deity of the highest number-one rank.[60] A supplicant would serve tea at the altar and pray for seven days for healing; a banner flag was offered to conclude the rite. As the text says, pilgrims and patrons from faraway places worshipped at the shrine. An edition entitled *A Convenient Guide on Shrines and Temples*[61] (1816) and focused on the Osaka area was published in the same format of listing temples and shrines and the customs surrounding these institutions. Kitano Megami no Hachimangū, a famous shrine, honored Megami no Hachiman, a Hachiman deity and healer of eye diseases.[62]

Some places specialized in medicinal waters. The use of waters from natural sources to harness their medicinal properties had been practiced for a long time. In Japan's classical period, bathers were mostly aristocrats, and baths fulfilled the religious purposes of ablution and ritual purification. Lee Butler's survey has established that Arima (in Kōbe city, Hyōgo prefecture today) was one place where bath waters[63] were believed to promote healing because of their steam and saline compositions.[64] Massive movement of people along pilgrimage routes and on adventures facilitated the fame of healing sites. Hot-spring resorts attracted more than their fair share of tourists: thousands of visitors stopped at some places.[65]

In Buddhist beliefs of healing, special waters blessed by deities were believed to open the eyes—a metaphor for clearing away impediments, healing vision, and enlightening the mind. *A Supplement to the Illustrated Gazetteer of the Famous Places of the Imperial Capital*[66] (1787), a survey of the region around Kyoto, lists important sites where the waters could perform wonders on the eyes. Ritsuganzan Yōkokuji (or Yōkokuji) had a reputation as one of those temples.[67] The temple, said to have been consecrated centuries earlier during the Heian period, was dedicated to the deity Thousand-Hand Kannon.[68] At the back of the main worship hall, a patron would find "willow-tree" water,[69] which was touted as water for cleansing and healing the eyes. "Vajra" water[70] flowed at the same site and, like "willow-tree" water, was said to be good for curing eye diseases. Elsewhere, at the temple Raigōin, "Vajra" water streamed out of the ground next to the rock shrine altar of the deity Kōjin.[71] A legend connected "Vajra" water to Kōbō Daishi (Kūkai), an illustrious Japanese Buddhist priest who lived from the late eighth through early ninth centuries. In the legend, he broke the ground at that temple with a *vajra* (a powerful and symbolic weapon in Buddhist rituals) and unleashed the water from its underground source. Pilgrims and visitors, especially if they had traveled to these sites from afar, could try to heal themselves and take some of the waters home as souvenirs for their families.

Religious supplications did not necessarily have any medical basis or explanation, but we may consider them to be an important facet of the multifaceted popular mindset about cure. Smallpox is an example of a disease—measles is another (see the next section on popular medical prints)—that causes visual impairment and whose treatment was steeped in a popular medical culture that blended ideas of medical cures and elements of what may seem to us as religion and magic. People feared the consequences of smallpox, with which they would have been all too familiar; texts made it clear that impaired vision from smallpox was one frightening consequence frequently witnessed in victims. Hartmut Rotermund's survey of magical treatments of smallpox highlights the diversity of these practices in daily life, from wearing talismans to inscribing codified spells on the belly, marking houses with red streamers (red was a symbolic color for protection from smallpox), or reveling in dance.[72] Rotermund also found that some believed that astrological timing could influence whether "poison" in the body would cause smallpox or measles.[73]

In local places, some ritual practices were centered on the worship of Hōsōgami (a smallpox deity), in whose honor permanent institutions such as shrines were erected. Outbreaks of smallpox inspired outbursts of fervor in worship, and the nature and frequency of rites reflected local patterns of worship. Gazetteers are important sources on these aspects, and Helen Hardacre's focused study of them sheds light on popular religious beliefs and practices.[74] As an example, the *Newly Edited Records of the Customs of Sagami Province*[75] tells us quite a lot about one smallpox shrine in Miura (in Kanagawa prefecture today). It was popularly known as Niibashigū, or "New Chopsticks" shrine.[76] The annual rite was performed to appease the deity so as to repel smallpox and protect the community. Every year, on the twenty-sixth day of the sixth month, a bowl of red bean porridge[77] was offered to the deity, together with a new pair of chopsticks fashioned from fresh straw grass, a material used for thatching roofs. This rite, as the text claims, was derived from an older rite conducted at that same site many centuries earlier in remembrance of Taira no Takakiyo (a warrior of the Heike clan, celebrated in *The Tale of the Heike*).

From a modern perspective, we know that measles, like smallpox, is highly contagious and can damage vision in some infected people. As chapter 1 explained, medical scholars in Tokugawa Japan understood that diseases with sores such as smallpox, measles, and syphilis could severely impair vision. Reconstructed profiles of blind people in the Tokugawa and Meiji periods suggest that measles was a significant cause of blindness in childhood (see chapters 4 and 6 for profiles of a couple of people blinded by measles in childhood). This also suggests that to some extent, the general population in Tokugawa Japan was familiar with blindness caused by measles.

Measles, as well as smallpox, was one of the diseases that was featured in late Tokugawa Japanese popular medical prints. Popular medical prints were essential sources of information for readers (see figure 2.1, a medical print about measles). Food was thought to be medicine for the body, and many prints were about food. The dietary regimen of prohibitions and recommendations, what to eat and what not to eat, was believed to enhance convalescence and recovery and to prevent the resurgence of "poison" from measles (see chapter 1, which discusses "poison" and visual impairment).

In some medical prints, treatments of measles are portrayed as imbued with elements of religious and magical therapies. In one example, measles is personified as disease demons with sinister features.[78] The text mentions the plant *Osmanthus* (holly *Osmanthus*), whose leaves Tokugawa Japanese believed to be associated with the power to expel evil spirits. On the night of Setsubun (the day before the calendrical start of spring), a person was urged to collect *Osmanthus* leaves hanging from the doors of thirty-three households, decoct those leaves, and feed the decoction to a child who had not yet contracted measles. This was said to help the child, who would develop only mild symptoms of measles and gain protection from the disease. It was also said that a person could mitigate the menace of measles by performing a holy incantation written on the leaf of a holly *Ilex* plant.

Perhaps the paucity of physical proof of efficacy of healing rituals and other customary therapies elevated the intriguing power of cure in

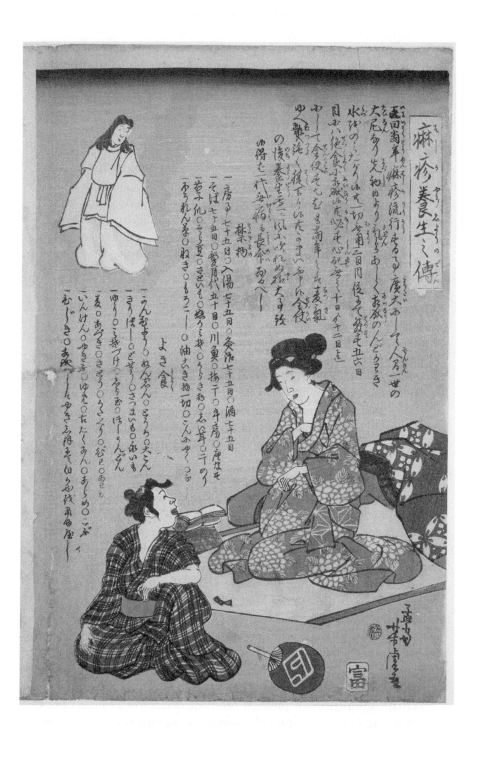

麻疹養生之傳

此度當年麻疹流行するは廣大おーて人万一世の...
大尾あり先知より...
水油のんどりへ...
目水あつき小米飯小を心そ...
かーて今俊女大をもあ南年さもて麦こ...
ゆ（難）洗くよまり以夜つまひ...
の俊養生そーに...
ゆ滑を二代兵病と...

葉物
一房るニ十五日○入湯○...
そば七十五日○賛月代...
茹子ねり○とうふ...
あられ茶○ねぎ○もろこ...

よき食
こんぶよう○れんこん○そうめん○大こん
きりぼし○ごぼう○さつまいも○かいも
ゆり○三つ葉づけ○うらう○ぜん
麦○あづき○きうり○うどう○ほーうん
いんけん○ゆきよ○さゝげ○むぎ○あをじ
むぎき○あめ─あづきゆき志摩こー日々代

子孙中...
芳虎...
富

the popular consciousness. What may appear to be religious or magical to us today was viewed and experienced in a context of medical cure by people in Tokugawa society.

Getting Involved in the Business of Cure: Physicians and Patients

PERSONAL RECORDS OF ILLNESS AND CURE

Sources such as letters and diaries had limited readership as they were written to be records of personal experiences, not as literature for printing and circulation. But it is important to remember that these sources are integral to understanding how popular medical culture was reflected in people's everyday lives. Authors of these records were physicians and patients who told accounts through their perspectives. They were literate people who read a lot and possessed adequate (in fact, often more than adequate) knowledge about their own health conditions or the conditions of people with whom they interacted. Their records can give us useful insights into people's experiences with everyday practices, including how some people struggled with visual impairment, sought help from physicians, and tried cures for eye diseases.

In the early Tokugawa period, physicians catered to the demands of the shogun and his closest aides.[79] Domain lords were high-ranking offi-

---

(*facing page*) Fig. 2.1. A popular illustrated medical sheet about measles from 1862, when the Japanese measles epidemic was proclaimed as the epic crisis of a generation. The text outlines the clinical stages of measles infection. At first, a person will start to feel terrible and suffer from unquenchable thirst. By the fifth and sixth days, the victim will lose the appetite for food and cease eating, causing much worry. From the tenth through twelfth days, the person's condition will significantly improve. However, even after the symptoms of measles have abated, the person has to follow a strict regimen in order to completely recover and avert a relapse. For seventy-five days in the convalescent period, the person has to abstain from certain actions and food items: sex, bath, moxibustion (a medical therapy involving the burning of moxa on meridian points on the body), wine, and buckwheat. Other taboo foods include burdock root, spinach, sorghum, eggplant, and taro, while the following are recommended to boost the person's constitution: daikon (radish), pickles, sweet potato, azuki bean, common bean, kelp (*arame*; sea oak is a type of kelp), lily, and others. From Utagawa (Mōsai) Yoshitora, *An Account about Recovering from Measles* (Japanese title: *Hashika yōjō no den*), 1862. National Diet Library Digital Collections.

cials who had privileges; leveraging connections with the shogunate to be seen by medical specialists was one of those privileges. A good example of a domain lord with connections is Hosokawa Tadaoki, lord of Kokura domain (in Fukuoka prefecture today) of the early seventeenth century and also patriarch of the Hosokawa clan. A staunch ally of shogun Tokugawa Ieyasu, the first Tokugawa shogun, Tadaoki was a zealous proponent of the regime's early anti-Christian campaigns to enforce Buddhism and stamp out Christianity from Japanese soil.[80] His political fealty earned him the shogun's trust and created goodwill between the Hosokawa clan and the shogunate. He was someone who had sound knowledge of current medical theories. For instance, when he learned that his grandson Mitsunao had been stricken with smallpox, he warned about eating abalones, which he believed aggravated the "poison" of smallpox.[81]

Tadaoki wrote letters to officials, and the letters, which documented some details of his life, reveal that he suffered from deteriorating vision in both eyes when he was in his fifties. This is perhaps one of the earliest written firsthand accounts of vision loss by someone of that period. Because the stages of impairment unfolded over some time, it seems likely that Tadaoki had been experiencing a slow degenerative eye condition with symptoms similar to those of macular degeneration or glaucoma. The impairment almost caused total vision loss sometime in early 1618.[82] He was seen by Yasuharu and Risai, two ophthalmologists in the area, but to no avail. We learn from the letters that at Tadaoki's request, a Majima ophthalmologist arrived from Osaka to treat him (see chapter 1 on the Majima lineage's specialization in treating complicated eye disorders). After the treatment, Tadaoki started to regain partial vision in his left eye and described being able to vaguely discern silhouettes. However, the improvement in vision was short-lived. His right eye, though, remained in the same state of poor vision.

Using his influential political connections, Tadaoki appealed to Doi Toshikatsu, Middle Elder[83] of the shogunate and later Senior Elder,[84] who promptly sent for a Majima ophthalmologist from Owari province.[85] The series of communications would suggest that the Majima ophthalmologists strategically employed their fame and boasted followers within the shogunate. Tadaoki's complaints about his prolonged distress also elicited a response from shogun Ieyasu's successor, Hidetada, who instructed Toshikatsu to assist with the arrangements for caregiving. In later years, with some help, Tadaoki enjoyed the luxury of taking trips to Kyoto, where he recuperated for periods of time to nourish his eyes.

However, it appears that Tadaoki's vision loss was irreversible.[86] Because of the relatively late onset of blindness, the impairment did not have much impact on his status. His high stature ensured that he had a good degree of material comfort. He did not have to worry about being provided for in his old age.

By the late Tokugawa period, medical services had become widely available, giving patients bargaining power. Compared with the early seventeenth century, when medical services for the populace were nascent, in the eighteenth century and thereafter, the medical infrastructure in cities, towns, and rural places had become well developed and well connected. The diary of village official Suzuki Heikurō of Shibasaki (in Tachikawa of Tokyo today) gives us some perspectives on the mobility and choices of well-connected patients in the nineteenth century. In the second month of 1850, Heikurō's son, Yashichi, started to feel unwell because of an eye disease.[87] Though the degree of impaired vision is not obvious from the descriptions or context, it is clear that Yashichi was gravely troubled by the symptoms. Nagata Naoko's analysis highlights that Yashichi chose not to go to his regular physician, who was a medical generalist, but instead traveled to the nearby village of Ishida to consult an ophthalmologist.[88] It was a patient's choice to see as many specialists as possible to get cured. Within a few days, he was seen by Itō Genbin of Hachiōji (in Tokyo today), an ophthalmologist whose training was in Dutch-method medicine, as Western-style medicine was known in Japan at that time. Genbin assured Yashichi that the symptoms did not seem serious. However, still feeling uneasy, Yashichi sought the expert opinions of at least three other ophthalmologists, who advised, to the contrary, that the matter of his eye disease was not to be taken lightly.[89] One of them was an ophthalmologist of the reputable Majima lineage. Nevertheless, as Yashichi trusted Genbin's expertise the most, he returned to Genbin to be checked and treated with medicines. By the early part of the fourth month, his eyes were almost completely healed.

Kyokutei (or Takizawa) Bakin, one of the most iconic writers in his time, was known to have suffered from blindness in the twilight of his life. His diary, written in the nineteenth century, tells us much about his literary activities. It is also a record of the mundane affairs of an ordinary household and, in this context, a record of the preoccupations of a writer and a family patriarch. Most important for our purpose is that his diary is a source that offers an intimate patient-centered perspective on his struggles with vision loss and the social experience of medicine. Living in the capital Edo, as Bakin did, had its advantages. It allowed a prolific writer like Bakin to keep up with literary trends and popular tastes in books. It also afforded certain conveniences, including a broad choice of medical services.

Bakin would have been considered an able-sighted person for most of his life. However, he started to complain about failing vision in the years leading up to 1839. That was the period when he was finishing the installments of *The Eight Dog Chronicles*,[90] which is widely considered to be the magnum opus of his literary career. His visual impairment not only got worse over time but also became unbearable.[91] He tried various eye medicines, but they did not work at all. Under pressure to proofread and correct the drafts of his text, he dictated instructions to his daughter-in-law Omichi (here, and in other contexts, the prefix "O-" expresses endearment). She assumed most of the editorial work under his direct supervision. Over time, he suspected that he was succumbing to "old eyes" or "aging eyes"[92] and described worsening blurring[93] in his vision. The symptoms he described seem to be associated with degenerative vision loss—perhaps cataracts, glaucoma, or macular degeneration—complicated by age-related factors. In 1840, he could barely read fine print characters without help.[94] As a temporary solution, he approached Hayashi Sōzō, an optician, and received a new pair of eyeglasses. With the eyeglasses, he was able to see things a little better. By the start of 1841, however, he could no longer see with his right eye. He wrote in an ironic jest that the right lens of his old pair of eyeglasses, which had been recently replaced, had become nothing but an ornament.

A regimen of self-medication and home therapies was quite typical for many families even in the late Tokugawa period. Such methods would commonly have been a first line of treatment for treating minor eye irritations. In Bakin's time, vernacular handbooks were invaluable, as were medical formulas and recipes passed along by word of mouth. Many drugs could be conveniently manufactured at home, and medicines from famous temples were readily available. One time, Bakin received an eyewash from the Nishiarai temple where his book publisher prayed on his behalf; that temple's eye medicine was said to cure eye diseases.[95] However, after years of poor vision and vision loss, he abandoned all hope of ever finding a cure. His daughter Osaki was periodically beset by eye afflictions.[96] The symptoms were mild and improved after she consumed an enhanced decoction of *Bupleurum* plant.[97] To get medicines and miscellaneous supplies, Bakin sometimes sent his grandson (Omichi's son) Tarō on errands to the Isoda pharmacy, a regular pharmacy of the family.[98]

For a lay person, Omichi became very knowledgeable about medicines because she handled them at home. She regularly brought home ingredients of a decoction that probably was a tonic for women to fortify the constitution.[99] Other common medicines that the family bought were "miraculous-response"[100] pills and "black"[101] pills; the latter were thought to be effective for treating abdominal pains.[102] On one occasion, Wasa, a friend from the Tomikura household, was troubled by an eye ailment and asked Omichi for her recommendations about eye medicines sold by the Kōshūya pharmacy.[103] Some items, especially rare medicines and ingredients, had to be specially ordered. In one episode, Tarō attempted to buy some powder of antelope horns from a pharmacy but was turned away because he had not placed an order in advance.[104] He returned later that same day and was able to purchase it. With that as an ingredient, Omichi made pills by following a family recipe.[105]

As Bakin's example highlights, the family was the basic unit of support in times of illness. Caregiving by a person's family was a crucial part of the experience of illness and often a shared domestic responsibility that demanded patience and sacrifice. Family members, and sometimes the community, were expected to find ways to provide care. Bakin mostly rested at home and was cared for by his family. With much support, and as a celebrated writer, he did not have to go to the trouble of finding work outside. Because he was old, blind, and in poor health, it would have been hard for him to manage the household by himself or venture into the streets alone. He learned to trust Tarō and especially Omichi for everything. On a day-to-day basis, Omichi waited upon Bakin and filled in diary entries on days when he did not feel well enough to write. One night, Bakin's illness overcame him. He was gasping for breath and could not lie down in bed.[106] No medicine seemed to be working. Omichi stayed up all night at his bedside to keep a close watch over him.

Home regimens worked in conjunction with routine home consultations by physicians. A family could call for a physician to check on a family member and get medical advice. Kusama Shūsen was the regular physician for Bakin's household.[107] In one incident after his health had deteriorated, Bakin was distraught when Omichi was suddenly stricken with a fever and an abdominal ache.[108] She tried a decoction of "five-rei"[109] powder, but by the next morning the symptoms had intensified and she was losing fluids because of severe diarrhea. Shūsen was summoned by the family and arrived the following evening to diagnose her illness. He put her on a soft diet of porridge and a regimen of peony decoction with extra ingredients, instructing the family to order and collect medicines. Tarō excused himself from his social engagements to stay at home with Omichi.[110] Despite minor setbacks, Omichi soon regained her strength and health. Within days, from the nineteenth day of the eighth month (roughly August-September) of 1848, she resumed her role of recording entries in Bakin's diary on his behalf.[111]

Diaries can also give us important perspectives on the activities and experiences of physicians. Kadoya Yōan was a physician who diligently kept records of his day-to-day activities from 1835 through 1869, documenting routine activities such as what he did to help his patients. His diary gives us clues to the developed state of medical care and infrastructure in a region distant from Edo in the nineteenth century and suggests that the contacts that he had with his patients were not too different from contemporary practices elsewhere (see the discussion of Bakin's diary earlier in this section).

Born in 1792, Yōan spent most of his career in the mining town of Innai Ginzan (in Akita prefecture today), where he took up residence in 1816 and was supported as a samurai physician.[112] He was granted permission by the local government to operate a lodge to house visitors to supplement his income from practicing medicine. He adopted a son named Taian, who was born in a neighboring village. Taian studied medicine in his youth. Because of his flair for medicine, he was enrolled in the domain academy of Meitokukan and was sponsored for further studies in Kyoto. Upon his return from Kyoto, he married Osuma, one of Yōan's two daughters. He assumed the duties of patriarch of the family after Yōan passed away and continued to practice medicine.

Several important points can be noted. Yōan was a well-connected personality in his home community. He cared about the well-being of his family and the community, recording births, marriages, and funerals.[113] He received a wide range of patients, whom he knew by name, from all around the area. Sometimes he traveled to the nearby village of Nagakura; at other times, he ventured a little further north to Yuzawa. He entertained visits by patients and guests from Kubota (the castle town of Akita domain) and Shinjō (south of Akita, in Yamagata prefecture today); those two towns roughly demarcated the geographical scope of his contacts, though he also had contacts in other places.[114] On some days, Yōan's own health suffered; for example, he suffered from eye affliction, and when he felt the attacks of "evil winds," he had to rest his legs.[115] When he was feeling well enough to travel, he checked on his patients by making house calls.[116] He also responded to medical inquiries from the local government.

Yōan was known as a physician of general medicine. He was not unlike other physicians who were broadly trained in medicine. His patients' frequent complaints included abdominal pains[117] and, periodically, smallpox and measles infections.[118] As part of his repertoire of therapies, he performed moxibustion and, occasionally, acupuncture.[119] When he encountered afflictions that he did not routinely treat, he deferred to the expertise of specialists. In ophthalmology, he tapped into his network of contacts, which extended to the surrounding hubs of Kakunodate and Yamagata (in Akita and Yamagata prefectures today).[120] For example, he was acquainted with Satō Junseki of Kubota,[121] an ophthalmologist who had completed a study tour in Nagasaki, and someone named Kōrin, a Majima ophthalmologist, of Yamagata.[122] The ophthalmologists traveled to visit patients and provide medical treatments. Yōan was not an ophthalmologist but that did not stop him from seeing patients with eye diseases who were keen to consult him for advice.[123] In one example, a regular patient named Sekiguchi Banzō arrived in the first month of the new year (1864) to offer gifts to Yōan.[124] As Banzō was experiencing some problems with his vision (minor visual impairment), he thought it opportune to seek eye medicines from Yōan.

Yōan was a well-informed, innovative healer who kept abreast of current medical trends. His grandson Ryōsuke had succumbed to smallpox at the age of three in 1850. Despite his best efforts at treating Ryōsuke with medicines to reduce the fever, he suspected that worm afflictions had affected the heart, rendering moxibustion, acupuncture, and medicines utterly useless.[125] Perhaps because of this heart-wrenching personal loss, Yōan was an ardent advocate of smallpox vaccination, which was new to Tokugawa Japan. As cowpox vaccines began to be distributed from Nagasaki and Edo sometime in 1865, he went to Yuzawa to collect the vaccine and inoculated willing patients, some of them children, in the fight against smallpox.[126]

Networks of trade in medicines across Japan included even remote places. Generally, the bulk of Yōan's supplies came from sellers in Osaka, a nexus of wholesale trade. Taguchi Tamesaburō, probably a pharmacist and a merchant agent, delivered goods to Yōan; sometimes, the goods were rerouted to Kubota and distributed from there.[127] Yōan also approached Shibata Chōkichi (Nagayoshi) of Ōmagari, a regular intermediary of the supply and distribution chain from Osaka.[128] Some of the supplies that Yōan purchased from the Shibata house were licorice, acupuncture needles, camphor pills, and crow-dipper (*Pinellia ternata*).[129] His inventory of purchases indicates that he bought not only ready-made medicines, such as pills, but also ingredients to mix and decoct his own medicines. In making eye medicines and other medicines, Yōan probably followed family recipes and other recipes that he had studied through his training and experiences.[130]

A patient like Banzō would have paid Yōan a fee for eye medicines. It seemed to be a common practice for the payment of medicines to be based on trust and agreement. Yōan's records suggest that making profits from practicing medicine was not his goal, but he conscientiously tracked payments.[131] When payments were overdue, he had to remind those delinquent customers of their obligations.[132] When he treated someone who had granted him favors in the past or someone who wielded political influence, he prescribed medicines for free as a gesture of his gratitude. This may be why he tried to decline a payment offered by Satō Shōichirō, a samurai vassal of Akita domain.[133] In the long term, however, he ran into financial difficulty and had to borrow money to buy supplies and pay off debts.[134]

REGISTERS OF PHYSICIANS

The eighteenth and nineteenth centuries witnessed the commercialization of medical services by physicians. Texts advertised medical services, targeting consumers interested in general and specialized medical consultations. *A Register of the Names of Physicians*[135] (1820) by Shiratsuchi Ryūhō was a directory of notable physicians who served at the domiciles of domain lords in Edo.[136] Ryūhō remarked that he did not rank physicians because the information was assembled from various sources; he did not want to judge those physicians' skills, instead offering practical information, such as their medical backgrounds and their locations in the city.[137] Most of the physicians were medical generalists,[138] or perhaps they chose that professional identity to widen their reach among medical consumers.[139]

Ryūhō's register sometimes furnishes details of a physician's expertise and genealogy to help readers choose wisely. One physician named Sawada Genryō was popularly acclaimed as a specialist in smallpox.[140] As if by clairvoyance, he was said to have been able to precisely discern from diseased lesions whether a patient's smallpox condition was curable. His wondrous treatments even were reported to have completely erased ugly pockmarks of smallpox, which are common in the aftermath of the disease. Many of the ophthalmologists had backgrounds in general medicine. For example, Matsuoka Dōen was a physician of general medicine with specialized skills in ophthalmology and external medicine.[141] He was known to be well versed in secret medical recipes of medical lineages and had imparted them to his son, Fumiyoshi. Another physician, Gyōtoku Genboku, had a background in general medicine and ophthalmology. He had studied medicine in Kyoto under two masters and was a well-respected pioneer in ophthalmology.[142] The public listings suggest that domain physicians were hired for medical services by samurai and non-samurai clients unconnected to their households.

MEDICAL CASE HISTORIES

Medical case histories are specialized case studies that were narrated and written by physicians. These sources were studied by medical scholars and though not circulated to most readers, they are important for our perspectives on the interface between physicians and patients in medical treatment, because medical services had become widely available in the eighteenth and nineteenth centuries. Some cases featured patients who were suffering from blindness and how they were treated. Medical cases were selected to provide instruction on clinical approaches to diseases. Each case showcased a physician's analytical skills and knowledge of medical precedents. Patients' circumstances differed from case to case, and sometimes there were surprising symptoms. Many factors could complicate diagnosis and treatment. Because of the physician-centered perspectives of the genre, illness was described through symptoms that were manifested to a physician; whether or not symptoms appeared, the facts had to be analyzed in the context of factors such as a patient's gender and personal medical history.

One case study by Hara Nan'yō, a reputed physician of Mito domain, focuses on a patient who was in great hardship because of vision loss and physical impairment.[143] All we know about the patient is that he was a peasant from the village of Morita; biographical information about patients is scarce in this genre. The unnamed patient had just recovered from what we may identify as chancroid,[144] a contagious sexually transmitted disease, and it appears that he was suffering from debilitating health complications. That patient complained about pain in his bones, had a twisted arm, and was limping around with numbness in one leg. He also was in a lot of distress because his eyes were red and stinging from pain. Nan'yō assessed that the patient had lost most of his vision and could barely see. Despite his suffering, and despite the available choices, the patient had postponed treatment because he was too poor to afford it. He had no savings—not a single cent of money, as described by Nan'yō— and begged to be treated. His plight might have reflected the distress of countless other patients whose visual impairment could not be cured, not because there was no cure but because they could only afford to prepare simple home remedies. To save him, Nan'yō prescribed pills, powder, and decoctions. After "some tens of days," the patient's vision slowly improved. Not only that, he began to regain the ability to extend and move his weakened arm and leg. Nan'yō was cautious about measuring the dosage and frequency of the medicines. Although the prescription was issued for short-term use, the patient became overly dependent on it and claimed that he suffered from headaches and vision loss when he discontinued it.

In a particular case study by Odai Yōdō, a physician of the influential Ancient Formulas medical scholars,[145] the patient was a woman in her thirties.[146] She had been troubled by painful visual impairment and irregular menstrual flow. Because she had not had her period for three to four months, she assumed that she was pregnant. However, just when she felt that she was doing well, her vision deteriorated so suddenly that within four or five days, she completely lost her vision. When Yōdō examined her, he found that her eyes were bloodshot. She was in so much pain that she could not even open her eyes. He recommended an aggressive therapy with medicines but warned her that even if she did not fear the disease, she could suffer from the intense effects of the medicines. Crying and pleading, she consented to the treatment. The underlying cause of her disrupted menstrual cycle turned out to be the same cause of her vision loss, which was a late symptom of the unknown disease. After more than half a month of treatment, her vision and menstrual cycle were finally restored.

Conclusion

Being blind meant being disabled by visual impairment and suffering from disablement. For that person, too, being blind could include the experience of being enabled by choices to locate and access cures. This insight is clear from the context of the eighteenth and nineteenth centuries, in which the medical industry, print culture, and commercial markets for medicines burgeoned.

General audiences were enabled as patients and as consumers in popular medical culture. Previously, in the seventeenth century, some of the earliest published Japanese medical texts disseminated information about easy household remedies to treat medical conditions. This dimension of medicine, focused on self-diagnosis and self-medication, compensated for the scarcity of medical resources and personnel. But beginning in the eighteenth century, the horizons of knowledge were broader than they had ever been before.

General audiences in the eighteenth and nineteenth centuries were consumers of print culture. In their reach, they were inundated with voluminous printed copies of gazetteers and other vernacular genres that fed the popular imagination of medicines and cures. Pharmacies and vendors laid claim to the types and genres of medicines that were being produced. Travels by tourists and pilgrims propelled the popularity of these medicines.

Where a cure came from really mattered. The miraculous origins and benefits of wonder drugs were advertised to engender the idea that a cure existed for all ailments, including eye ailments. Popular eye medicines were regarded as no less significant than medical prescriptions by physicians and ophthalmologists. A dearth of physical evidence that popular drugs actually cured eye conditions did not deter people from believing that their eye illnesses could be cured. As the examples of Yōan, Bakin, Yashichi, and other nineteenth-century medical case histories tell us, physicians entered into productive social relationships with their patients to treat eye diseases; so, too, did consumers, as patients, exercise their discretion in making choices.

In the social and cultural contexts of popular medical culture, medical knowledge was constructed as vernacular knowledge, and medical services were accessed by general audiences. People suffering from blindness were enabled by choices to consider ways to address their conditions, even if they were not completely cured in the end.

CHAPTER 3

The Blind Guild

Status and Power

———— ❧ ————

Historical sources from the Tokugawa period used a range of words to refer to blind people. Adjectives such as *mō, meshii,* and *mekura* mean "blind." *Katameshii* specifically means "blind in one eye," while *akimekura* and *akijii* mean "clear-blind"[1] (a reference to cataracts). General nouns such as *mōjin* and *kosha*[2] mean "blind person" or "blind people." In some contexts, the gender-based noun *zatō*, the name of a rank of the Kyoto guild (to be discussed in this chapter), can also mean "blind man" or "blind men." The gender-based noun *goze*,[3] a word for "blind female musician" or "blind female musicians" (to be discussed in chapter 4), can also mean "blind woman" or "blind women."

This remarkable array of vocabulary may lead us to believe that historians must know a great deal of specific information about many different aspects of blind people's medical conditions and personal experiences in Tokugawa Japan. That is only partially true, and chapters 1 and 2 explored some answers. Medical records reveal more about eye diseases and ailments, but less about whether patients with eye diseases were actually cured; and while we can imagine that people suffering from blindness had choices to get cured, it is less clear how many of them continued to live with blindness even after trying treatments. There is also no consistent way for historians to tell the extent to which a blind person was visually impaired.

78

Even though we hardly have documentation of blind people's own words about their experiences, we have broad information that gives us a good sense of how Tokugawa Japan's social and political contexts shaped disability identity and how those contexts had consequences for a blind person's choice of livelihood, status, and social membership in society. The rich references to blind people in historical sources allow us to reimagine what it meant to be blind from a blind person's perspective: that being blind could mean assuming a distinctive disabled identity, one validated by visual impairment. So, what did some blind people do, and how did they benefit from their identities?

This chapter focuses on the Kyoto guild (or the guild) and the blind men who were guild members. As previously described in the introduction, the guild was established as an elite musical academy in Kyoto sometime in the thirteenth century or early fourteenth century (the medieval period of Japan's history) and trained blind male musicians to perform *The Tale of the Heike* (*Heike* music), the guild's traditional genre. Beginning in the early seventeenth century, the shogunate governed Japan through the system of status rule, which classified and governed people according to their statuses; commoners were diverse but, as a whole, made up the largest status group.[4] Under status rule, the shogunate empowered the guild with special political authority to govern Japan's blind population categorically as the blind status group.

Lacking a proper definition of sight, vision, or blindness in the Tokugawa period, I use "blind people" as a translation of the references to them in the historical sources of that period in this chapter, as well as in all other chapters (an approach that I explained in the introduction). Blind people in Tokugawa society were visually impaired people, and we can say that they were different from sighted people and were made out to be different also because of status rule. We do not know the level of vision sighted people had, but we may think of them as members of the majority of Tokugawa Japan's population: that is to say, they were people with sufficient functional sight to perform work and tasks in everyday life that involved sight. As we consider the context of the guild, we may also think of sighted people as people with sufficient functional sight that they did not need disabled identity and did not need to be associated with the guild.[5]

Blind people made up a status group because blindness was the common impairment among them and also because the guild had a long history as the institution that served blind people, even though it maintained an exclusively male membership throughout the Tokugawa period and discriminated against some blind people. (Why or how some blind people were excluded from the guild is the subject of chapter 4.) Though the shogunate validated the guild's medieval heritage, the guild's mandate to protect blind musicians' traditions became less important than its new political role. The guild still continued to teach *Heike* music to guild members in the ensuing centuries, albeit because of the historical legacy, but it also embraced a range of existing and new professions, including music, acupuncture, and massage. (Those professions are the subjects of chapter 5 and chapter 6.)

This chapter's focus on guild members demonstrates that the guild was an important source of identity. Guild membership enabled disabled identity, allowing some guild members to earn appointment to high positions in the guild's hierarchy. The networks of local guilds extended across Japan and operated under the Kyoto guild's comprehensive command; through their local guild groups and leaders, guild members engaged with the Kyoto guild's political authority.[6] Historical sources make it clear that in the eighteenth and nineteenth centuries, low-ranking guild members, who constituted the majority of guild membership, used the guild as a platform to protect their welfare and interests.

Guild membership also came at a price. It disadvantaged those guild members who did not have wealth or connections. Despite being protected by the guild, many guild members led precarious lives because the guild imposed great responsibilities and financial obligations on them. Some had to engage in moneylending activities, and many more made money by collecting alms. In short, disabled identity legitimized by guild membership was enabling and opened some doors for guild members, but the significant hardships that guild membership caused could prove socially and economically disabling.

The Medieval Legacy of the Guild in the Tokugawa Period

MUSIC AND RITUALS

Blind people in Japan have been known for performing music. The medieval history of *The Tale of the Heike* provides some context for understanding why blind people became musicians in that era. Composed sometime in the thirteenth century,[7] or a little earlier, the tale is remembered today as an epic historical fiction about the rise and fall of the noble Taira clan (the Heike), who vied with the rival noble Minamoto clan (the Genji) for power. As the story goes, the Heike had ambitions to the imperial throne and scored early victories, but the Genji faction won over important allies and turned the tide in the conflict, deposing the embattled Heike from power.

Musicians of *Heike* were blind men. They narrated verses of the tale with music (*Heike* music) in solo performances before live audiences. Their blindness appeared to have enhanced popular ideas about the sanctity of their musical performances. In the popular imagination of Japan's medieval period, blind musicians were believed to easily cross the imagined boundary between the mortal and the supernatural realms through music and rituals. Because *Heike* was performed with the *biwa* (a type of Japanese lute), and also because it was thought that their performances were imbued with religious power,[8] those blind musicians were popularly known as *biwa hōshi* [琵琶法師] (*biwa* priests). These ideas about blind musicians' musical gifts endured in the Tokugawa period.

We do not have the exact date when the Kyoto guild was founded, but its founding would probably have coincided with blind musicians' early success in performing *Heike* music. To enter the musical profession, a blind man joined the guild as a disciple of a master, who taught him *Heike* music. As a disciple progressed in his training, he earned ranks in the guild's hierarchy—in the medieval period, the guild awarded ranks to recognize a guild member's professional achievements in *Heike* music. Literary scholars today consider Kaku'ichi, an early leader of the guild, to be one of the most influential blind musicians in that period.[9] With a strong following among aristocratic audiences (primarily the court nobility), *Heike* music peaked in popularity sometime in the late fourteenth century or early fifteenth century. The fifteenth-century source *Diary of Things Seen and Heard,*[10] written by Gosukōin, who was a courtier and a patron of *Heike* music, gives us some names of the guild's reputed blind musicians.[11]

In view of the importance of *Heike* music to the guild's musicians, it is surprising that we do not have definitive, historical accounts of the origin of *Heike* music. Stories about its origin can be traced to the medieval period, but they are speculative. One pioneer was supposedly a blind man, perhaps a priest, named Shōbutsu. Not much is known about his life or his relationship with the guild, but Yoshida Kenkō's *Essays in Idleness,*[12] a fourteenth-century collection of essays on miscellaneous topics, offers some clues.[13] It seems that Shōbutsu lived in the thirteenth century, predating Kaku'ichi's lifetime, and led a provincial life in eastern Japan. He learned *Heike* from former court official and priest Yukinaga of Shinano (in Nagano prefecture today), who some say was the com-

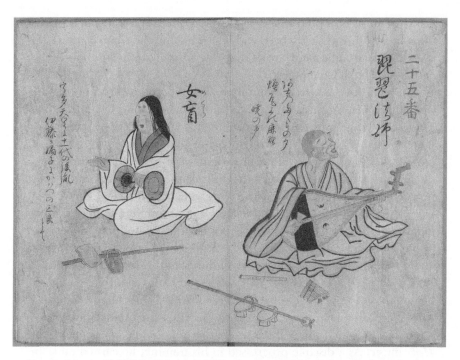

Fig. 3.1. Image of blind musicians. *Left:* The female musician is described as a *jomō* (blind woman; *jomō* reverses the usual word order of *mōjo*)—the Japanese *kanji* characters are glossed as *mekura* (dark eyes), a reference to her blindness. Less is known about blind female musicians of the medieval period than about blind male musicians, but it is likely that blind female musicians performed music with drumbeat, as seen here. *Right:* The male musician is described as a *biwa hōshi* (blind male musicians who played the *biwa* and specialized in *Heike* music). His head is shaven, and he is dressed like a Buddhist cleric, a physical appearance consistent with the image that early blind male musicians were musical, religious performers. The verse next to the man narrates the scene from *The Tale of the Heike* about the Heike's retreat from Fukuhara, the clan's capital, with smoke rising as the palace goes up in flames. The verse next to the woman honors the ancestry of Iwazu Saburō, the father of the Soga brothers and the male heir of the Itō clan with links to Emperor Uda, who ruled in the late ninth century. This verse comes from *The Tale of the Soga Brothers* and suggests that blind female musicians had a role in performing the tale. From *Poetry Contest of All Kinds of Artisans and Professionals* (Japanese title: *Shokuninzukushi utaawase*; undated manuscript likely produced in the late medieval period or early Tokugawa period). National Diet Library Digital Collections.

poser. (The literary history of *Heike* is much more complicated, as chapter 5 will explain.)

That blind people were unique, distinguished both by their blindness and by their special fates, has been a common motif in Japanese literature and culture since the early days—Zatōichi, briefly surveyed in the preface, is one example of a fictional, blind, superhuman swordsman and icon in contemporary Japanese popular culture. From early records, we know of a blind musician named Semimaru, though authoritative information about him—when he was born or when he lived—is slim, and historians regard him as an enigma. Records about him have survived in fictions. In *A Collection of Tales Present and Past*,[14] which was compiled in the eleventh or twelfth century, the story about Semimaru says that he lived alone in the Ausaka pass of Kyoto.[15] Despite his lowly birth, he was admired for possessing extraordinary skills with the *biwa*. Through his impeccable musical performances, he mesmerized courtier Minamoto Hiromasa. In some musical and religious traditions, itinerant performers such as Buddhist preachers claimed Semimaru as their founder; so, too, did the guild celebrate him in its myths.[16] Susan Matisoff's literary analysis of texts about Semimaru tells us that the fascination with him continued through the medieval and Tokugawa periods. A late medieval *nō* drama (a theatrical genre) attributed to Kanze Motokiyo Zeami recast Semimaru as a blind prince—a son of Emperor Daigo—and a tragic hero.[17] Tokugawa-period playwright Chikamatsu Monzaemon also adapted Semimaru for the genre of *jōruri* (puppet theater), interweaving the theme of blindness into the plot.[18]

Understanding the guild's myths and rituals is essential for understanding how the guild constructed its authority in the medieval period—those medieval myths and rituals were reimbued with authority in the Tokugawa period for the guild's ideological purpose of creating identity. The guild depended on narratives about illustrious blind people to corroborate its ideological claims of a time-honored heritage. The genealogy described in *The Essential Collections of the Guild*,[19] an eighteenth-century source that was likely circulated much earlier, was quite typical of genealogies that had constructed fictive profiles of founders with unverified links to actual historical figures.[20] The guild's founder, Saneyasu Shinnō (posthumously deified as Amayo no Mikoto), was said to have lived sometime in the ninth century of the Heian period.[21] As the guild told his life story, he was born to imperial consort Fujiwara Sawako and was Emperor Kōkō's younger brother. At age twenty-eight, he lost his vision due to an unknown eye disease. He was well versed in music and poetry and received the transmission of the secret melodies of the *biwa*—knowledge that was reserved only for the most impressive, distinguished musicians. Emperor Kōkō granted ranks, setting up the guild's hierarchy, to honor Saneyasu.

The guild created religious rituals in the medieval period to celebrate its founder, Saneyasu. According to one account, Emperor Kōkō ordered blind people from various provinces to gather annually on the sixteenth day of the second month in Kyoto to participate in a sacred rite called *shakutō*, which was named after the symbolic act of stacking stones in honor of Saneyasu (see figure 3.2).[22] For her devotion to her duties, Saneyasu's mother was also honored by the guild annually in a parallel ceremony on the nineteenth day of the sixth month.[23] The stone-stacking rite brought guild members together and was central to the ritual life of the Kyoto guild. The rite would have commenced at the guild's headquarters with guild members making special offerings to the deities worshipped by the guild.[24] Low-ranking members had to pay respects to high-ranking members, as dictated by the guild's laws. The event climaxed with the revelry of *Heike* music and concluded with selected guild members stacking stones at the riverbank. Though likely discontinued by the eighteenth century, from the medieval period through the early part of the Tokugawa period, the rite solidified the ideology of the guild's ruling tier by staging an elaborate performance that amplified hierarchical privileges and differences in ranks.

In keeping with blind musicians' historical traditions, during the Tokugawa period many local guild groups continued to worship Myōon Benzaiten, the patron deity of music.[25] The Myōonkō was a religious confraternity (a religious association) formed by local guild groups (and also by local groups of blind female musicians) to celebrate the deity. This gathering had functions analogous to those of the stone-stacking rite of the Kyoto guild: to highlight hierarchical differences and to instill an individual's sense of belonging to the guild. Because the Myōonkō rite was organized around each local guild group's traditions, and was not coordinated with the Kyoto guild, the presentation had a strong local orientation and was a source of each group's identity. It appears that local guild members continued this practice through the nineteenth century. Though the origins of worship are unclear, the dates and protocols of gatherings varied from place to place.[26] Permutations of ritual elements were common. In Nagoya, for example, some local guild members gathered annually on a special day in the tenth month, reciting the Buddhist *Heart sutra*[27] and praying for the longevity of donors (see figure 3.3).[28]

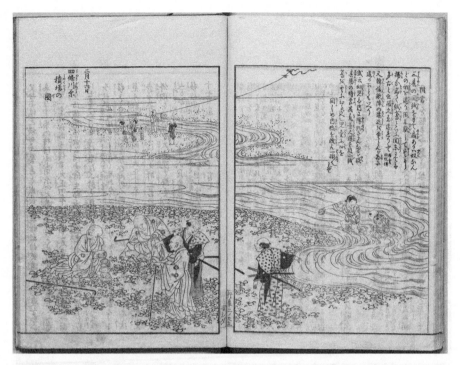

Fig. 3.2. Image of the guild's stone-stacking rite, as imagined by the illustrator.
The protocols of the guild's rituals can be reconstructed from *Records of Enpekiken*
(Japanese title: *Enpekiken ki*), a seventeenth-century source written by Kurokawa
Dōyū under his literary pseudonym, and from Hayami Shungyōsai's *The Illustrated
Compendium of Festivals of Various Provinces* (1806) of the late Tokugawa period.
Left: Three blind men are gathered at a riverbank at Shijōgawara. Their heads are
shaven, and each person has a walking staff. The leftmost person is stacking stones,
the blind man next to him is gathering stones, and a third blind man (perhaps the
oldest) stands in the foreground. Two samurais bearing swords may be observers of
the rite and serve the blind men as sighted guides. This ritual activity would have
followed a grand performance of offerings and music at the guild's headquarters.
Illustration by Hayami Shungyōsai from *The Illustrated Compendium of Festivals
of Various Provinces* (Japanese title: *Shokoku zue nenchū gyōji taisei*), vol. 2 (1806).
National Archive of Japan Digital Archive.

The gazetteer *Questions and Answers about the Customs of Awaji Province*[29]
tells us that in that province (in Hyōgo prefecture today) the rite was
routinely held in the tenth month.[30] Guild members from all over the
province arrived on the day of the rite; they performed duties according
to their ranks and played music all day and night. In Higashiyanagi (in
Hiroshima prefecture today), local guilds congregated annually on a day

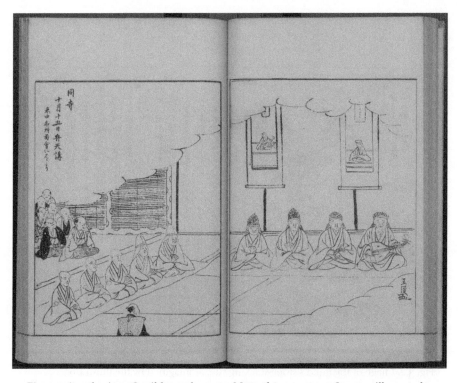

Fig. 3.3. A gathering of guild members at a Myōonkō ceremony, from an illustrated travel guidebook typical of the late Tokugawa period. This illustration shows a local guild group at Nanatsudera (a temple) conducting the ritual of Myōonkō (also called Bentenkō) to honor the patron deity of music. The text says that the rite was held on the fifteenth day of the tenth month. The blind musicians are sitting on the floor around a central space in an L-shaped configuration. The arrangement is determined by the men's ranks. *Left:* Three men with their heads shaven are low-ranked members (this is clear from their lack of headgear; the higher the rank, the more elaborate the dress code). *Right:* The blind musician playing the *biwa* appears to be a senior guild member, presumably playing *Heike* music, the music of choice at ceremonies. Scrolls showing venerated blind musicians hang in the background. Sighted onlookers have been invited to the venue to observe the rite— the participation of sighted people as audience members was probably common. From Okada Kei et al., *Illustrated Gazetteer of the Famous Places of Owari* (Japanese title: *Owari meisho zue*), edited by Wakayama Zenzaburō (Nagoya: Nagoya Onkokai, 1933). National Diet Library Digital Collections.

in the ninth month and allowed members to be excused only if they were too ill to attend.[31]

THE GUILD'S HIERARCHY

Hierarchy was the most important feature of the guild, so guild members who held high ranks had great privileges. In the medieval period, high ranks and appointments empowered the guild's elites, granting them the prestige to perform *Heike* music to aristocratic audiences and receive recognition for their performances. The guild used religious rituals, which have been discussed, to emphasize the distinction of high ranks from low ranks in its hierarchy. Even in the Tokugawa period, ranks were so important that the guild did not alter its hierarchy, and guild members were required to earn ranks and promotions. Each rank of the hierarchy was divided into grades, which were still more finely divided into subgrades,[32] making the guild an elaborately structured, bureaucratically cumbersome institution.

The *sōkengyō*[33] or *shokukengyō*[34] was the guild's top leader.[35] Historically, this office was known by either designation and was filled by one person. Seijuan, near Bukkōji in Kyoto, was the guild's headquarters. For a brief period, from the late seventeenth century through the early eighteenth century, the two offices were filled by separate leaders—the *sōkengyō* was relocated to Edo, while the *shokukengyō* remained in Kyoto. But they were merged and became one office again in Kyoto sometime in or around 1736. After that time, the Edo officeholder was named as *sōroku*.[36] Based in Edo, he served as a proxy head of the Kyoto guild. This person held the rank of *kengyō* (see the description below). He had broad-ranging powers and acted on behalf of and under the authority of the main Kyoto guild leader. He was given executive rights by the Kyoto guild to pass sentence and implement orders in Edo.

The guild had four basic ranks. The highest of those ranks was *kengyō*.[37] The ten most senior members of this rank were elected to join the Council of Ten Elders (*jūrō*[38]), and the guild's top leader was chosen from among them. The next highest rank was *bettō*.[39] This rank was named after the Buddhist clerical rank of abbot. Next was the rank of *kōtō*.[40] Senior guild members often held this rank, which was respectable but less prestigious than the top ranks. A guild member of this rank could be appointed to a minor position of leadership in a local guild.

The fourth, and lowest, rank was *zatō*.[41] This was the guild's most common rank (also mentioned in historical records as *shubun*[42] or *shibun*[43]). It confirmed a guild member's official induction into the hierarchy. A guild member started his career with the guild as an unranked novice (*mukan*[44]) and a disciple of a master. He had to rise through the grades of *shoshin*[45] and *uchikake*[46] before becoming approved as a *zatō*.

In the seventeenth century, the guild systematically expanded its membership and commanded a wide base of blind subjects, uniting peers and leaders across large geographical distances in an interlinked "national" community.[47] The guild in the Tokugawa period had a much broader reach with local guild groups across Japan than it did in the medieval period when its scope was limited to Kyoto. Guild leaders of local guilds represented the national (in the sense of countrywide) authority of the Kyoto guild in the communities where they lived. An early, invaluable glimpse into the organization of the guild appears in a book by German physician-naturalist Engelbert Kaempfer, who visited Japan in the late seventeenth century. He commented that the guild functioned like "a common-wealth" with a broad scope of jurisdictional autonomy:

Whoever is once admitted a member of this Society [the guild], must remain such for life. They are dispersed up and down the Empire, but their General resides at Miaco [*miyako*; Kyoto], where the Cash of the Company is kept. He is called Osiok [probably *o-shoku*, an abbreviation of *shokukengyō* and a deferential address], and hath 4300 Thails a year allow'd him for his maintenance by the Dairi [possibly a named proxy of the shogunate]. He governs the common-wealth, being assisted by ten Counsellors call'd Siu Ro [*jūrō*; Council of Ten Elders], which signifies Elder Men, Alder-men, of which he, the General himself is the eldest. They reside at Miaco, and have, jointly with the General, power of life and death, with this restriction however, that no person can be executed, unless the Sentence be approv'd of, and the dead-warrant sign'd by the Lord Chief Justice of Miaco. The Council of Ten appoint their inferior officers, who reside in several Provinces: Some of these are call'd Kengio [*kengyō*], as it were, Father Provincials, being each in his Province, what the General is with regard to the whole Society. . . . Every Kengio hath his Kotos [*kōtō*], as they are called, to assist and advise him. . . . The Kengio's and Koto's have many other inferior officers subordinate to them, who are call'd Sijbun [*shubun*, a grade equal to the rank of *zatō*], and are again subordinate to one another. . . . The main body of the Blind are comprehended under one general name of Mukwan [*mukan*; unranked novices].[48]

In Tokugawa Japan, as guild membership became diverse, ranks became open to members who had no background in *Heike* music. In the medieval system, guild members proved their proficiency in *Heike* music and paid fees to elders of their musical lineages and sects to gain the right to be promoted. By the Tokugawa period, the sale of ranks had become an even more significant source of revenue for the guild. Fees[49] for ranks were dictated and imposed by the guild. The guild's wealth was managed by the guild's elites, and money collected from the sale of ranks was paid out as dividends to guild members in amounts commensurate with their ranks. Low-ranking guild members were much less likely than high-ranking guild members to benefit from direct income from the guild.

As we are told anecdotally by *Drops of Japanese Hop: Gossips from Here and There*,[50] a nineteenth-century source, it cost 1,000 *ryō* (a gold currency unit) to rise to the elite rank of *kengyō* in the guild.[51] Paying this sum would have caused the financial ruination of most blind people. The moderately prestigious rank of *kōtō* could be purchased with 300 *ryō*, which was not a modest sum of money by any standard. The sums were probably exaggerated through hearsay, but stories about these exacting payments were the stuff of conversations about blind people even after the Tokugawa period. Basil Hall Chamberlain, famed British professor of Japanese at Tokyo Imperial University, had heard enough about the guild to write in *Things Japanese* in the late nineteenth century that "for the highest grade to which any ordinary blind mortal could aspire—the grade next under that of a provost—a fee of $1000 was exacted."[52]

Throughout the Tokugawa period, one aspect of being a guild member meant honoring the lifelong commitment to stay with the guild. In any guild member's career, becoming a master marked a milestone, because it meant that he had attained a position of authority. A master profited from his disciples: he could extract fees for training them and for securing ranks from the Kyoto guild on their behalf. Such financial relationships could place an enormous burden on a disciple's resources. For example, according to *Records of the Customs of Aizu*,[53] a gazetteer about the customs of the area around Aizu (in Fukushima prefecture today), after a disciple was admitted into the local guild, he had to offer a fee to his master.[54] Also, while training as a musician, he had to defray his expenses. When he was promoted by a grade in rank, he owed his master one *bu* in cash (one *bu* was a quarter of one *ryō*). The practice described in that source was not too different in other places, and a disciple might have paid fees to multiple masters of the guild, such as the local guild leader, his own master, and the lineage master.[55]

A sighted person had less incentive than a blind person to become a guild member. Because niche professions that hired blind people tended to favor blind people, sighted people would have more easily found jobs in a broad range of livelihoods. The costs of ranks also did not justify the limited choices of employment.

LAWS AND STATUS RULE

The Kyoto guild had laws that dated back to the medieval period. The laws suggest that the guild in the medieval period discriminated against other itinerant, musical professions so as to justify its distinctive identity and mandate in society. The guild at that time also drew on the authority of the Koga clan of court nobles, who were patrons of *Heike* music, to bolster its own authority to confer ranks upon its elites; in return, the Koga clan demanded financial dues from guild leaders.[56] Starting in the seventeenth century, however, as the guild strengthened its ties with the shogunate, that clan was sidelined to a nominal role.

At the beginning of the Tokugawa period, blind people stood out because the Kyoto guild had already demarcated blind people's identities in the medieval period. Status rule (highlighted in the introduction) was a unique form of political rule in Tokugawa Japan that categorized people by their social statuses and granted status groups certain autonomy in governing their affairs: samurais, commoners (including peasants, townspeople, and merchants), and temple and shrine clergy were major status groups in society. For guild members, the guild's rituals and hierarchy framed and legitimized their individual disabled identities and their special blind status identities in Tokugawa society, while other disabled social groups were granted no such special status since they had no parallel or preexisting institutions to represent them.

Members of status groups had work responsibilities that can be thought of as their occupations. David Howell's analysis of the status system demonstrates that occupation was a defining feature, an obligation to that system. For Howell, occupation means "the economic activity linked to a household's formal status,"[57] while livelihood means "the economic means by which households actually supported themselves."[58]

As Howell also points out, as the Tokugawa Japanese economy developed over the eighteenth century, the range of livelihoods expanded to the extent that people could pursue their livelihoods independently of their occupations. To use Howell's example, a male peasant was expected to engage in agricultural production because that was his occupation tied to his status, or the duty of peasants as "land tax-paying cultivators,"[59] but he was also free to make a living (his livelihood) in other industries that were not directly related to his occupation.[60]

There were conditions under which a person could adopt a new status and assume the responsibilities of that new status—what Howell calls "a new occupationally defined status identity."[61] Maren Ehlers identifies artisans and entertainers as status groups with occupations not based on "productive land"[62] and also as status groups with members who could move between occupations to assume multiple status identities. The status system had evolved to become quite flexible over time, and the occupations of commoners and those of marginal status groups contributed to the dynamic, diverse mix of overlapping status identities.

We may think of the Kyoto guild as an occupation-based status institution. But compared with other status groups, the guild was less accommodating toward nonmembers in order to preserve an exclusive status identity. By becoming guild members, blind men of different backgrounds acquired the same blind status identity and pledged to be identified by that status. This was a disabled identity that was bound to guild membership. This disabled identity was different from that of a blind person who was not a guild member, because it came with the obligations of guild membership discussed earlier, such as participating in religious rituals, paying for ranks, and paying fees to masters and elders. In the case of a blind male who claimed his disabled identity based on his blindness, as long as he did not join the guild, he still retained his original status identity and did not officially become a member of the blind status category, which was governed by the guild. This arrangement could be the best of both worlds for such a blind person: he could be employed in a livelihood but avoid his duty to the guild. This also became a problem for the guild's authority, as chapter 4 will discuss, since the guild regarded blind people who were not guild members to still be included in the blind status category and hence subjects of the guild's rule.

There was flexibility in the work that guild members could do, and this flexibility is important for our understanding of guild members' livelihoods. Music was the guild's oldest profession, with roots in the medieval period, and certainly the guild's main profession early in the seventeenth century, but over the next centuries the shogunate and the guild focused on demanding that eligible blind men join the guild and fulfill their duties—leaving it to blind individuals to choose their livelihoods. Because guild members usually ended up in niche professions and pursued their livelihoods as their occupations in the guild's context, the general idea that a guild member's livelihood included his occupation is adequate.

When status rule was introduced in the early seventeenth century, the shogunate expediently constructed the guild's authority based on the existing foundation of the guild's medieval laws. The shogunate reorganized the guild's legal codes and inscribed them with new authority to give substance to the legal framework that encouraged, but also restricted, the guild's autonomy. The executive powers of the guild's top offices were enshrined in the *Ancient Legal Code*,[63] the guild's first legal code (1634)[64] of the Tokugawa period. It was updated as the *New Legal Code*,[65] which was introduced in 1692. In both legal codes, the laws were divided into sections about various facets of the guild's internal government, such as the regulation of ranks, the appointment of masters and disciples, everyday conduct, formal etiquette at ritual and religious ceremonies, behavioral prohibitions, and punishments for criminal acts.

The Kyoto guild defended its laws to carry out status rule, enabling its leaders to possess the autonomy and right to exercise power over guild members. Guild members had to abide by the laws if they wanted to remain with the guild. Though focused on guild members, the guild broadly interpreted its laws as applying to the blind status category, with the implication that they could be applied to any blind person who claimed a disabled identity. Also, by implication, the guild considered any blind person who was working in a niche profession to be involved in an occupation and hence to have the duty to serve the guild.

In their early forms in the seventeenth century, many of the guild's laws focused on guild leaders' exercise of jurisdictional authority. For instance, if a guild member brought forth a lawsuit, the Council of Ten Elders could decide the outcome by majority vote. If the elders reached a deadlock, the lawsuit had to be deferred to the guild's top leader; difficult lawsuits were turned over to the shogunate. If judged to be guilty by the guild's judicial system, defendants were summarily expelled from the guild. Guild members who failed to fulfill ordinary obligations could also face the threat of expulsion, and if expelled but later allowed to rejoin the guild they would not be reinstated to their original ranks.[66] The *New Legal Code* of 1692, while preserving the essence of previous laws, made Edo a co-headquarters of the guild; this would explain why a proxy head of the Kyoto guild (introduced earlier through the guild's hierarchy) was installed there in Edo to bolster the guild's rule.[67]

The Kyoto guild over the next centuries often interpreted its political autonomy through the legal frameworks of local guild groups' domains and local status governments. Local guilds, while being under the higher authority of the Kyoto guild, had to also work with the authorities of their home communities. For instance, this means that a local guild of blind males based in a rural, predominantly agricultural community made up of peasants had to respect the authority of the Kyoto guild and that of the status government of that place (the local status government). Because a local guild's membership could span several different communities, the local status governments of those places could become involved in the political process. Other status groups in Tokugawa society also moderated their autonomy to accommodate the rule of their domains and local status governments. Among the things a local guild group could do was to operate an office;[68] but to establish one, guild members had to get approval from their local status governments.[69] High-ranking guild members and guild leaders in local areas who had been authorized by the Kyoto guild to receive income from the guild because of their ranks would have claimed what was due to them through their local guild offices.

There is reason to believe that as the networks of local guilds grew in the eighteenth and nineteenth centuries,[70] the Kyoto guild became more flexible in dealing with local guilds and increasingly entrusted them with duties that involved local status governments. As examples from nineteenth-century Higo and Kumamoto domains (both in southern Kyūshū) highlight, even as the Tokugawa regime was nearing its end, the Kyoto guild still maintained communication with local guilds to make important decisions, such as promotions and appointments.[71] After a guild member paid for his rank, the fee was conveyed to his local guild leader and passed through political intermediaries before it reached the Kyoto guild. This invisible route of cash remittance to the Kyoto guild, a route that also conveyed the Kyoto guild's approval of ranks back to local guild groups, traversed large geographical distances and was part of an extensive national system of communication that bound a guild member in the far-flung corners of Japan to the Kyoto guild. Financial exchanges between parties and intermediaries were based on mutual trust that the money would reach the intended recipients and not be misappropriated along the way.

A guild member trying to take up a leadership position in his local guild had to be approved for promotion by the Kyoto guild, and it was not uncommon for him to also seek the approval of his local status government. For instance, while a local guild group was entitled to elect a leader, the choice might have to be endorsed by the home community's leaders and by the main administrative office of the domain;[72] as part of the protocol, the domain office was informed of the short-listed candidates and the impending vote. Through the nineteenth century, these channels of authority that co-opted existing government structures at each location allowed the Kyoto guild to efficiently extend its rule via local guild offices with minimal disruption.

Guild Membership: Who Could Join the Guild?

Guild membership was a marker of the blind status category, and becoming a guild member meant giving up one's former status to adopt the blind social status identity and agreeing to be governed by the guild. As a disciple, a guild member could acquire vocational skills and start a career. He also earned the right to be recognized by his rank wherever he lived in Japan. While these were compelling reasons for a blind man to join the guild, guild membership was not advantageous for every blind person. For example, a blind samurai who had the privilege of receiving a stipend from the domain government because of his samurai status would probably have been less willing than a poor, blind commoner to give up his status, only to trade it for the blind social status. Gerald Groemer's analysis of disability suggests that in a situation in which disability was a limiting factor, "Edo-period warrior-class individuals with poor eyesight or little brawn who did not engage in productive labor were far less likely to be belittled by the community than identically constituted commoners who could not toil at or above the 'normal' rate or accomplish certain preordained tasks."[73] Yet, for a blind man with little means to support himself and his family, guild membership could have paid off—or at least it would have been justified by the possibility of becoming socially mobile.

Gender was also a significant factor in guild membership: blind men, not blind women, were admitted into the guild. The guild's exclusively male identity was inherited from the medieval period. Yet this did not mean that blind women were excused from the guild's rule, as will be discussed in chapter 4 (which will also discuss why blind women usually trained to be musicians and how those musicians organized themselves into kinship groups). The guild was generally open to new members so long as they had the funds to pay for membership and did not belong to the outcast status group (see the section on charity later in this chapter, which discusses the outcast status group). A blind male had to find a guild master to accept him as a disciple. While mastering vocational skills, a disciple attempted to earn the first formal rank of *zatō*. He could earn the privilege to adopt a personal name with a "Jō-" prefix or an "-ichi" suffix—this was decided by his master. At no time in the Tokugawa period did the guild set any rules about the degree of visual impairment required for guild membership.

The Kyoto guild also generally did not fix a legal limit on the minimum or maximum age for membership. In late Tokugawa-period sources from places like Hata of Tosa domain (in Kōchi prefecture today), there are reports of an age limit for blind people hoping to be accepted by local guilds.[74] As a general rule, blind males under the age of fourteen were eligible to train as guild members, probably because any male under that age was not considered an adult and was presumed to have the time and potential to learn new skills. The age limit also applied to blind females who were looking to join organized groups of blind female musicians.

The Kyoto guild devolved autonomy to local guilds in matters such as age limit and the length of professional training so that local guild leaders could decide what was appropriate. The degree of autonomy seems to have increased as more local guild groups were formed across Japan throughout the seventeenth century and as they deepened their relationships with the Kyoto guild and with local status governments. It appears that a blind master could decide the skills that would be taught to his disciple. The basic training program was usually broad, spanning the niche professions of music, massage, and acupuncture. A disciple developed his specialty based on his talent and his master's specialty.

In general, blind males had a significant advantage if they started with the guild at a young age: as soon as they completed their training, they could enter a profession and make money to support themselves and to ascend the guild's hierarchy. As chapter 4 will also highlight, the guild's broad authority could not be thoroughly enforced, and it became clear that not every working blind male joined the guild.

The Costs of Ranks: Blind Moneylenders and Their Activities

Because the guild exploited guild members by making them pay for ranks, a guild member incurred significant expenses to progress through the guild's hierarchy. This would explain why guild members could end up in debt. The financial demands of the guild were constant and perpetual no matter when—in which decade or century—a guild member was accepted by the guild. Examples abound of guild members getting loans and trying to make ends meet. Incidents of dishonesty made things worse. In one episode, Hirayanagi, a ranked guild member, accepted a deposit of sixteen *ryō* from a disciple and agreed to act as that disciple's proxy to get approval for a rank from the Kyoto guild but allegedly squandered more than half of the deposit.[75] (He was accused of embezzlement.)

Reports about blind moneylenders were common starting in the eighteenth century. It is reasonable to imagine that many blind moneylenders were desperate guild members whose financial debts to the guild forced them to resort to moneylending. Moneylending was a means by which guild members could make money, though it was probably not their main livelihood. Rumors about blind moneylenders obscured the real stories about guild members' plight. Consumer culture had transformed spending habits in the eighteenth and nineteenth centuries, and in the Japanese economy, cash and credit circulated widely. Excoriating the culture of profligacy of his day, Buyō Inshi recorded hearsay accounts about blind moneylenders in his nineteenth-century work *Affairs of the World: An Account of Things Heard and Seen*.[76] "They [blind moneylenders] take 10 or 20 percent interest, plus another 10 or 20 percent in so-called service charges. When they lend out a certain sum, they subtract the interest and the service charges from the basic amount. They make the contract as being for a deposit without interest. If a borrower fails to meet the deadline for repayment, they use the authority of that deposit contract to collect the loan."[77] This anecdote alleges that blind moneylenders deceived their clients by unreasonably inflating interest amounts and lending sums that were significantly less than what had been promised. It is no surprise that in that age of inexorable consumerism and fluid credit, personal greed was a theme in many moralistic accounts, which unfairly overstated the threat of blind moneylenders to society.

The shogunate was not opposed to the idea of moneylending, but feared that unregulated practices of moneylending would create problems for government authorities and borrowers; bad loans could trigger a chain of defaults involving multiple parties. In the early to mid-eighteenth century, as more and more reports of moneylending surfaced, the shogunate clarified its position through decrees that vilified blind moneylenders and portrayed them as the most visible symbols of moneylending. Blind people were strongly discouraged from becoming moneylenders, but because many of them were already deeply involved in moneylending, they were warned to act discreetly and be aware of the "proper" conditions of moneylending. For example, blind moneylenders were prohibited from acting as intermediaries in business.[78] Those decrees accused blind moneylenders (guild members) of borrowing money from people and then illegally lending the borrowed money to other people to generate service fees, which they allegedly used to buy ranks.

The incentives to keep the vicious cycle of moneylending going did not seem to end. One injunction of the shogunate in 1765 censured the guild, charging that in recent years, guild members had grown brazen, threatening debtors and resorting to violence.[79] The shogunate maintained that blind moneylenders swarmed the gateways of samurai households, kept up their raucous calls, and refused to leave. The injunction acknowledged that these blind moneylenders had every right to seek repayment but criticized that their allegedly disorderly behaviors reflected badly on them and also disgraced their samurai debtors. Blind moneylenders were urged to stop the practice of passing loans from others as their own money; instead, they were to earn fees for ranks by engaging in proper livelihoods.

Through moneylending, blind creditors were bound in relationships with their clients and with political and legal institutions. Many loan agreements were likely based on verbal contracts—in other words, they were likely verbal agreements between borrowers and creditors, sealed by the stamp of trust and integrity. Illegal interest rates were the grievances most often cited by debtors. In one lawsuit from the early nineteenth century, for example, the defendants were three blind moneylenders, Hisa'ichi, Jōkichi, and Jōshun.[80] They had charged an initial interest rate of one *bu* for a loan of twenty *ryō* and had given their client three or four months to repay the loan with interest. However, they demanded service fees and compounded the principal sum with additional interest charges without consent. Hisa'ichi was accused of raising the original interest rate severalfold, collecting two *bu* for every seven *ryō*, while Jōkichi and Jōshun were accused of extorting one *bu* for every nine *ryō*.

In accordance with the legal statutes of the Kyoto guild, and consistent with its autonomous power, blind moneylenders who were charged in Edo and found guilty of extortion would have been turned over to the

Edo proxy head for sentencing. Unless the crime was heinous and punishable by death, the office of the city magistrate[81] (a senior office representing the shogunate) routinely delegated the Edo proxy head of the guild to mete out justice.[82] From the founding of the office in the early eighteenth century, the Edo proxy head had authority over Edo, but it seems that his jurisdiction did not extend too far beyond that city. For example, in a place like Sunpu (in Shizuoka prefecture today), where the local guilds' practices probably reflected those of most places outside Edo, a blind person guilty of a crime had to be brought before his local guild leader.[83] After conducting his own investigation, the local guild leader could decide whether to defer the matter to the Council of Ten Elders at the Kyoto guild for further action.

Exile was an extreme form of punishment in cases usually involving grave offences. The guild's top leader proposed updates to the guild's laws in 1792 to the shogunate and the office of the magistrate of temples and shrines[84] (a senior office representing the shogunate and tasked with overseeing religious administration). The laws discussed categories of exile.[85] If sentenced to harsh exile, a guild member would be expelled by the guild and banished from Edo, Kyoto, Osaka, his home province, and the domain where he was accused of committing the crime. Whether or how the sentence of exile was imposed is less clear; but what is clear is that the guild had the discretion to withdraw guild membership and to refuse to reinstate former privileges. It seems that the Kyoto guild or local guilds did not punish blind moneylenders most of the time. That was why through the nineteenth century, despite repeated warnings from the shogunate, blind moneylenders did not discontinue their moneylending activities.[86] The shogunate periodically reprimanded the Edo proxy head, instructing the office to step up the surveillance of guild members and promptly report wrongdoings.

It is unfair to generalize blind moneylenders as being avaricious and cunning. Instead, through no fault of their own, many blind moneylenders became victims. They were easily exploited by the guild because they were desperate to make money. In fact, as moneylenders, they operated on a limited scale and could not compete with other lenders who had access to deep pools of credit, such as rural elites and large-scale financiers and bankers. Because the risk of loan default by a borrower was real, the day-to-day existence of a blind moneylender was quite precarious. He could not simply depend on moneylending as his sole source of income.

Defending Guild Membership: Charity as a Right

Guild members ordinarily had the right to receive charity because of guild membership, and perhaps it was this right to income—and for many, this was a reliable source of income—that outweighed the disadvantage of struggling to pay for guild membership. Receiving charity could mean receiving remuneration for services to donors on special occasions or getting material (food and financial) assistance due to poverty. *A Record of the Dividends of the Guild*[87] of the Koga clan suggests that from the earliest days of the Tokugawa regime, the shogunate had given blanket authority to guild members to receive alms from major status groups and institutions, such as the Tokugawa shogunate, samurai lords and vassals, temples and shrines, and commoners.[88] Whether it was in the seventeenth century or the nineteenth century, guild members could try to support themselves by seeking alms. This basic right to income from charity was attendant on disabled identity—blind people did not have to be guild members to earn this right, but because the guild claimed a monopoly on blind people's historical roles in performing music and rituals, it gave guild members greater access than nonmembers to patrons and donors. Blind musicians of various genres, as well as those whose repertoire included performing religious rituals, accepted alms as payment for their performances. Blind people without skills could appeal to donors' compassion.

Most blind people, including guild members, benefited from charity through their home communities and by seeking sources further afield. In Edo, when the shogun celebrated an auspicious event, the shogunate distributed alms to blind people.[89] High-ranking guild members who had close ties to the shogunate were mentioned by name in *The Veritable Records of the Tokugawa Shoguns*, the official historical annals of the Tokugawa shoguns.[90] Communities also commemorated certain days or periods of the year by giving out alms. The start of a new year was a significant event, as were events that marked the stages of life: birth, marriage, and death. In some parts of Aizu, blind people conducted rites at households to welcome the new year.[91] For this purpose, many blind people traveled to faraway villages and towns and were still on the road even as late as the second or third month of the new year. At other times, when death befell a family member, blind people showed up at the deceased person's household to collect alms. Collecting alms in any domain, and in any local community, was a competitive business. There also were reports through the nineteenth century that sighted people had appropriated blind people's right to conduct rites at donors' households.[92] This development was neither unexpected nor unusual; government authorities could do little more than issue decrees to stop sighted people from supplanting blind people in these traditional roles.

In the status system, disability did not mean equal treatment of disabled people, even though it enabled their access to charity. Discriminatory attitudes and practices were openly directed at certain disabled people. The blind status category and leprosy status category (briefly discussed in the introduction) are two examples of disabled social groups with different statuses. In fact, leprosy, the disease alone, would have given cause for discrimination. The signs of physical impairment and disfigurement associated with leprosy unjustly deepened society's revulsion of sufferers of leprosy and their families. Blind people, on the other hand, were generally not shunned by society. They were much less likely to have to deal with the stigma of disease—unless leprosy was the cause of their visual impairment, and, in that case, physical symptoms of leprosy might also have been noticeable.

Under status rule, the blind status group and the leprosy status group would have argued to be differentiated from each other and from outcasts. Daniel Botsman's discussion of the outcast status highlights that outcasts owed specific duties to the shogunate and fiercely guarded their own self-governing rights.[93] The occupational work to which outcasts had economic rights was stigmatized by medieval ideas of ritual pollution.[94] Historical perceptions of outcasts, which denigrated their social backgrounds, pedigrees, and work, were armed with the force of law through visible institutional forms of discrimination in the status system. Leaders of the outcast status asserted authority over the leprosy status category and, as Groemer shows, also over some professions, such as itinerant musical performers,[95] but outcasts' rule over the blind status group was challenged by the guild.[96]

The shogunate did not regard outcasts as a disabled social group, insofar as their collective or individual status was not identified by or united by a common bodily impairment, disease, or illness. An individual could be both blind and an outcast but would ordinarily have been treated as an outcast and excluded from the blind status category, because the outcast status identity trumped that person's disabled identity. As Howell notes, in the status system, "membership in an outcaste group was generally determined by birth"[97] and "it was nearly impossible for *eta* to escape outcaste status."[98] Blind people of non-outcast groups, by contrast, were less constrained by birth or by their social backgrounds. They had better chances at social mobility by joining the guild or finding sponsors for their livelihoods.

In some important respects, domain leaders and local status governments dispensed charity to poor people to display their benevolence in the predominantly patriarchal social order. The domain lord was expected to embody the moral principle of benevolence and burnished his image as a compassionate, sympathetic ruler through public acts of relieving hardships.[99] Devolving authority to local status groups was a pragmatic strategy of the domain government to minister to the poorest subjects. But charity did not always have to be compensation for disability or material deprivation. As Ehlers demonstrates in her study of Ōno domain (in Fukui prefecture today), beggars performed essential work, such as policing vagrants, and in return asserted the right to seek alms.[100] As blind musical and religious performers collected alms, it may appear that they were not too different from beggars, but beggars were identified by their activities as outcasts. Begging was a legitimate status occupation, and local beggar guilds were organized by local outcast leaders.[101] Guild members were protected from being absorbed by beggar guilds because they were shielded by the guild's authority.

The fact is that from the beginning of the Tokugawa period, blind men and women, regardless of guild or group membership, were thought to be part of society's vulnerable, disabled population on account of their blindness. Their disabled identities were often understood through public perceptions that linked physical disablement to the entitlement of aid. For example, in routine seventeenth-century reports from Kaga domain (spanning Ishikawa and Toyama prefectures today), such as one dated the third month of 1675, village officials monitored the welfare of starving blind people and ordered that food relief be issued to them.[102]

Evidence also comes from Tottori domain (in Tottori prefecture today) in western Japan. Early in the seventeenth century, Tottori domain authorities worked to construct a safety net to assist their vulnerable, indigent subjects but were also circumspect in limiting access to alms. This precaution prevented the system of charity from becoming overwhelmed. Blind people were allowed to travel to collect alms, but were not allowed to travel to places located more than a day's journey away on foot; this distance served as an approximation of the perimeter of their collection rights.[103] In 1677, the domain revised its restrictions on travel, allowing blind people to travel beyond their home bases if they had a travel pass—a pass bearing the name of Teiichi,[104] most likely the name of a guild leader. As a protective measure, in 1692, government authorities limited the alms that blind people from outside provinces could collect in the domain in one duration or season.[105] The measures were adjusted over a period of time according to demands. In 1753, when the domain experienced a surge in the number of mendicant blind people and religious performers, government authorities introduced new restrictions to discourage itinerant livelihoods.[106] People who were physically impaired[107] had to obtain prior written permission to seek exemption from labor—it is less clear, however, if blind people were excused simply on the basis of their blindness or if a similar process of documentation was required. In the broader context of local village economies, the authorities believed that many able-bodied peasants were so focused on their livelihoods that they were neglecting their occupations: many had signed up to be disciples of physicians or had migrated and removed themselves from village registers.[108] These were systemic problems that the domain attempted to solve through the nineteenth century, though with little success.

As early as the seventeenth century, in those places where local guild groups were active, a guild member could leverage a local guild leader's authority to increase his share of alms. As one example from 1688 indicates, several guild members from the area of Sanuki province (in Kagawa prefecture today) traveled with some blind women to entreat Ichise, a guild leader in nearby Tokushima domain (in Tokushima prefecture today).[109] They argued that because shogun Tokugawa Tsunayoshi had peacefully outlasted an inauspicious year, blind people had the right to celebrate by collecting alms. With Ichise as a guild delegate, they presented their argument to the supervising government officials. The outcome was a success, achieved through the working relationship between local guild groups and their local status governments. The amounts to be awarded to blind people were determined based on past practices and rates in neighboring areas: each guild member who held a rank received a sum according to his rank; blind women, since they were not guild members and did not hold ranks of the guild, were paid according to their seniority.[110]

Over the eighteenth century, almsgiving continued to sustain durable, reciprocal relationships between blind people and their communities. However, these relationships were not without problems. Sometimes there were disagreements over territorial limits of collection rights, but more often the main problem was that communities simply could not keep up with demands for alms by itinerant people, such as blind people. This problem, discussed earlier in the context of Tottori domain in the seventeenth and eighteenth centuries, was common[111] and persisted into the nineteenth century, as the later example about Kariya domain will show.

Okayama domain (in Okayama prefecture today) experienced the same problem in the eighteenth century. In the early 1740s, villagers in that domain complained about the steady stream of blind people arriving at their homes to collect alms, prompting the district magistrate[112] to gather advice on how to regulate the incoming traffic of blind people.[113] Someone named Okamura,[114] who was presumably the head of the local guild, mediated in communication with the Council of Ten Elders of the Kyoto guild and with the district magistrate and village headmen to find a solution. They decided that blind people could travel but only with a pass issued by Okamura—that is, with the express permission of the local guild. (A similar measure was adopted in Tottori domain.) This was a sure way of confirming a local guild leader's direct authority over guild members and other non-allied blind people. Blind people, though, were not to travel in large groups but could travel only in pairs, perhaps so as to reduce the number and also the frequency of requests for alms. Also, the alms that blind people would receive were pegged to villages' assessed wealth and productivity, with large villages having to give more money than small villages. Still unable to cope with the stress, villagers asked for a reprieve again in 1744 and negotiated a deal with the officials to further lighten their burden.

It is easy to imagine that a crisis of staggering magnitude and prolonged duration could put an enormous and disproportionate strain on scarce resources and that this could create a situation in which blind people who needed alms were more desperate to travel. One crisis in the late eighteenth century, the devastating famines during the Tenmei era (1781–89), tested the readiness of government authorities to react appropriately and opportunely to a sudden increase in the needs of the affected populations. Take, for example, Tosa domain, which was one of many domains that suffered through the Tenmei-era famines.[115] The authorities of Hata in Tosa introduced temporary regulations that halted the travels of blind people through the area.[116] Instead, blind people were to be supported by provision of rice at home by their own villages; they were also given aid proportionate to factors such as their gender and ranks in the guild.[117] According to the principle of top-down patriarchal, benevolent rule by government authorities, blind people, who received relief during hard times, could expect to get further support in this crisis. Guild membership was not a prerequisite for aid, though guild members could leverage their ranks for greater support. For guild members, the cash amounts they received decreased commensurately with each lower grade or rank; blind women received the least. In future years (1793–97), following the famines, the officials reviewed measures to streamline the process of coordinating relief.[118] A village maintained the authority to dispense cash and rice to blind people under its jurisdiction, and village headmen could help to feed blind people from villages that had shortfalls in supplies.

While guild membership gave some stability to guild members' lives, it could not shield them from the vicissitudes of the nineteenth century that were felt all across Japan. The shogunate and all levels of government were under the tremendous stress of mounting financial debts due to political administration cost overruns, which were complicated by factors such as responses to famines, price inflations, and the riots of the Tenpō era (1830–43). Pressures in foreign diplomatic relations in the mid-nineteenth century[119] deepened the mood of looming internal social, political, and economic crises. The Tenpō-era reforms by the shogunate could not reverse the economic downturn of the earlier decades. For example, in Kaga domain before that time, finances had run aground.[120] In 1814, village officials of Hakui and Kashima in Kaga domain implored their respective superiors to intercede and save blind people under their jurisdiction.[121] While quite a lot of blind people made a living in niche professions, others had become too physically impaired and too ill to find work. Recent poor harvests had exhausted the available resources of village officials; extreme poverty exacerbated the difficulties of village administration.

Even through the nineteenth century, home communities of guild members honored guild membership and felt obliged to help guild members living among them meet their financial obligations to the guild. This means that a guild member could ask his home community for financial assistance, especially if he did not want to be involved in moneylending or if earnings from charity or from his livelihood were inadequate. Records from the *Notes of Meetings of Village Cluster Headmen*[122] of Kurume domain (in Fukuoka prefecture today) provide some evidence.[123] The infrastructure of support in Kurume was developed well before the nineteenth century, as was the infrastructure in many rural areas. It was a system that depended greatly on complex coordination of local offices and leaders. The village cluster leader (the leader of a cluster of villages and headmen)[124] was a prominent official in the

upper hierarchy of rural society, chosen from among influential peasant families. As an intermediary between villages and higher authorities,
he represented village officials under his charge. He was delegated the
authority to manage important matters, such as the collection of annual
taxes and the resolution of legal disputes; for his service, he was entitled
to receive regular rice stipends from the domain.[125] In one instance (in
1817), Jū'ichi of Iwazaki village, a guild member, could not afford to pay
the local guild and needed a loan.[126] The village cluster leader ordered
seven village units to contribute equal amounts to make up a portion
of the loan to that blind man. In another instance, a blind man named
Mika'ichi had difficulty paying his dues to the local guild's religious confraternity (Myōonkō; see the section on rituals earlier in the chapter)
and approached officials in his home village for help.[127] He was approved
for a loan. (Upon the village cluster leader's orders, loans could be dispensed through a bank of funds,[128] which village units managed.[129])

Blind people and guild members were not the only ones who experienced great financial need during the nineteenth century, as many local
communities were struggling with financial troubles. This was a problem that was also discussed in earlier examples from the seventeenth
and eighteenth centuries: communities recognized that itinerant people
such as blind people had the right to collect alms but they did not have
the resources—in fact, they had even fewer resources in hard times—to
provide alms. For example, government authorities of Kariya had introduced austerity measures through reforms of the 1830s and 1840s, including measures to curb the influx of itinerant people seeking alms.[130] However, the measures to relieve the economic burden on communities did
not meet with much success because they could not be strictly enforced.
In the years after 1854, Kariya suffered from torrential downpours that
caused damage to temples around the area. Temples hired itinerant
performers to raise funds for reconstruction, compounding an already
dire financial situation for communities. No matter what the situation
was, local guilds still wielded some authority to help guild members seek
recourse. In another part of Japan in 1843, the leaders of four local guild
groups in Shinkawa of Kaga domain voiced their grievances about recent
changes that had resulted in a reduction of alms.[131] Pleading to reinstate
previous rates of almsgiving, the blind leaders submitted their petition
to guild leader Kasamatsu, who represented them to request that the
supervising government office intervene favorably. In the end, whether
in crisis or in peaceful times, incomes of blind people who depended on
alms were tied to the financial stability of local populations.

Conclusion

For a blind man, being blind could mean having to make the choice to serve the guild. This was not disadvantageous, depending on his circumstances, because it could mean being enabled by guild membership to become trained for a profession and to collect alms. At the same time, being a guild member could mean being disabled by the guild's social and financial obligations.

Disability in the checkered social and political landscapes of Tokugawa society was constructed around politics of power. Guild membership was heterogeneous, as was the composition of the entire blind population. As an autonomous status institution, the Kyoto guild empowered its elites and also, to some extent, average guild members. Though their disabled identities were strengthened by guild membership, the majority of guild members paid a high price. It was not easy for guild members to support themselves, even though the guild and local guild groups afforded a sense of community.

The fact remains that guild members and other blind people had to stay resourceful to make a living. Music (see chapter 5) and acupuncture and massage (see chapter 6) were niche professions of blind people. Moneylending seemed like a quick way to make money, but it was a risky livelihood. If blind people did not work, they could seek alms. Relief programs were coordinated by government authorities and often involved local guild groups. Guild membership did not determine whether a blind person was eligible to receive charity, but in some situations, guild members had a significant advantage over unaffiliated blind people.

As a result of major developments, the guild had an enduring influence on blind people's lives even after the Tokugawa period. It had firmly established a system for training blind people for work and bequeathed to Meiji Japan a sound, credible framework for setting up vocational programs in music, acupuncture, and massage for blind people (see the epilogue). Yet, despite its seemingly charitable functions during the Tokugawa period, the guild was not guided by an overarching altruistic, noble, philanthropic mission to save guild members or blind people—at least not consistently. The guild did not help to advance the careers of poor guild members. But it was a dependable institution with the autonomy to represent the collective membership. Guild membership offered some degree of security but never guaranteed equal opportunities for everyone.

CHAPTER 4

Nonmembership and the
Challenge of Authority

⎯⎯⎯ ✤ ⎯⎯⎯

The previous chapter profiled the Kyoto guild, the enablement—as well as struggles—associated with guild membership, and how in the early seventeenth century the shogunate reshaped the medieval legacy and reset the legal framework of the guild. By the start of the eighteenth century, however, with more guild members dispersed across Japan in local guilds, the guild had to adapt to new challenges. Not every blind person needed the guild.

With a focus on the eighteenth and nineteenth centuries, this chapter explores what it meant to be blind and not have guild membership. Who were some of these blind people, how did they live, and in what contexts did they live?

For various practical reasons, which will be explained later in this chapter, eligible blind men who should have joined the guild did not do so but instead found other sources of identity. This complicated the guild's role in the government of the blind status category. As the problem of nonmembership deepened from the eighteenth century onward, the shogunate took important steps to increase the guild's authority and delineated some criteria to coerce blind men to become guild members. But neither the shogunate nor the guild could fully control blind people's activities. The guild's ability to exercise its authority declined, because blind people found alternate arrangements that made guild membership less essential to them.

Music was an important profession of blind people in Tokugawa society, and in that profession, blind female musicians[1] organized themselves into social (kinship) groups to form their own identities. Considering some examples in this chapter of blind female musicians who lived and worked in the early twentieth century will let us draw some general conclusions about their predecessors' lives and experiences during the Tokugawa period. There is evidence to suggest that while the guild existed, before it was dismantled in 1871, it tried to extend its power over blind female musicians, even though they were excluded from guild membership because of a long history of gender discrimination.

Religion was another profession in Tokugawa society in which blind people worked and formed local groups. "Blind priests"[2] were noted for being lay performers of music and religious rituals. Although many blind priests maintained distinctive identities through groups linked to Buddhist temples, the guild attempted to diminish their legitimacy to engage in certain work that was dominated by guild members. But it seems that the guild had little success in this regard, because it could not restrict nonmembers' autonomy to act.

All of these examples point to the broader argument that no matter how blind people organized their disabled identities, they were implicated in the guild's rule.

Filial, Honest, and Virtuous: Finding and Making Model Blind People

WHAT TO DO WITH BLIND PEOPLE?

For much of the seventeenth century, the shogunate did not clearly articulate the types of work that blind people could do. Blind people were traditionally employed as musicians, but they also were starting to explore professions in acupuncture and massage from the seventeenth century onward. By remaining open to a range of professions, the guild could greatly expand its membership. Government authorities also early in the Tokugawa period rarely found fault with blind people who did not join the guild but were taken care of by their families, hosts, or patrons.[3] This option of forgoing work was more likely a viable choice for blind people from above-average and well-to-do families than for those whose families were poor. Blind people who found adequate support at home were less likely to publicly claim their disabled identities, because they did not have to leave home to beg for alms or to find work to support themselves. Regardless of what blind people chose, their choices did not appear to impede the guild's operations.

In the eighteenth century, however, the shogunate began to waver from its original position. On the one hand, the social argument to keep blind people at home alleviated to some extent the problem of blind people's dependency on charity. The onus and expenses of care fell upon the family and community. On the other hand, the shogunate had to justify the guild's existence. Growing numbers of blind people were traveling for work without the guild's permission, and the shogunate was aware of this. Many of them were likely also capitalizing on their disabled identities to collect alms and find jobs without joining the guild.

The shogunate feared losing its grip on the status rule of blind people, so it paid close attention to the guild. The guild's rule could have been interpreted by some blind people, and likely also by some of the populace, to apply only to guild members. This would explain why the shogunate continually issued decrees through the eighteenth and nineteenth centuries to stress the guild's authority over the blind status category—essentially, anyone who claimed to be blind could fall under the guild's authority. A series of decrees by the shogunate (such as the decrees of 1776–77) marked the shogunate's renewed political commitment to the guild.[4] The shogunate made important concessions to try to close the gap between disabled identity and guild membership. For example, blind sons of samurais and samurai vassals who resided in towns and cities and made a living as musicians, acupuncturists, and masseurs were, by default, considered to be subjects of the guild even if they were not yet guild members. If they lived in Edo, they had to submit their names to the Edo proxy head of the guild (see the discussion of the guild's hierarchy in chapter 3). If they had previously accepted disciples, though they were not supposed to do that, their disciples were similarly bound to the guild.

The decrees were not clearly understood by everyone. Sponsors of blind people preferred to err on the side of caution. In one case, a samurai sought advice from the shogunate about a blind acupuncturist he had been supporting.[5] Although the blind acupuncturist rendered services mostly within the samurai's household, he took leave every now and then to attend to other patients. The shogunate determined that those external visits provided sufficient grounds to regard the acupuncturist as a practicing professional and, hence, a subject of the guild. In a similar inquiry, a samurai asked about the status of a blind acupuncturist who was his personal physician. Because the blind acupuncturist did not perform any professional service for a livelihood beyond his required duties at home, and had not accepted any disciples, he was considered to be beyond reproach and did not have to serve the guild.

It seems that so long as blind men performed tasks in nonprofessional roles—that is, not as livelihoods—they were not accountable to the guild. Blind men who were employed in livelihoods, particularly in the niche professions of the guild, were considered to be involved in occupations that were bound to the guild (see the discussion of occupation in chapter 3) and hence should have become guild members. Nonetheless, those who did not join the guild were not punished. Furthermore, there was little consistency in how the guild applied its laws. Status rule gave the guild the autonomy to rule but also created ambiguity about nonmembers. The flexibility of claiming disabled identity allowed blind people to decide what worked well for them in their circumstances. Blind women were routinely excluded from the guild and had to seek their own support. Even among blind men, not everyone could afford the fees of guild membership—guild membership was expensive because guild members were required by the guild to earn and purchase ranks. It took a lot of time and money to be promoted through the guild's hierarchy. There was even less justification for blind men to join the guild if they had sufficient material support from family members or if they could secure their own means to learn vocational skills without the stress of completing the guild's formal discipleship.

MORALISTIC STORIES ABOUT BLIND PEOPLE

Accounts about exemplary blind people offer additional perspectives on what government authorities expected of blind people. These brief accounts, which are scattered across mundane reports compiled by government authorities, portray the ideal blind person: someone who never neglected responsibilities despite being blind and poor. For example, an early eighteenth-century report (1713) from Kurume domain (in Fukuoka prefecture today) provides a fleeting profile of an impoverished, old blind woman who lived in Kajiyamachi.[6] For the record, her outcast status was an essential detail, because it indicated her marginalized place in society. Because she embodied compassion and moral spirit and fulfilled her status duties, the magistrate rewarded her.

The shogunate could not depend on blind men to voluntarily join the guild, nor could it count on blind people to accept the guild's authority. Aware of this reality, the shogunate identified blind people in its scope of the populace whose social mores and behaviors were to be policed. The increased surveillance starting in the late eighteenth century coincided with the Kansei reforms of the 1790s, a series of programmatic political reforms named after the Kansei era (1789–1801) to reorient society toward the shogunate's reenvisioned paradigm of social values. Matsudaira Sadanobu, Senior Councillor[7] of the shogunate, was the chief architect of the Kansei reforms. As Noriko Sugano's analysis of that era tells us, "The Kansei reforms represent the shogunate's second attempt to rejuvenate itself by returning to its founding principles, with emphases on reviving the economy, restoring the morale of the samurai administrators, and promoting the practical application of Confucian ethics."[8] The somber mood was reflected in didactic advice in moralistic literature.

Blind moneylenders were singled out for representation in moralistic literature as people who were cunning and greedy, even though, as chapter 3 highlighted, many of them were likely guild members who were victims of the guild's exploitative system that incessantly demanded payments. For example, in *Tales of Yoshino*,[9] a collection of hearsay accounts by samurai author Mizuno Tamenaga,[10] an anecdote warns readers of blind moneylenders. An unnamed vassal who was entitled to an annual stipend that provided enough for a comfortable life made the mistake of borrowing twenty-four *ryō* from blind moneylenders.[11] The moneylenders returned without fail every fourth month to extort eight *ryō* from him, even though he had supposedly paid twenty *ryō* to offset the loan. (A loan of four or five *ryō* was said to have easily accrued enough interest charges to swell to fifty or sixty *ryō* in a short period of time.) In the end, the moneylenders were charged in court and handed over to the Edo proxy head for trial. For Tamenaga, whether this story was factual was not particularly significant; what was more significant was that by scapegoating and vilifying blind moneylenders, he could exploit the story as an exhortation for necessary reforms to fix the ills of society.

Even if blind people did not (or perhaps could not) become guild members, they could become model subjects. That was what the shogunate wanted people to believe and strive for in their everyday conduct. *The Official Records of Filial Piety*,[12] an ambitious work of the late eighteenth century that recorded stories about filial subjects from domains across Japan, is an important source on the shogunate's moral ideology in the era of the Kansei reforms.[13] The exemplars—men and women alike—in these stories were everyday people, including blind people. These characters were chosen to embody certain motifs so as to inspire audiences' feelings of sympathy, pity, and compassion and, more important, to invoke a call to act virtuously. In fact, many of the stories about blind people hardly ever mentioned guild membership, but they stressed that blind people shared moral attributes that transcended birthright, gender, and predestination. As Marcia Yonemoto's analysis of gender in the stories tells us, it is hard to find "distinct patterns of filiality according to class or status, for although enforcement of filial obligations and principles tended to be more rigorous in the samurai class, values of female sacrifice and daughterly duty were disseminated widely and were generally consistent across status groups."[14] Blind women experienced their fates like long-suffering sighted women did and in that regard were little different from sighted and blind men: all blind people endured a great deal but were contented in the end, the stories declared. Blind people's own perspectives were not represented, but the stories cast blind people in the active roles of surmounting physical disablement in order to amplify the virtue of self-sufficiency and purpose in the context of disabled identity. Though the stories were prescriptive, the veracity of them was never meant to be doubted by readers.

In one story from *The Official Records of Filial Piety*, Sayo was a sighted woman from Fukagawa (in Tokyo today).[15] Her father, Shunyō, was blind. When he was able, he worked as hard as he could to earn a living as a masseur. (The story does not say whether he was a guild member.) Because of the family's impoverished circumstances, Sayo found work doing errands for samurai families to make ends meet and helped out at home to look after her blind father. Fueled by a keen desire for self-improvement, she tried to pick up new skills in her spare time, such as learning to play the *koto* (a stringed instrument; figure 5.1 in chapter 5 features the *koto*). She parted with what little remained of her earnings from work to buy Confucian classics, which she voraciously read. As a good-hearted person, she gave back to her community by teaching girls to perform music and to read and write—cultural pursuits that were consistent with the image of desirable, refined feminine demeanors. She refused to marry, arguing that marriage would distract her from her filial duty to serve her parents.

In another story from *The Official Records of Filial Piety*, Seiden was a blind caregiver originally from Yama of Aizu domain (in Fukushima prefecture today).[16] He grew up without a mother and contracted a disease that left him blind at the age of four. There is no indication that he joined the guild. When he came of age, he took care of his father, Yasubē. He assumed his role as a dutiful son and did what was right. Yasubē started to suffer from poor vision as he aged; his health was also attenuated after a crippling stroke. In view of the combination of disabling factors (old age and blindness), both men, father and son, were exempted from village duties. (The text does not say this, but this type of exemption was probably quite common for blind and physically disabled people elsewhere in Japan, too, and this was another good reason why disabled identity was useful.) At first, Seiden tried to train to become a musician. He later learned acupuncture and roamed the streets day and night in every season looking for clients. A steadfast and dependable son, he diligently waited on his father and never wavered in his commitment. Without inconveniencing his neighbors, he occupied himself with household chores just as any able-bodied (and able-sighted) person did, persevering without letting blindness interfere with his ability to smoothly manage things.

The two stories about Sayo and Seiden and their families have common motifs that emphasize hard work, filial piety, and responsibility. The stories make it clear that blind people were expected to work independently as breadwinners and caregivers. They were capable of working hard. Even if they were unable to work, they could still act honestly and responsibly to bring out the best qualities of the family's or community's character. The political overtone that the family, in its multiple configurations, was the core structural unit of society is unmistakable. When blind people were too incapacitated to work, they had to be properly cared for and supported by their families and communities.

The two stories, like others featuring blind characters,[17] hint at the shogunate's acknowledgment, and perhaps even approval, of various situations in which blind people worked but were not guild members. The shogunate did not excuse working blind men, such as Sayo's father and Seiden, from having to join the guild, but because it could not ensure that every person heeded its decrees, it created an expedient moral argument using stories that, by deliberately leaving out reference to guild membership, explained what any blind person could do to lead a purposeful life. What the stories presented here do not say is that blind people could expect to receive charity if they could not work, had no family or community, and were helpless. In fact, receiving charity was a right that blind people could claim, and many blind people, through the guild or not, worked to collect alms for their livelihoods (see chapter 3).

Excluded by Gender: Blind Female Musicians and Their Social Groups

THE PROFESSION OF MUSIC

Blind female musicians (*goze*) were prominent among blind people in Tokugawa society because they were professional musicians and belonged to their own organized groups. In the broadest sense, *goze* referred to blind women, just as *zatō* referred generally to blind men (and not only blind men of the guild). In strict usage, the scope of *goze* was limited to blind female musicians. The etymology of the word, however, has been the subject of much speculation. *An Overview of Amusing and Entertaining Details*,[18] which essayist Kitamura Nobuyo compiled in the early nineteenth century as an encyclopedia of Japan's customs and cultural practices, explains that the word probably originated as a highly deferential term that was later shorn of all trappings of nobility.[19]

The genealogies of blind female musicians' groups were largely derived from the mythical lore of the Kyoto guild of blind men. These tales, likely apocryphal in nature, were stitched together from the tapestry of oral histories, with themes and timelines that stretched back to the eighth or ninth century. They were told by blind female musicians to counter biases against their gender and profession. A myth recorded in Abe Masanobu's *Miscellaneous Essays from Sunkoku*,[20] an early nineteenth-century source about the area of Sunkoku (in Shizuoka prefecture today), claimed that the ancestor of blind female musicians was Sagami no himemiya, a daughter of Emperor Saga of the ninth century. She was born blind and stayed blind despite fervent prayers by her parents to cure her blindness.[21] As the story goes, at around age seven, she had a vision of Nyoirin Kannon (a bodhisattva in Buddhist traditions) of the Kumano Nachi shrine (a famous mountain worship site in Wakayama prefecture today). Nyoirin Kannon instructed Sagami to help blind women and faithfully serve the Kamo clan (a noble clan based in Kyoto). Because Nyoirin Kannon's true identity was Myōon Benzaiten (the patron deity of music), blind female musicians, like the blind men of the Kyoto guild, honored the same deity of music. This tradition of worshipping the patron deity of music, for example, endured in early twentieth-century Nagaoka (in Niigata prefecture today), where blind female musicians gathered in the spring to celebrate with rituals and songs.[22]

The organic ties between music and religious rituals may explain why early textual and musical genres such as *Heike* music in which blind male musicians were heavily involved were infused with religious aura and incantatory qualities.[23] The music of blind female musicians, as musicologist Gerald Groemer highlights, also had ritual functions.[24] In religion, blind and sighted women found roles as shamans. Scholars have demonstrated that blind female shamans, who were known by different designations according to local and regional customs, performed functions related to their blindness—sighted shamans fulfilled different roles.[25] Some of the most well-known blind female shamans were the *itako* of northern and northeastern Japan. Typically, their parents had sent them away at a young age to train as shamans.[26] Many blind people learning skills in professions, such as blind female musicians and guild members, usually spent some periods of time away from home, training as disciples or apprentices and then traveling in search of work and income.

Starting in the seventeenth century, it was common for blind musicians to become proficient with the *shamisen* (a stringed instrument; see figure 4.1) to launch their careers. The *shamisen* was a late addition to Japanese musical traditions. It gained popularity because it was performed by blind and sighted musicians for popular musical and lyrical genres. Blind male musicians, who traditionally played the *biwa*, crossed over to new genres of *shamisen* music. Blind female musicians also adopted the *shamisen* to develop their new repertoire[27]—it appears that in the medieval period, they played drums to perform lyrical verses from *The Tale of the Soga Brothers*,[28] an epic and historical fiction that paralleled *The Tale of the Heike* (see figure 3.1 in chapter 3). *A Collection of Gleanings*,[29] an early eighteenth-century source by Daidōji Yūzan on miscellaneous subjects, explains how there was a surge in interest in *shamisen* music in the Genroku period (1688–1704) as female commoners were learning to perform songs of the *shamisen*.[30] It was said that before the boom, only blind female musicians were associated with *shamisen* performances. This observation would be an understatement of popular trends, since blind male musicians were also experimenting with new genres of music at around the same time. Every now and then, samurai households hired blind female musicians and hosted musical ensembles, but we do not know anything about the backgrounds of these blind musicians. As the popularity of the *shamisen* spread, families were said to be eager to recruit tutors, hoping that their sighted daughters could be trained in music and dance and then be employed by wealthy and influential samurai families as entertainers.

Blind female musicians traveled across Japan to perform music and seek alms (see figure 4.1). Daunting as this would have been for any

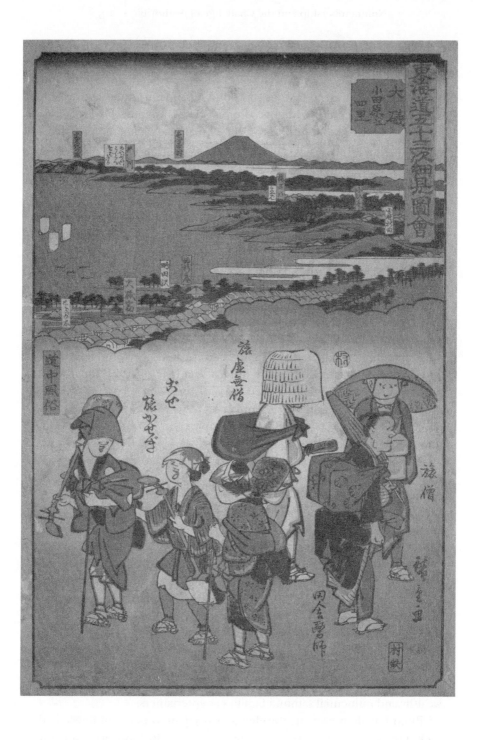

sighted, able-bodied traveler, the perils of long-distance travel were especially real for blind people. For reasons of mutual security, companion-
ship, and ensemble performances, blind female musicians traveled in
groups. Traveling alone was dangerous. For example, an anecdote by late
eighteenth-century literary essayist Katō Ebian recounts a blind female
musician's mishap. Colored by dramatic storytelling, this anecdote can
be read as a fictive interpretation—and also as a cautionary tale—of the
actual depredations that awaited vulnerable blind women on their journeys.[31] The unnamed musician in the story, who was around twenty-four
years of age, was wandering in the streets in Fukagawa (in Edo) when a
robber stalked her. The robber lured her to a nearby temple, where he
mercilessly assaulted her. He robbed her of all her belongings, including
her *shamisen*, and sneaked out of the temple premises through a side
fence—but not before gagging her and tying her to a stupa so that she
could not scream for help or try to escape. However, his plan to abscond
was foiled when he aroused the suspicions of city guards. They were puz-
zled because he was acting surreptitiously around the temple in broad
daylight and had in his possession a worn-out *shamisen*. They followed
the trail of clues to the temple cemetery where they discovered the vic-
timized woman, bound and helpless, and promptly arrested the robber.

Blind women had limited prospects if they were not musicians. As
commercial print culture and consumer culture proliferated across cities and rural areas in the late seventeenth century, opportunities became
available for sighted women to learn to read and to get an education.[32]
However, blind women were disadvantaged because they were not taught
to read and write but instead had to train for a profession. Massage,
which required some training and less technical skills than acupuncture,

---

(*facing page*) Fig. 4.1. Illustration of blind female musicians and other travelers by
Utagawa Hiroshige, from *Illustrations of Detailed Views of the 53 Stops of the Tōkaidō*.
The scene is Ōiso, one of the stops in the series. The three women huddled in the
foreground are blind female musicians (the characters say *goze tabi kasegi*, or blind
female musicians traveling to earn their livelihoods). They wear blue cloth shades
over their heads, probably to shield their faces from sunlight. The women each
have a *shamisen*, the musical instrument associated with their profession and musical
genres, and at least two of the women walk with staffs and with cloth rucksacks tied
around their torsos. Next to them are two traveling priests and a village physician.
From Utagawa Hiroshige, *Illustrations of Detailed Views of the 53 Stops of the Tōkaidō*
(Japanese title: *Tōkaidō gojūsan tsugi saiken zue*, late Tokugawa period). National Diet
Library Digital Collections.

emerged as a popular profession of guild members and blind men (see chapter 6). From what we can tell from fragmentary evidence, there were no laws that excluded blind women from the professions of acupuncture and massage, but blind women would have faced intense competition and discrimination.[33]

The gender bias favoring male masseurs appeared to be a characteristic of the profession, but stories about masseuses suggest that blind women were hired. In one account, a blind woman named Tsune lived in Kawasaki along the Tōkaidō highway (the major highway connecting Edo and Kyoto).[34] As a recent widow, she was dealt another crippling blow in life when an eye disease destroyed her vision. She became disabled. She found work as a masseuse without much difficulty, it seems, and did other jobs to help her younger brother provide for their aging and disabled mother. She was commended for her perseverance in carrying out her duties. The context of this story is important. By the late eighteenth century, at around the time of the Kansei reforms discussed earlier, the shogunate was keen to promote paradigms of impeccable conduct, work ethics, and filial piety. Moralistic accounts express the shogunate's ideological slant in ideas about disabled identity and gender roles: it seems that the shogunate did not object to the kinds of work blind women did as long as the work was respectable.

KINSHIP GROUPS

In the context of status rule, a blind female musician's disabled identity depended on her group membership and livelihood (or occupation as a musician). When a blind woman began her training as a musician, she joined a group of blind female musicians. These were usually small local groups that emphasized seniority and discipline. Each group was configured as a kinship group like a stable family. Over time, kinship groups were recomposed and reorganized as old members passed away and new members were recruited as disciples and successors. The blind men of the Kyoto guild formed relationships between masters and disciples that were akin to genealogical bonds; but these relationships were mainly regulated by the Kyoto guild. Because blind women lacked an umbrella institution like the Kyoto guild, they had less support than guild members in representing their rights to their home communities or to the shogunate. But this disadvantage was also an advantage, insofar as it gave blind female musicians' kinship groups the autonomy to manage their affairs, as they were not bound by obligations to groups beyond their immediate locales.

The localized nature of blind female musicians' groups means that hierarchies, ranks, and discipleships in each group were determined by local or regional historical precedents. As remnants of traditions show, some groups borrowed the structures and laws of the Kyoto guild of blind men.[35] It seems that the highest position a blind woman could aspire to attain in her group was the position of First Elder[36]—the same deferential term used for the most senior elder on the Council of Ten Elders of the Kyoto guild (who was also the guild's top leader). As the name suggests, the position was probably reserved for the most senior woman, a group's matriarch. Generally, a blind woman had to be at least forty years old to earn this appointment. The appointment below First Elder was Middle Elder;[37] initiates or novices made up the bottom of the hierarchy. Group members paid fees for ranks and were punished by demotion if they violated the code of conduct.

What seems to be true across the groups is that their ranks were less elaborately defined, and less widely recognized, than those of the Kyoto guild. But like local male guild leaders, matriarchs had authority over their local groups. Group members pledged their loyalty to their matriarchs and were not permitted to stray from their routines and training. How musical sects were formed in these women's groups, or whether sects were developed from associations with musical genres, is less clear. The blind men of the Kyoto guild inherited the system of sectarian and lineage membership of *Heike* music from the medieval period and could have passed on some of those institutional features to the women's groups.

The process of inducting a blind female musician into a group was part of the context of status rule in her home community. In Hata of Tosa domain (in Kōchi prefecture today), a rule introduced in 1833 required a blind woman seeking to be a disciple to first secure permission from her village headman's administration.[38] Village leaders could grant or deny permission, and these decisions limited the autonomy of blind women in choosing their groups. This rule probably aimed to control the number of blind female musicians so as to reduce the villagers' burden of giving alms to them and to other itinerant people. Its introduction implies that in the past, blind women had more autonomy to exercise their choices—and this would have certainly been true in other places where similar restrictions did not exist. In another case from Hata in 1859, the village headman of Iwata interceded with the ruling district office[39] for a woman under his charge named Tatsu, who had turned fourteen and was blind.[40] Born into a poor family, she could not find employment, and her age might have made her too old to start training with blind female musicians; her financial hardships were compounded by other physical impairments. A blind man named Hisaoichi, whose name suggests that he was a guild member, took her in as a student while she was awaiting news about her future.

Blind men and women made up separate gender groups in the blind status category, but they were free to interact with one another and form professional relationships. Hence, the relationship between His-aoichi and Tatsu, which crossed gender lines, would have been common among blind male and female musicians in the nineteenth century and even before then. They supported one another if they had good reasons to do so. According to mid-nineteenth-century essays such as *The Ways of the Floating World,*[41] which amused readers with commentaries on the sights and sounds around Japan, city authorities tried to separate the livelihoods of blind musicians based on gender differences, but no matter how hard they tried, blind female musicians still taught music to men and women to make money.[42] Blind male musicians, not surprisingly, had been engaged in the same practice for a long time.

THE EXAMPLE OF ISO

What the next example from 1846–47, documented and analyzed by Japanese historian Yamada Kōta, tells us is that a local male guild group could arbitrarily prevent a blind woman from joining a blind female musicians' group. This practice involving a local male guild's assertion of authority over blind female musicians can be seen as an institutionalized form of gender discrimination against blind women—and as a political validation of the Kyoto guild's broad power to govern any blind person who was considered to be in the blind status category. Examples of guild members receiving more alms than blind women (discussed in chapter 3) indicate that blind women were treated unequally, and while it is hard to tell what circumstances led the guild to curtail the autonomy of blind female musicians' groups, it seems that even before the nineteenth century, blind women had already learned to adjust to the dictates of patriarchal power.

Iso was a blind woman from the village of Tōjio in Matsushiro domain (in Nagano prefecture today),[43] whose father, Heisuke, made a living as a confectioner. As in most villages, agriculture was the mainstay of the local economy. Blinded by smallpox at age five, Iso lived with her family. Someone like Iso could have helped with household work but would have had a difficult time finding work on her own in the labor force due to prejudices against blind women. Heisuke was eager to prepare her for a career. Harboring hopes that she could secure a livelihood as a musician, he made her take lessons in music from age ten. However, when he tried some years later to enroll her as a disciple of a senior blind female musician in the area, he encountered strong resistance from the local male guild.

Local male guild leaders interfered in the matter and spoke for blind female musicians, denying Heisuke's request on the grounds that he was engaged in a base profession—and that fact alone, according to their argument, undermined the local guild's good standing, even though Iso could not have become a guild member. Fiercely defiant, Heisuke refuted their argument. The dispute had to be mediated by a local official, who transmitted the arguments from both sides to the magistrate's office. It was resolved only after much acrimony had poisoned relations among the various parties. The local male guild was found guilty of illegally inflating fees for admission and overcharging disciples. Iso was finally granted permission to train with a group of blind female musicians. In light of this outcome, it would seem that the argument by the local male guild was premeditated and served as a pretext to discriminate against Heisuke and his family. The tumultuous start was, in retrospect, a foreboding of Iso's prospects. Perhaps incited by rivalries and ill will, she was accused of lacing a fellow musician's meal with mercury; as punishment, she was banned from playing music.

SUGIMOTO KIKUE'S STORY

Oral histories of blind female musicians from the early twentieth century can reveal much about the generation of blind female musicians who grew up in an era when the Tokugawa period was still fresh in Japan's cultural memory. Musical traditions from the Tokugawa period largely survived through the late nineteenth century and into the early twentieth century because of these musicians, whose stories hint at their diverse lived experiences.

The life story of a musician named Sugimoto Kikue, as well as stories of other musicians, was meticulously documented by Saitō Shin'ichi.[44] Born in 1898, Kikue belonged to one of the remaining groups of the former Takada domain (in Niigata prefecture today). She recounted vivid, intense memories of her anguish upon becoming blind and her anxiety over being separated from her birth family. In her early childhood, at age five, she was stricken with measles. Due to misdiagnosis and a delay in treatment, her loss of vision became irreversible. Desperate for a miracle, her mother traveled to the temple Sōshōji and returned home with its famed medicinal powder. (There were many religious sites across Japan that advertised their powers to heal diseases; see chapter 2.) Local residents claimed that the medicine from that temple had the potency to cure pediatric diseases, but it did not work, leaving the family in despair. Such experiences of getting treatment were probably common among families of blind children in the Meiji period, as well as in the Tokugawa period.

How Kikue became a musician probably mirrors other blind girls' experiences earlier in the Tokugawa period. Parents of blind girls in that era probably felt compelled to conform to traditional ideas about blind girls, and those ideas still held sway in the Meiji period. The pressure that Kikue's parents faced could have forced them to make the heart-wrenching decision to send Kikue away to be trained for a livelihood in music. She was too young to know that she was going to be separated from her family for good or that she wanted to become a musician. She left home at age seven and was welcomed as an adopted daughter by a senior blind female musician named Mase-san (the suffix "-san" was a deferential address).[45] In the first month after Kikue moved into Mase-san's household, her mother trekked across villages while carrying Kikue's baby sister to visit her. No matter how eagerly Kikue anticipated her mother's visit each time, the contact between the two of them became infrequent and then ceased altogether because Mase-san had assumed the guardianship of Kikue and was entrusted to take good care of her. Living under Mase-san's roof, Kikue was considered to have severed ties with her natal family. (In this regard, blind males in the Tokugawa period who became guild members were also considered to have, socially and symbolically, left their households and given up their original status identities.) Known to be a strict teacher, Mase-san supervised all aspects of Kikue's grueling training. Kikue's other instructor, Katsu of Akakura, was a senior member and, in the group's configuration of kinship, was also considered to be her mother.

Like in the Tokugawa period, blind female musicians in Kikue's time routinely traveled to perform music. It took time for fledgling blind female musicians like Kikue to get used to these long-distance travels.

On her first trip, Kikue could barely keep up with the physical toil of traveling on foot. As she grew accustomed to the routine, she spent all of her days committing songs and verses to memory and rehearsing them at home and on the road. Through conscientious rote learning and practice over time, she expanded her repertoire. She reached a milestone at age thirteen (about six years after her adoption into the household) when she acquired her stage name, Haruko, which acknowledged that she had advanced in her career; and at age sixteen, she earned a promotion and was entitled to accept her own disciples.[46]

Kikue's blindness fell along the spectrum of visual impairment, as it does for many blind people in any culture and period—a fact that is easily overlooked and underappreciated due to stereotypical understandings that starkly contrast blindness and sight. Because Kikue was born with sight, she retained impressions of colors she had seen during her childhood, especially those of flowers in bloom. After the loss of vision, she could still roughly describe colors. Even at age twenty-two, Kikue was still hopeful that she could be cured, that her vision would be restored. After visiting the Nogami ophthalmological clinic in Saitama prefecture, however, she completely gave up hope on a cure. For most of her adult life, Kikue's blindness did not completely incapacitate her, but she was used to traveling with a sighted guide. Reminiscing about her journeys, she confessed that she was seized by terrible feelings of trepidation during pitch-dark, moonless nights.[47] Moonlit nights were somewhat reassuring to her and brought her joy because she could sense her eyelids fluttering in response to the gentle light of the moon. In the day, the sun's intense glare made travels easier than in the nighttime; she could make out the shadows of her sighted guide dancing and flittering on the ground as she gingerly trod narrow mountain paths. When horses and dogs passed her, her visual sense was stimulated by movements of their shadows. However, by the time Kikue turned sixty, the sensitivity to light upon which she had relied most of her life had completely failed her. Left with a keen sense of hearing, she was still able to discern from the footfalls of her sighted guide the types of terrain underfoot—she could tell whether obstacles like potholes or rocks were ahead. Bereft of material support, she did not retire early and continued to travel until well into her seventies.

The nexus of Kikue's network was Mase-san, who was born in the late Tokugawa period in 1845 and was in her early twenties when the Tokugawa regime collapsed. As matriarch, Mase-san managed her household.[48] She worked tirelessly all her life to lead the disciples whom she had taken under her wing. Early in life, she had a close brush with death when she suffered from smallpox. Though she recovered from that episode, the disease left her badly disfigured and caused significant permanent vision loss. At a young age, she was instructed by Mito-san, a blind female musician of the Miyashita household, who had found her to be a likeable, gifted child with a strong aptitude for music. When the time came, she was chosen to succeed Mito-san. At age eighty, Mase-san retired and left the errands to her disciples. One day, she suddenly suffered a stroke. Kikue, who was away on her travels at the time of the incident, returned home and diligently attended to Mase-san by her bedside. Mase-san passed away at age eighty-seven in 1932. At the funeral, Kikue learned that a middle-aged woman in attendance to pay her final respects was, in fact, Mase-san's biological daughter, who had been born out of wedlock from Mase-san's union with a local fisherman many years earlier. Mase-san had not shared with others the fact that she had a partner or the fact that her partner had died. She had also kept the birth of her daughter a secret, perhaps because of the social and cultural taboo dating back to the Tokugawa period against improper relationships between men and blind female musicians.

Not all female musicians associated with Kikue were blind. Chino, Kikue's confidante, was sighted, and she would have been the sighted guide for her blind companions on their travels together. She had entered the profession to escape crippling poverty—she was proof that sighted women could train and live with blind female musicians. This practice was probably already accepted in the Tokugawa period and could have been more common than we think. What Chino's experience also suggests is that sighted women had more choices than blind women. Chino quit the profession after she met someone from Nagoya and settled down with him.[49] She embraced a life that was the envy of many blind female musicians, who probably were denied marriage because of the same social prejudices that Mase-san had faced in her lifetime.

The Politics of Religious Affiliations: Blind Priests

THE ORIGIN OF BLIND PRIESTS

Some blind male religious practitioners in the Kyūshū region and in the environs of the ancient imperial capital of Nara[50] were known as "blind priests"[51] in Tokugawa-period historical sources. We do not know much about the early history of blind priests, but religious scholars suggest that from the classical period onward, blind priests were active in groups in those regions.[52] They were said to have performed music and religious rituals, and it is possible that in the early days they were not too different from the blind male musicians (*biwa hōshi*) of the Kyoto guild. Contemporary scholars have examined blind priests' traditions and music, but studies of their origins are inconclusive.[53] We do know that blind priests' religious repertoire included incantations of a genre called *Sutra of the Earth Deity*,[54] which existed in many variations among blind priests. That genre had religious and ideological contents: it glorified blind priests' unique heritage, tracing the origins to Buddhist deities and divine manifestations.[55]

Blind priests in the Tokugawa period performed roles that were thought to be suitable for blind people in music and in religion at that time. Their groups, like the Kyoto guild, had exclusively male membership. As musicians, blind priests recited songs from musical genres,[56] and those genres were influenced by local and regional musical traditions. As religious practitioners, they served parishioners and patrons by conducting rites of the hearth;[57] they also prayed for bountiful harvests,[58] safe passage, blessings at childbirth, and the coming of age for young adults.[59] In return for these services, they collected alms, a practice that guild members and blind people engaged in (see chapter 3). A blind man trying to decide whether or not to earn his livelihood as a blind priest likely had to consider a combination of factors, such as his personal preference and finances, the choices of the blind people around him or in his social circle, and the availability of other blind masters to accept disciples. A blind man who was contemplating joining the guild would have had to consider these same factors.

Information about blind priests is dispersed, but there is evidence that many blind priests, because they had no affiliation with the guild, maintained status identities that were separate from those of guild members. For example, Nagai Akiko's analysis of nineteenth-century census records indicates that some local communities recognized blind priests as forming a distinctive category of blind people.[60] It is less clear, however, whether those local communities regarded blind priests as having an equal standing with guild members. For many blind priests, not having guild membership meant having to find security by organizing their own groups, as well as not having to obey the guild's orders or pay fees to the guild. But the lack of representation by a national institution like the guild made blind priests more likely to depend on their local ties and less likely to move out of their local communities, because they had little protection or representation beyond their local communities.

In the early Tokugawa period, as the guild extended its network of local guild groups across Japan, it treated blind priests as competitors. For example, historical records from the late seventeenth century tell of one episode in which the guild enforced its political mandate to oppress blind priests.[61] The tensions of that episode were politically motivated as guild leaders sought to expel blind priests from professions that the guild dominated. The guild prevailed over blind priests by exploiting its authority over the blind status category to force them to accept the outcome, which undermined their claim to an equal disabled identity or social status. Blind priests were ordered to stick to their traditional repertoire of Buddhist incantations. They were banned from earning the ranks of the guild, and anyone who impersonated a guild member could be incarcerated. Blind priests were also prohibited from playing the *koto*,[62] *shamisen, kokyū* (a stringed instrument played with a bow), and *zatō biwa* (the variety of *biwa* commonly associated with guild members and used in *Heike* performances).

While the guild's orders may suggest an antagonistic relationship between blind priests and the guild, blind priests were free to conduct their activities as they wished, and that autonomy could even include the choice to join the guild. A late eighteenth-century source on the guild, *The Great Records of the Guild*,[63] offers the important detail that the guild allowed blind priests to become guild members.[64] The guild could have been open to accepting blind priests as guild members even before the late eighteenth century, and even thereafter, but the guild's openness belied its persistent discrimination against them. The guild clearly indicated that those who had become guild members had to give up recitations of their traditional genre if they wanted to rise above the basic rank of *zatō*. The guild's stance implies that blind priests who continued recitations of their genre remained at the bottom rungs of the guild's hierarchy and could not acquire privileges. It is unlikely, however, that a blind priest who was already with a group would have also wanted guild membership. Though concurrent membership was possible, the obligations were not only onerous but also expensive—chapter 3 discussed the costs of guild membership, and the next sections will say more about blind priests' duties to Buddhist temples.

TEMPLES AND BLIND PRIESTS

Blind priests who did not join the guild had to find ways to legitimize their disabled identities. One way was to seek ties with Buddhist temples.

In fact, a Buddhist temple was often the institutional nexus of a group of blind priests. By forming ties with a Buddhist temple (their home temple), blind priests could earn the right to collect alms from that temple's parishioners. Blind priests of a group appointed their group leaders to represent them in dealing with their home temple. A survey of the Kyūshū region, for example, shows that some blind priests served the historic temple-shrine complexes of the sacred mountain Kōrasan in Kurume domain through the nineteenth century.[65] Historical records sometimes documented the genealogies of blind priests—with information on age, predecessors, parishioners, and household members.

A consequence of blind priests' association with a Buddhist temple was their subordination to the temple's clergy on routine matters. Take, for example, the matter of discipleship, which temple clergy supervised and authorized. Shōkai was a blind priest who, in 1834, was promoted as a leader and assumed responsibility for his parishioners.[66] His household consisted of eleven members—three men, five women, and three disciples (who were blind priests). Shōkai succeeded his master, Kōkai, and as it appears, was later succeeded by Ukai.[67] Having risen in rank, Ukai earned the authority to appoint disciples.[68] In one instance, a blind teenage person whose blindness could not be cured was hoping to become a disciple. Though Ukai was inclined to agree, he had to first obtain the consent of his home temple. Also, as later examples from the nineteenth century will demonstrate, many blind priests' groups could not even recruit enough blind people to ensure their continuity.

Blind priests of a group carved out their niche status identities as subjects under their home temple's authority. They argued that because they were detached from the blind status category, they had no obligation to take orders from the guild. However, it seems that perhaps because of their disabled identities, and probably also because they were not considered to be formally ordained by Buddhist temples, blind priests did not have the same status as ordained clergy. In the clerical hierarchy, blind priests were ranked beneath temple clergy. Even within a group, blind priests had a hierarchy—their ranks paralleled those of the guild, with distinct levels to confirm the roles of leaders, but with much less complexity.[69] Like guild membership, group membership for blind priests could be economically disabling for poor, lowly ranked group members because of the responsibilities expected of them.

In exchange for the benefits of temple affiliation, which included the right to collect alms, blind priests were made to pay dues to the clergy. For a home temple, this meant that when blind priests accepted more disciples, they could bring in more revenue. Temple clergy routinely extracted fees from blind priests to endorse promotion in the hierarchy. When a blind priest was conferred a ceremonial robe in recognition of his promotion, he had to offer a payment to the abbot and to each assistant cleric; a new leader was also expected to honor the abbot.[70] These financial demands remind us of the exploitation of guild members by guild leaders. Also, in times of disaster, demands for financial contribution trickled down the hierarchy to blind priests. For instance, when a fire broke out in the samurai lords' residences in Edo in 1856, some blind priests had to raise cash and remit the funds to the magistrate of temples and shrines.[71]

Collecting alms was not the only means of making money, as other ingenious, legitimate means can be noted.[72] A bill of purchase from 1846 highlights that a blind priest's rights to parishioners were, in fact, tradable commodities. In this instance, a blind priest named Seisei had agreed to sell his rights to Honsei for two *ryō*. Honsei acquired Seisei's parishioners—a total of twenty-four households—who were scattered across the parish. As the new legal proprietor, Honsei could keep the rights, unless he chose to relinquish them or negotiate a separate deal. As a transaction from 1862 also reveals, it was possible to pledge such rights as a form of collateral in a loan. A blind priest named Myōshō (Meishō or Myōsei), who owned a total of thirty-five parishioner households, promised his creditor, Usaemon, that he would use the earnings from his parishioners to pay off the accrued interest charges by the following year. If Myōshō neglected to honor the agreement, Usaemon could exercise his right to take over Myōshō's parishioners.

THE LATE STRUGGLES OF BLIND PRIESTS

Despite tensions over rights to livelihoods, it seems that the guild mostly did not interfere with blind priests' everyday activities through much of the seventeenth and eighteenth centuries. However, beginning in the late eighteenth century, as discussed in an earlier section in this chapter, the shogunate grew concerned about the guild's authority over blind people. As part of its agenda to strengthen status rule, the shogunate acted to shore up the guild's political bases. Amid these changes, Shōren'in, a Tendai-sect Buddhist temple located in Kyoto, saw its opportunity. In 1783, by repeatedly issuing decrees, Shōren'in declared its ambition to subjugate blind priests, targeting areas across western Japan where, it seems, the guild had less political influence than in areas closer to the guild's head offices in Kyoto and Edo.[73] Shōren'in did not face any challenge to its authority from the guild or the shogunate. This was likely because Shōren'in had a powerful reputation as an eminent temple[74] of the court nobility and also likely because the guild had devolved so much autonomy to local guild groups, especially those in far-flung territories, that it could do little to halt Shōren'in's advances.

As we can imagine, Shōren'in's political agenda had a financial motive.[75] Blind priests paid to be affiliated with their home temples, and the clergy of Shōren'in would have known that by exploiting blind priests there was potential for financial gain. The plight of blind priests in Chōfu domain (in Yamaguchi prefecture today) is evident: once they agreed to be bound to Shōren'in, duties were imposed upon them.[76] They were expected to pay for new appointments and promotions, and in return, they probably hoped that Shōren'in's reputation could lend some authority to their livelihoods. Isolated blind priests became easy targets and were particularly vulnerable to the burgeoning ambit of Shōren'in. In this regard, blind priests faced immense pressure to confirm existing affiliations with their home temples or form new ones with Shōren'in. While using previous rulings to justify blind priests' submission,[77] Shōren'in also acted cautiously and preemptively to avoid conflict, ordering existing guild members to be left undisturbed so as to respect the political will of the guild and the shogunate.[78]

Shōren'in's ambition was alarming to the clergy of temples with blind priests.[79] For example, some of the temple clergy disputed the legitimacy of Shōren'in's actions and indirectly invoked the shogunate's authority for protection by claiming to have historical and religious ties to the temple Tōeizan, which was a funerary temple of Tokugawa shoguns.[80] However, despite the threats, blind priests had no obligation to obey Shōren'in's decrees. A blind priest could continue his activities without interruption because there were no reprisals for refusing to be part of Shōren'in. Also, because that temple was located far away from where most blind priests lived, it made more sense for blind priests to choose to ally with local temples or even to migrate to join local guild groups to find better prospects.

It is worth highlighting that Shōren'in's intervention in the late eighteenth century came at a time when, it seems, local groups of blind priests had been experiencing a slow decline in numbers. That decline could have been a sign of the steady erosion of traditions. The problem of cultivating blind successors deepened in the nineteenth century. An injunction dated 1858 criticized the recent trend in which sighted disci-

ples were assuming the professional roles of blind priests without permission.[81] In fact, it seems that starting in the late eighteenth century, more
and more sighted people worked with blind priests to form reciprocal
relationships with parishioners and provide religious services. Sighted
people were free to intermingle with blind priests, and their relationships with blind priests only deepened. Because of a dearth of blind
disciples, many blind priests were accepting sighted disciples and nam-
ing them as successors. Temple clergy expressed concerns that sighted
appointees were not properly inducted into blind priests' traditions; not
only that, allowing sighted people to profit from financial relationships
with patrons had the potential to undermine blind priests' livelihoods.

Other problems involving discrimination surfaced in reports—as if to
make things more dire than they already were.[82] Groups of blind priests
were accused of refusing to admit some blind people into their groups
on account of family background and genealogy. As such, blind men of
different status groups, who would have qualified as blind priests, were
deprived of livelihoods.

Conclusion

Being blind could mean being enabled by disabled identity without having to depend on the guild. This aspect of enablement for blind people
who were not guild members did not go unnoticed. Starting in the late
eighteenth century, the moralistic themes of stories and decrees circulated by the shogunate point to the real problem of how the guild could
properly deal with blind people. The shogunate worked in concert with
the guild and with government authorities to dictate guild membership
through the end of the Tokugawa period. However, numerous blind
people and groups did not bow down to the guild. For example, blind
people with the luxury of means stayed at home, while those who were
working tried to evade the guild.

Blind female musicians were among the most visible blind women
in Tokugawa society. They drew attention to the precariousness of blind
women working in a niche profession under patriarchal authority. Gender oppression, however, did not end with the collapse of the Tokugawa
regime. In the Meiji period, the social system that had sustained the
cohesion of communities of blind musicians suffered. New political ideologies that reinvented gender ideas and reinscribed differences onto
women's bodies further marginalized disabled women. The population

of blind female musicians nationwide dwindled. So too did records of their lives, and their musical and performance traditions gradually faded into oblivion.

Blind priests formed autonomous groups that were centered on Buddhist temples. Temples that gained control of blind priests collected fees from them as tributes of loyalty. Like guild members, blind priests were beset with political pressures and financial challenges of their own. While disabled identity was given institutional legitimacy through the guild, it also assumed other organized forms that were central to the lives of some nonmembers, such as blind priests and blind female musicians.

Like blind female musicians, blind priests outlasted the guild and lived into the twentieth century. The newly installed Meiji government that succeeded the Tokugawa regime overturned the former bases of power of the shogunate and dismantled the guild in 1871. Because blind priests had a history of ties to Buddhist temples, the head temple office of the Tendai Buddhist sect was given control of them. In the overarching framework of religious administration, the Tendai head office established offices at two core temples in Kyūshū to govern blind priests there in two groups: the Gensei group and the Jōraku'in group.[83] All blind priests elsewhere who did not belong to either group fell under the authority of the Tendai head abbot. This streamlined administration displaced previous local networks and institutions but achieved expediency in overseeing the mundane affairs of appointment, promotion, and instruction.

A further change came when laws that were enacted in 1904 and 1905 recognized that inadequacies in regulation before the Meiji period had allowed sighted instructors to be appointed among blind priests; only those named, sighted instructors—and no other sighted instructors— were approved to perform their functions alongside blind priests.[84] In supporting the creation of self-sufficient communities, these restrictions also accelerated the downfall of historical traditions.

CHAPTER 5

Texts and Performances

The Significance of One Blind Musician's Career

———— ❧ ————

By the dawn of the Tokugawa period, performances of *The Tale of the Heike* (or *Heike* music) had become a well-established and highly esteemed genre of entertainment through the patronage of connoisseurs from ruling elites.[1] During the medieval period, highly respected blind male *Heike* musicians were showered with honors and gifts. This was one reason why blind male musicians of that period specialized in *Heike* music. But a life of luxury or distinction was not a common fate. Certainly, over the seventeenth century, as a sign of the changing tastes of audiences, new and fashionable musical genres eclipsed *Heike*.

This chapter expands on the discussion of *Heike* music in chapter 3 to explore what it meant to excel as a blind male *Heike* musician. A centerpiece of the chapter is an analysis of the career of Ogino Chiichi (1731–1801) and his major composition, *Heike mabushi* (*Correct Tunes of Heike*). The discussion focuses on the eighteenth century but also casts the analytical gaze both ways onto the centuries before and after the eighteenth century to contextualize the importance of Chiichi's life and composition. *Heike* texts, music, and performances were bound together through their respective histories and were also intertwined with the lives and interactions of blind musicians.

In view of the scarcity of specific biographical information about blind musicians and autobiographical accounts written by them in the Tokugawa period, this focus on Chiichi reveals much about his privileged position. A revealing portrait of a self-aware individual emerges through historical and literary perspectives—a portrait that reflects particular details as much as it refracts broad realities through these details.

Chiichi embodied what was exceptional among blind musicians of his time. He was a senior member of the Kyoto guild by the time he gained preeminence in his field. His exceptional rise to prominence illuminates the networks to which he had access as a blind musician. Through his connections and charisma, he reached the coveted echelons of the guild. He also secured a platform beyond the guild to elevate his profile. His most promising students were proficient in new genres, as were many blind musicians.

Blind musicians found work in music, and some of them, such as Chiichi, played significant roles in developing musical traditions. *Correct Tunes of Heike*, the literary work Chiichi became known for, not only serves as a primary source about his life but is also one of only a few surviving documents to open a new window onto the contexts of composing and performing *Heike*. The analysis of *Correct Tunes of Heike* and other *Heike* texts exposes gaps in the common narrative that *Heike* was an oral genre owned exclusively by blind musicians. Chiichi's circumstances tell us that the genre was a protean living tradition that was also defined by literate sighted people in literary production and connoisseurship: these people were self-financing students of blind masters, self-proclaimed copyists and hobbyists, and resourceful peers of other trained and amateur musicians who coalesced around a core of common interests. In other words, these were sighted audiences—many of whom are anonymous to historians today because of the limitations of sources—who were so interested in *Heike* that they wanted to participate in blind musicians' activities. By subverting the ease of positing clear-cut ownership of textual production in literary activities, the discussion locates the contents of oral and written traditions in the realm of shared knowledge.

In short, the narrative about Chiichi can be reanalyzed to shed new light on the literary and social contexts of a blind, well-connected professional musician whose work was characteristic of his erudite learning and high stature.

Biographies: A Micro-Historical Approach

Blind musicians can be found all over the world today. One abiding reason is that in many cultures, the popular imagination still associates visual impairment with heightened sensitivity to auditory cues and sensations—and hence equates visual impairment with enhanced ability and with certain stereotypes.

For example, Terry Rowden writes in his study of blind African American musical culture that "the idea of the special attitude of blind people for music has been all but taken for granted since the beginning of organized education for the blind."[2] This association of musical affinity with visual impairment is not new in contemporary Japanese society and in Tokugawa society. The idea that blind people had an intuitive sense of touch, and hence worked well with their fingers and could play musical instruments, is also a possible factor favoring the compartmentalization of blind people in the musical profession in Tokugawa society.

There is much more to this convenient explanation that draws on ideas about visual impairment, musical affinity, and touch. Historical conditions would offer more compelling reasons for the professional roles and careers of blind musicians. Every society is different; so too are the conditions that turn blind people into musicians.

AN INTRODUCTION TO HEIKE

The *Heike* genre was the most symbolic genre of the Kyoto guild. Even as the popularity of *Heike* declined among audiences, *Heike* characters, stories, and motifs were kept alive in the cultural memory of the Tokugawa period through literary adaptations in print and on the theatrical stage.[3] Even for twenty-first-century readers, the *Heike* narrative lives up to its reputation as a grand work of historical fiction. The main plot follows the waxing and waning of the fortunes of the formidable Taira warrior clan (also called the Heike), a branch of the royal family, through the tumultuous years of the twelfth century. The chief character is patriarch Taira no Kiyomori, who had pretensions to the throne. He schemed to raise the clan from the status of lesser nobility to an unprecedented position of political power in the imperial court. He manipulated relationships with the court and exacted vengeance on his opponents, especially his archenemies of the Minamoto clan (or the Genji). His grandiose strategy of usurping power also involved the move of the capital from Kyoto to Fukuhara and the arranged marriage of his daughter Tokuko (who was given the title of Kenreimon'in) to the reigning emperor Takakura. While the tale celebrates Kiyomori's daring, ambitions, and charisma, it also warns of his fall from grace amid the impermanence of earthly existence. As the authority of the clan wavered, rebellious warriors entered into alliances with the Minamoto faction led by two brothers, Yoritomo and Yoshitsune. Together, they fought against their Taira rivals and reclaimed power. The conflicts culminated in the infamous sea battle of Dan-no-ura in which Kiyomori's widow Taira no Tokiko and the child emperor Antoku (who was Kiyomori's heir) were drowned. The rest of the narrative describes the consequences—the fates of imprisonment, execution, torment, and religious atonement—that befell Kiyomori's vanquished supporters.

Heike was performed with music, and *Heike* musical scores were texts that were written to be recited.[4] These texts made up a subset of the whole corpus of texts about the *Heike* narrative. The intricacies of musical performances of *Heike* can be gleaned from existing handwritten Tokugawa-period texts, which presented lyrics written with overlays of musical notations. *Heike* was performed with the *biwa* (a type of Japanese lute) by a blind male musician in a solo performance before a live audience. The narrative was divided into verses (called *ku*); with the accompaniment of *biwa* music, a musician recited some verses, and not the narrative in its entirety, in each performance. Each performance was complex and interwove episodes of the narrative according to its chronological logic.[5] Japanese musicologist Komoda Haruko explains that each melody had its own combination of tones and made up a "melodic formula," which could be applied to various sequences.[6] The varieties of melodies increased as the styles of narration acquired nuanced and blended lyrical textures.

BLIND MUSICIANS' NEW GENRES

Diaries of Japanese courtiers and literati from as early as the sixteenth century suggest that blind musicians did not just perform *Heike* music but also played the *shamisen* (a stringed instrument; see figure 4.1 in chapter 4) for *jōruri* (puppet theater),[7] a genre that blossomed in popular entertainment later in the Tokugawa period. With new musical genres came new opportunities for blind musicians. In the seventeenth century, literary master Matsuo Bashō took notice of a blind musician's rendition of *okujōruri* (a regional variant of *jōruri*) at a stopover in Shiogama (in Miyagi prefecture today). Bashō was intrigued. As he explained in his words from *The Narrow Road to the Deep North*,[8] "I must confess that the songs were a bit too boisterous, when chanted so near my ears, but I found them not altogether unpleasing, for they still retained the rustic flavors of the past."[9]

For blind people who were trying to become musicians, their choice of musical instrument was important, because it determined what kinds of musical genres they would perform and also what kinds of audiences they could attract. Certainly, in the seventeenth century, and thereafter, most blind musicians chose to acquire proficiency with the *shamisen* and the *koto* (another type of stringed instrument; see figure 5.1). Enterprising blind musicians became popularly associated with *jiuta* and *sōkyoku*, new musical genres performed with the *shamisen* and the *koto*, respectively.[10] *Sōkyoku* (a *koto* genre) and *jiuta* (a *shamisen* genre) delighted audiences and were characterized by styles that were thought to be livelier and more entertaining than *Heike* performances. In ensemble music, blind musicians were accompanied by musicians of the *shakuhachi* (a bamboo flute) and the *kokyū* (a stringed instrument played with a bow).[11] The two genres of *sōkyoku* and *jiuta* had relatively shallow roots traced to elite guild members such as Yatsuhashi, Ikuta, and Ishimura.[12] In the late Tokugawa period, Kitamura Nobuyo's *An Overview of Amusing and Entertaining Details*,[13] a nineteenth-century encyclopedic work about miscellaneous Japanese cultural topics, comments that *koto* music was so popular that blind people everywhere were learning to play the instrument and become musicians.[14] Another anecdotal source, *Miscellaneous Stories of Yoshiwara*,[15] describes *shamisen* music in the pleasure district of Yoshiwara in Edo, one of the places where blind musicians entertained audiences.[16] Apparently, one blind musician named Tsuruyama, who pioneered the Tsuruyama style of *shamisen* music, was banned from performing there because the somber tones of his music were discordant with the general mood of excitement and revelry.

Over the eighteenth and nineteenth centuries, government authorities across Japan acknowledged that blind musicians depended on new genres and new professions to make a living but also recognized that *Heike* was the traditional genre of blind male musicians. For example, in Kaga domain (in Ishikawa and Toyama prefectures today), the ruling authorities approved of blind people who were performing *koto* and *shamisen* music.[17] The authorities not only encouraged these musical genres but also gave permission for blind people to find employment in other suitable professions. Further afield, at one point in 1827, blind musicians in Hata of Tosa domain (in Kōchi prefecture today) were accused of contravening the laws and traditions of the guild[18] because they did not perform *Heike*.[19] The order probably used this pretext to keep blind musicians away from genres that were also performed by sighted musicians. There was no clear, consistent argument anywhere that blind male musicians had to perform only *Heike*.

Heike music was remembered by general audiences of the Tokugawa period more for its ritual, historic importance than for its entertainment appeal. The diary of wealthy wine merchant Yao Yazaemon of Itami (in Hyōgo prefecture today) points to evidence of the popular mindset that associated *Heike* music with ceremonial and religious music. *Heike* music seemed to be rarely performed by blind musicians in public anymore. On one occasion in 1734, Yazaemon was excited about the Buddhist ritual ceremony at the temple Dairenji, which had attracted crowds of pilgrims and worshippers.[20] In the atmosphere electrified by exhilaration, a blind musician, whom Yazaemon had heard much about, was supposed to perform *Heike* music, but for unknown reasons, that musician's performance did not live up to expectations. Later in the evening, another blind musician who was just passing through arrived in town. However, again much to the disappointment of everyone, he did not seem to be trained in *Heike* music and instead conducted routine religious rites.

Despite competition from new musical genres, blind male musicians did not abandon *Heike* music (although over time an increasing number of blind people chose the more profitable profession of massage—masseurs were in great demand[21]). Though steeped in a time-honored decorum, *Heike* music had become distant from the esoteric tradition that it once was. Yet, through musicians like Chiichi, the guild continued to instruct new musicians in the art of *Heike* music, which the guild's elites respected as the most important genre of traditionally trained blind male musicians.

OGINO CHIICHI'S CAREER

A micro-historical approach that examines Chiichi's life exposes the imbrication of disability in the social, political, and literary relationships that were central to his musical pursuits, and to his profile, in Tokugawa society.[22] Whether Chiichi was learned has little to do with his ability to read and write—acts that proved to be difficult due to the limitations of his visual impairment. Instead, the emphasis here is on the breadth and depth of his elite learning. He was conversant with the textual traditions and performance styles of *Heike* because of the knowledge he had acquired through a lengthy period of formal, rigorous training with the guild. His erudition among guild members, and among blind musicians, was by no means ordinary, as the guild had strayed from its founding mission of cultivating talent and incentivizing merit in *Heike*. As chapter

3 discussed, the guild deemphasized *Heike* and expanded its role as the status institution of blind people in the seventeenth century, increasing its revenues by selling ranks to members. With his background in performing *Heike*, and by engaging in textual studies with sighted intermediaries, Chiichi would have realized that texts were more than just an underpinning of performances: they outlived performances as permanent records.[23]

A micro-historical approach also shows us that Chiichi contributed to the orthodoxy of *Heike* in late Tokugawa Japanese culture that involved sighted audiences. Cultural developments, particularly from the late seventeenth century onward, changed the reception of *Heike*. The proliferation of print culture was one catalyst that sped up the devaluation of proprietary knowledge related to *Heike*. (Chapter 2 discussed some examples of how printed materials such as popular travel literature spread news among consumers.) In that environment conducive to the consumption of knowledge, *Heike* texts were shared, circulated, modified, reproduced, and adapted for personal endeavors by blind and sighted people. The mediation of *Heike* through written cues and musical notation was part of the larger transformation in the modes of information in Tokugawa society, corroborating recent studies about the popularization of genres and the vernacularization of elite forms of knowledge.[24]

The fabric of discussion of Chiichi's life and career sets in context the seemingly paradoxical relationship between literate blind musicians and written texts. It is paradoxical at first because blind musicians did not use sight—so, why did blind musicians need texts, and what could they possibly do with them? But a logical relationship emerges, too, because "secret tunes,"[25] or tunes that were taught exclusively to top, distinguished disciples of a lineage by their masters via the oral transmission of knowledge, were overtly codified through written transmissions in print and in manuscript by sighted people. Almost everything that was to be orally transmitted in lineages was openly recorded in their texts.

Lineages of *Heike* recall the *iemoto* system of the traditional arts and music in the Tokugawa period.[26] In that system, which was typical in that period, the head of a family or a lineage passed down prized knowledge about a subject to promising disciples and controlled the contents and styles of instruction. There are some similarities between *Heike* lineages and the *iemoto* system in aspects such as discipleship and hierarchical routes of imparting knowledge. However, the analysis of *Heike* lineages is complicated by the open nature of the genre: the circulation of texts, blind musicians' connections, and the collaboration of blind lineage members and sighted non-lineage amateurs and musicians. In a repetitive cycle of mutual learning and cooperation, blind musicians recited songs from memory. They depended on sighted audiences to narrate to them textual contents and intertextual references from sources in circulation and also to record by hand melodic elements for sighted musicians and reading audiences.

Chiichi did what many young blind men in his time did: he joined the guild. His motivation was not too different from that of many blind peers, which was to learn vocational skills and ascend the hierarchy. It appears that Chiichi did not have the luxury of growing up in an affluent family.[27] But he found sufficient means to buy his way into the guild, starting as a lowly guild member in his birthplace in Hiroshima domain.[28] He was blind at age six because of an eye disease, the details of which are unknown.[29] In his early career, when he became a guild member (likely in his early teens), he was trained in different genres of music by Tanizaki,[30] a local guild leader. Chiichi could have studied medicine and acupuncture concurrently, as guild members did as part of their broad training; but there is no evidence to suggest that he aspired to become a professional acupuncturist.

Chiichi found success by bolstering his disabled identity through the privileges of guild membership. After his basic training in Hiroshima, he moved to Kyoto, where he found connections through the networks of the Kyoto guild to train with expert musicians of the Maeda and Hatano lineages. These two lineages enjoyed significant influence in *Heike*, and through the Hatano lineage, Chiichi received verbal instruction of the secret tunes.[31] He used his influence to perform music for elite audiences, and his influential clientele was said to be from powerful temples and noble families.[32]

Chiichi eventually moved from Kyoto to Nagoya, and one likely motivating factor was the vibrant literary culture in the latter city. Recent scholarship on Tokugawa society informs us that the spread of economic wealth across regions, the shifting profiles of landholders, and the concomitant rise in literacy through the eighteenth century were part of the constellation of factors in the growth of literary cultures beyond Edo and Kyoto. Nagoya was a cosmopolitan regional hub of literary and artistic activities.[33] By the late seventeenth century, local guild groups were established across Japan. Yoshizawa Kōichi was one exemplary blind musician from Nagoya before Chiichi's time about whom scant records exist.[34] He was awarded the elite rank of *kengyō* in 1660 and trained a blind disciple named Itahana Kitsuichi, who studied medicine and later served shogun Tokugawa Ienobu. Like Chiichi, Kōichi rose to power because of strong political connections through guild membership. He consolidated his position in Nagoya through a solid relationship with Tokugawa Mitsu-tomo, lord of Owari domain (in Aichi prefecture today).[35] Another blind musician of the guild roughly contemporaneous with Kōichi was Kiri-yama Yun'ichi.[36] By age eighteen, he had mastered the entire repertoire of *Heike* and in 1687 was promoted to *kengyō*. He moved to Nagoya, pre-sumably sometime in the early eighteenth century. He returned to Kyoto to assume the leadership of the guild and was one of the *Heike* perform-ers who earned accolades from retired emperor Reigen in 1713.[37]

Another important and more significant factor in Chiichi's relocation to Nagoya was the support he received from a samurai family.[38] That fam-ily was the Ozaki clan, whom he likely got to know through his career. Some interpretations of sources suggest that Chiichi officially earned the rank of *kengyō* only after composing *Correct Tunes of Heike* and that before moving to Nagoya he held the rank of *bettō* but was nonetheless regarded as a *kengyō*.[39] In any case, Chiichi's situation was unusual, not only because he attained the highest rank but also because most blind musicians did not have the same kind of support that he had. The decision by the Ozaki clan to welcome Chiichi was a practical, well-calculated one. The head of the household had passed away suddenly without designating an heir, leaving the future of the clan in jeopardy. For the time being, Ozaki Tadataka had been left in charge of domestic responsibilities, despite temporarily relinquishing the ownership of the estate.[40] Tadataka con-vinced the local magistrate to allow the family residence to be converted into a venue for Chiichi to conduct lessons. It is unclear whether Chiichi drew a stipend from the guild or, if so, what the amount was—guild laws would have stipulated an amount for someone of his rank. The proposed agreement of support was a win-win arrangement for both Chiichi and the Ozaki clan. Chiichi could earn income from *Heike* enthusiasts and would also be assured of a home base for his professional role. In return, Chiichi could lend his reputation to the Ozaki clan by attracting audi-ences of sophisticated learning. For Chiichi, the Ozaki clan's unwavering support provided a bulwark against insecurity. There is little published information about Chiichi's family, but it appears that in 1781, perhaps as an act of reciprocity, Chiichi betrothed his daughter Suzu to Tadatatsu, the future Ozaki patriarch.

CHIICHI: FROM DISCIPLE TO MASTER

Who could join the guild, as well as what he gained by doing so (the value of guild membership), is a subject that was discussed in chapter

3. Although Chiichi specialized in *Heike*, his experiences as a disciple and, later, as an instructor probably paralleled those of other guild members. His discipleship reflects the general structure of discipleship in the guild. In the early seventeenth century, the guild expected professional blind male musicians to perform *Heike*. The legal codes—the ancient and new codes—of the guild (discussed in chapter 3) protected the relationship between masters and disciples of *Heike*. For example, a ranked guild member was not legally entitled to claim disciples as his own while his own master was still alive.[41] By the mid-Tokugawa period, the legal framework would have applied more broadly to address all the professions represented in the guild.

The guild's terms of a master-disciple relationship probably did not change much by Chiichi's time. Before gaining admission into the guild, Chiichi had to be sponsored by a master from the guild. Once accepted by the guild, a new guild member was duty-bound to obey his sponsoring master—a relationship little different from that of a parent-child genealogical bond. According to Katō Yasuaki's study of the guild's structure, a master was not randomly assigned but was appointed from a pool of available guild members living in close proximity; a master had to hold a rank to be eligible to accept disciples.[42] Although Chiichi moved to Nagoya, he was always considered to be a disciple of his first master in Hiroshima, under whom he started his career, for as long as they belonged to the guild.[43] The process of entering the musical profession would have looked different for a blind person who chose to learn and perform music without becoming a guild member.

Since one key obligation of a master was to oversee promotion, the practical implication of this arrangement was profound. The guild confirmed a master's right to assert his authority over a disciple's appointment.[44] A master could also make money by keeping a portion of his disciple's payment for rank. No matter who his master was, a disciple was permitted to pay to be a student of other instructors to expand his professional training—this means that a disciple could be a student of multiple instructors while maintaining exclusive ties with his master. This would explain how Chiichi was enabled to learn *Heike* music from blind musicians of different lineages; this would also explain how Chiichi was enabled to teach *Heike* music to other musicians. Because local guild groups were bound by the authority of the Kyoto guild, Chiichi's local guild group in Hiroshima would have abided by or adapted the laws of the Kyoto guild.[45] However, it is less clear how many blind students became Chiichi's direct disciples—that is, how many students had him as their master—whether in Kyoto or in Nagoya.

Chiichi's top students who were blind musicians advanced their careers by leveraging their personal connections with him and also by learning music from instructors with other musical specialties. These students represented the guild's elite tier and were renowned for their performances of *koto* music. Hoshino Yōichi was taught by Chiichi, and by 1801, after Chiichi's passing, he was made an elite guild member. From that time until around 1813, he was actively involved in promoting Chiichi's *Correct Tunes of Heike* in Edo. He won recognition as an accomplished *koto* musician under the tutelage of his instructor Fujii.[46] Also trained as Chiichi's student, Nakamura Ju'ichi was Yōichi's contemporary and owed his expertise with the *koto* to another instructor, Fujita.[47] According to a mid-nineteenth-century collection of essays on geographical names, genealogies, and trending news in Nagoya, Ju'ichi surpassed his peers and seniors in political achievements. He was made an Edo proxy head of the guild and, on the basis of his political power and experiences, returned to Kyoto to take over the highest office of the guild.[48]

By accepting both blind and sighted students, Chiichi likely followed an approved practice among blind instructors of musical genres—a practice so commonplace that it did not meet with the disapprobation of the guild or government authorities so long as it did not upset the social hierarchy. Although it is hard to tell how many blind and sighted students Chiichi mentored in his lifetime, the preface included in Chiichi's *Correct Tunes of Heike* suggests that at least two of his best students, perhaps his direct disciples, progressed to the highest level of their professional training and were taught the secret tunes by the master himself, while another two students advanced to the next highest level.[49] Sighted students pursued their interests in *Heike* by studying with blind musicians, organizing social meetings with peers in their networks and writing or copying musical notations in *Heike* texts in their free time. Komoda's study further explains that blind and sighted students paid fees for their lessons.[50] Students were, moreover, instructed through methods with different emphases. Sighted students had the benefit of following through a lesson while reading and studying texts, but blind students were better off training by verbal instruction and memory.

Perhaps it would be worthwhile to ask, Were sighted amateur musicians of *Heike*, such as Chiichi's sighted students, allowed to perform professionally after their training, either on their own or alongside blind musicians? While the available evidence does not point to any ready answer, most sighted amateurs did not graduate from training courses to become professionals. It is possible that in the mindsets of most audiences and contemporaries, sighted performers did not command the same status and respect as blind musicians, at least on ceremonial occasions, and were less convincing as performers than blind musicians. This was true in the seventeenth century, but that had changed by the late nineteenth century, when sighted musicians tried to save blind musicians' vanishing musical traditions from extinction. According to *The Veritable Records of the Tokugawa Shoguns*[51] (the shoguns' historical annals), seventeenth-century shogun Tokugawa Ietsuna was an avid patron of *Heike* and hosted performances. One of his favorite blind musicians was Iwafune, an elite guild member (a *kengyō*) who is mentioned by name many times in that source in the decade or so between 1658 and 1670; he performed for the shogun and received alms on special days.[52] He was also a familiar figure to the Koga clan of court nobles in Kyoto and supported that clan's efforts to control the guild. He wielded his political influence to represent the guild in disputes with rival "blind priests" (see chapter 4) and asserted the guild's authority to perform *Heike*.[53] Other elite blind musicians of *Heike* garnered favors from the shogunate.[54] From what we can tell from the shoguns' records, it seems that no sighted performer found comparable success with *Heike*—or with an exclusive audience.

KUZUHARA SHIGEMI'S MUSICAL CAREER

By comparison, Kuzuhara Shigemi is an example of a guild member and a blind musician who did not specialize in *Heike* music but who, like most blind musicians, was known for his skillful playing of the *shamisen* and *koto*. (As he is mentioned in the records as Kuzuhara, with the rank of *kōtō*, I refer to him under that name.) What made him unique among blind musicians (and among blind people, more broadly) was that he kept a diary. In his mid-twenties, he customized a set of wooden blocks of Japanese characters and wrote by inking and stamping them onto paper. This personal feat of writing was the culmination of his trial-and-error efforts, which predated the braille system adopted by Japanese schools in the 1890s.

In Kuzuhara's early career, he had much in common with Chiichi: they both became blind in childhood, trained with the guild, and ascended the guild's hierarchy. Born in 1812 to village headman Shigetomo of Yahiro village in Fukuyama domain (in Hiroshima prefecture today),[55] Kuzuhara lost his vision after contracting smallpox at age three. When he was around the age of nine, a blind female musician named Kiku in a nearby village taught him to play the *koto*. Despite traditions that separated the livelihoods of blind men and blind women, this arrangement that transcended gender differences—his instruction by a blind female musician—was not unusual and provided an expedient route for a potential guild member to equip himself with musical skills so as to shorten his training period with the guild.

We do not know when exactly Kuzuhara became a guild member—it was probably sometime after he became Kiku's student—but at age eleven, and by a leap of faith, he moved to Kyoto, where he became a student of Matsuno, a guild member.[56] Kuzuhara's relocation to Kyoto, like Chiichi's, was probably justified by opportunities to be connected with the networks of the Kyoto guild. Through Matsuno's connections, Kuzuhara was introduced to other elite blind musicians, such as Yaezaki and Kikuoka. After three years, Kuzuhara earned the rank of *zatō*. He returned to his hometown at age fifteen. He traveled periodically to Kyoto from his home and, at age twenty-two, was conferred the next rank of *kōtō*. He married at around age thirty and had two sons and a daughter. It seems that blind male musicians like Kuzuhara and Chiichi experienced less discrimination than blind female musicians in choosing to get married.

Kuzuhara's diary is useful for its insights into his activities as a blind musician. For much of his life, Kuzuhara was an instructor of music, teaching others to play the *koto* and *shamisen*. It is likely that he taught both blind and sighted students. His diary mentions some of his blind students by name: Jōsei, Jōsō, Teruno'ichi, Jōkitsu, and Hō'ichi,[57] all names that suggest guild membership. Many of the diary entries focus on his literary and musical interests, but he also wrote about travels to nearby places like Kanabe, Obe, and Onomichi.[58] Throughout his career, he was an avid poet. He composed poetry recreationally and embraced different styles and occasions—poetry that matched the tunes he played and poetry that he dedicated to friends as sentimental gifts.[59] While he probably assumed responsibilities at some point to oversee the local guild, as a career choice, he stuck to communities he knew well and did not travel very far. He retired without aiming for prestigious appointments in the guild and without chasing the allure of a glamorous life.

HANAWA HOKIICHI'S CAREER

Not all blind students who trained in music had an aptitude for it. That was why guild members started their careers by learning a range of skills. Hanawa Hokiichi, who was about fifteen years younger than Chi-ichi, is an example of a blind person whose early career with the guild included musical training but who later pursued a nonmusical career. Late in life, Hokiichi won acclaim for his encyclopedia, *The Collected Records of Various Subjects.*[60] A short biography[61] of Hokiichi was written by Nakayama Nobuna, a sighted scholar and Hokiichi's student and editorial staff member. A micro-historical reading of Hokiichi's life is instructive. Though an embellished tribute to Hokiichi, the biography reveals that Hokiichi conformed in many respects to Tokugawa society's general expectations of blind people.

It is believed that Hokiichi suffered from a mysterious liver disease at age five and became blind two years later.[62] (In Sino-Japanese medical thought, the liver's health was thought to affect sight and vision; see chapter 1.) He obtained his father's permission to move to Edo to seek a livelihood. At age thirteen, he traveled with a sighted companion, who was said to be a textile merchant. Perhaps through contacts of the guild in Edo, he was assigned to a blind master named Ametomi Suga'ichi. As a disciple, Hokiichi started his training in *shamisen* music and also attempted to master acupuncture and massage. As if to accentuate Hokiichi's destiny to be an author, Nobuna's biography of Hokiichi describes that he routinely forgot—almost overnight—the tunes that he had been taught, much to his master's dismay. Not only was he unable to play a complete tune, but he also could not harmonize musical sounds. But his prodigious memory served him well in some other regards. The text says that although he was mediocre in the clinical practice of acupuncture and massage, he had a superb ability to repeat verbatim what he had learned from the medical classics. When he was eighteen and still a struggling disciple, his master approved him to earn the basic guild rank of *zatō*. His endeavors in scholarship, as we are told, had just begun.

Hokiichi's career paralleled Chiichi's: they both used the privileges of guild membership to build relationships with influential sighted contemporaries with similar interests. Nobuna's biography of Hokiichi details Hokiichi's breadth of scholarship. Hokiichi was taught ancient imperial laws[63] by a scholar named Yamaoka Myōa. With a distinguished Buddhist priest, he studied *The Yellow Emperor's Inner Classic of Medicine*, a touchstone of classical Chinese medical thought.[64] At age twenty-four, he learned poetry from a well-known samurai poet named Hagiwara Sōkoku. Through the inner circles of connections, he was introduced to Kamo no Mabuchi, who was a well-regarded nativist scholar and intellectual, and acquired the essential knowledge of nativist scholarship. At age thirty, Hokiichi rose to the guild's next rank of *kōtō*. The promotion would have been forestalled had it not been for an opportune financial gift bequeathed to him by a deceased guild member named Hō'ichi. With his master's permission, Hokiichi used money from the bequest to pay for the rank. He gained the attention of Jōshōin Ryōen, who became a contributor to the encyclopedia and supported Hokiichi's proposal to found an academy[65] for Japanese studies.[66] It is said that the site of the academy was awarded to Hokiichi by the shogunate. As Hokiichi's personal fame spread, so too did the fame of his scholarship. Among the students who traced their learning to Hokiichi was nativist scholar Yashiro Hirokata, whom Hokiichi had trusted to assist with his work on the encyclopedia.[67]

It becomes clear from Nobuna's biography that Hokiichi's rise to the pinnacle of the guild's hierarchy had a lot to do with the fact that the guild highly valued senior guild members, especially those of repute. In this regard of securing political honor, Hokiichi was more successful than Chiichi. Hokiichi tapped into the elite platform of the guild to elevate his stature, and at around age thirty-seven, he was promoted to the top rank of *kengyō*.[68] In his fifties, he was ordered by the shogunate to review the guild's laws and was appointed in 1803 as the Edo proxy head of the guild. Another source about the timeline of Hokiichi's achievements[69] tells us that Hokiichi waited until age sixty-one before being inducted into the prestigious Council of Ten Elders of the Kyoto guild, the guild's council of the most senior guild members.[70] But instead of relocating permanently to Kyoto, as dictated by precedents, he continued to reside in Edo, perhaps because of his responsibilities at his academy. He was committed to overseeing the completion of the encyclopedia and solicited funds to finance the printing of it. At age seventy, exclusive privileges were bestowed on him that granted him a personal meeting with the shogun. At age seventy-three, he was recognized as the guild's Second Elder and was next in line for the top leadership position, which he filled three years later. But he did not last long in office and resigned on account of his poor health.

Musical Lineages of the Guild

Lineages of *Heike* were centered on *Heike* texts. The discussion of lineages hence begins with how or why *Heike* texts were produced and takes us back to earlier debates about textual continuities carried over from the medieval period. In traditional literary discourses, it is often argued that the split in *Heike* took place as the oral and written traditions of the genre began to diverge. To clarify the genealogies of *Heike* texts, scholars have posited two important categories—"recited texts"[71] and "read texts"[72]—and assigned texts to their respective places in this binary classification according to their general characteristics.[73] The distinction between "recited" and "read," though, should be treated cautiously to avoid the mistaken idea that the two categories of texts evolved along independent tracks.[74] "Recited texts," which would have included musical scores such as Chiichi's *Correct Tunes of Heike*, have received more attention from literary scholars, because texts from this group were thought to underpin performances by the guild. However, because not all "recited texts" were marked with musical notations, it is hard for us to tell how those unmarked texts were used in recitations.

The study of *Heike* remains important for scholars today because *Heike* had the longest continuity as a genre from the time of the guild's founding. The genre was a continuous historical record of blind musicians' literary activities and musical performances—more so than can be said of any other genre.[75] In terms of genealogy, Chiichi's *Correct Tunes of Heike* was distantly linked to an early seventeenth-century *Heike* text that we know as the *Rufu-bon* (the circulation text), a text that was printed and circulated (which explains the name we give it).[76] The circulation text did not bear musical notations and could have been read differently by sighted audiences as a narrative text, but this does not mean that it was not used in recitations.

The political context of the early decades of the seventeenth century may explain why the circulation text was significant to the guild. The timing of its textual production is important. At that time, the guild was implicated in bitter feuds between the rival samurai clans of Ōkubo Tadachika and Honda Masanobu.[77] Following accusations of treason made by the Honda clan, the shogunate acted swiftly to eliminate the Ōkubo clan and its allies. In 1613, several top-ranking guild members who had been supported by the Ōkubo clan were purged. As a result, there was a vacuum in leadership and a need to rebuild the guild's bases of authority. The guild tried to reestablish the legitimacy of *Heike* with the circulation text—as a text associated with the guild and as a text circulated in print to be read and appreciated by sighted audiences. The literary enterprise to produce that text was led by the Ichikata lineage (the parent lineage of the Maeda and Hatano lineages), which had dominated the guild. From that time on, however, after the publication of the circulation text, the priority of transforming the guild into a political institution to rule blind people overshadowed the guild's duty to protect *Heike* traditions. It became even more imperative for guild leaders, and for the shogunate, to focus on setting up a system of laws. Having solid laws could prevent the kinds of factional quarrels that had rent the fabric of the guild. Hence, in that context in 1634, a legal code of the guild was proposed and established under shogunate orders.[78]

The conflicts were not resolved, however, after the initial political fallout had destabilized the leadership of the guild. The early Tokugawa-period primary source *A Collection of the Remnant Drops of the Western Sea*,[79] attributed to the Maeda lineage, casts the struggle between the Maeda and Hatano lineages as one instigated and stoked by a long-standing rivalry that had deeper roots than mere disagreements over musical arrangements and textual permutations.[80] As we are told, tensions erupted between Maeda Kyūichi and Hatano Kōichi, two elite blind musicians with competing loyalties in the guild and who were said to be *biwa* virtuosos.[81] Kyūichi started his career in Kyoto and gained repute through the sponsorship of a powerful samurai lord named Oda Naga-masu.[82] Not expected to become the top leader of the guild, he moved to Edo (in or around 1658) to find new opportunities. He secured the political support of Tokugawa Yoshinao, who was lord of Owari domain and an ardent fan of *Heike* music, and made Nagoya his home base. His relocation to Edo and Nagoya and his relationship with the Owari lord were instrumental in broadening the patronage of blind musicians of the Maeda lineage in the area around Edo. By contrast, Kyūichi's rival Kōichi spent most of his life in Kyoto. In 1634, he was appointed to be the guild's Third Elder and later became the guild's top leader.

At around the same time, in the mid-seventeenth century, blind musicians started to compose *koto* and *shamisen* music and mix music in new ways.[83] Genealogies at that time linked various genres of music to *Heike* and the guild. Those records attributed to blind male musicians the common origins of certain genres, accentuating those blind musicians' ingenuity in systematizing musical lineages and their diligence in perfecting performances of secret tunes.

The genealogy of *sōkyoku* (a *koto* genre) is an example. It was steeped in tales that traced the lives of the pioneer Yatsuhashi, a blind musician of the guild, and his predecessors as far back as legendary times. The written narratives infused oral traditions with elements of historicity. The timing of Yatsuhashi's career appeared to coincide with the reorganization of *Heike* lineages early in the Tokugawa period. This suggests not only a new vibrancy in musical genres and performances but also the conscious reworking of storylines and themes by storytellers to narrate the textual histories of *koto* music and *Heike*. *Records of the Koto Tunes of Yatsuhashi Kengyō*,[84] which was written in 1695, identifies *koto* music with the divine qualities and sanctity of the imperial court.[85] According to the putative timeline of events, sometime in the late seventh century, during the reign of Emperor Tenmu, *koto* music so moved the heavens that it caused the skies to open up and a goddess to descend from above as the skies parted. Almost two centuries later, under Emperor Uda's rule, a musician from Tang China transmitted the secret tunes of the *koto* to Japan. It is said that many centuries passed before a priest in Chikugo province (in Kyūshū) mastered the tunes and taught them to Kenjun, a sighted, traveling priest of Hizen province (also in Kyūshū).[86] Kenjun traveled to Kyoto, where he impressed the court nobility with his performances. Hōsui, another sighted priest, tried to emulate him and fill his role. However, disappointed with his own musical abilities and the reception of his music, Hōsui departed Kyoto and recanted his monastic vows. Yatsuhashi, who was blind, became Hōsui's disciple and also, fortuitously, studied under a sighted priest named Genjo. This abbreviated narrative timeline, of course, implies that Yatsuhashi was one of the earliest known blind musicians of the *koto*.

Another primary text, *Records of the Main Contents of Koto Tunes*,[87] dated almost a century after *Records of the Koto Tunes of Yatsuhashi Kengyō*, highlights periods in the history of *koto* music.[88] The ancestor of Yatsuhashi's lineage was believed to have emerged from a series of musical lineages during the ninth century, at around the time when Semimaru, one of the mythical founders of *Heike*, was said to have lived. This claim was significant to blind *koto* musicians because it legitimized *sōkyoku* as a genre of the guild equal to *Heike*.[89] (As chapter 3 explained, we have very little information about Semimaru.)

We know that Yatsuhashi had a distinguished career through the guild. Descending from the Yatsuhashi lineage were lineages such as the Shin-Yatsuhashi (New Yatsuhashi), Ikuta, Yanagawa, and Sumiyama lineages. Yatsuhashi was a creative musician who also became an expert of the *shamisen*.[90] Following his instincts and natural flair, he reinvigorated and reinvented ceremonial court music with the colorful textures of *shamisen* music.[91] He not only expanded the repertoire of *koto* and

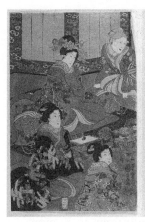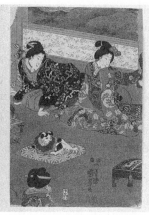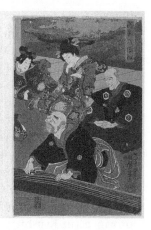

Fig. 5.1. An artist's depiction of a blind musician's *koto* musical performance. The *kanji* inscription at the top right says *o-oku* (possibly referring to a samurai's inner chamber of women) *hizikome* (this is the first *koto* performance of the new year). At the start of the new year, blind musicians were known to travel around cities, towns, and villages to perform music and also to conduct rites, which were accompanied by musical performances. From Utagawa Kuniyoshi, *A Blind Musician Plays the Koto to a Gathering of Women Dressed in Ornate Kimonos* (1849/1852; exact year unknown). From the Wellcome Collection.

shamisen music performed by blind musicians but also adapted existing elegant tunes and recomposed them in a vernacular style better suited to common audiences' taste.[92]

Lineages of *Heike* were thought to emphasize performative dimensions to enhance lyrical readings of the *Heike* narrative. It is likely that ideological meanings were grafted onto lineages' identities retroactively because of the primacy of written texts. The evidence from the corpus that has come to light, however, suggests that differences among texts were not at all straightforward.[93] For example, blind musicians of the Hatano lineage, compared to their Maeda counterparts, were believed to have been more liberal in interpreting musical and performance styles.

While a comparison of texts may point to real differences between the two lineages in their styles, it perhaps says more about the process of writing texts: it tells us that word accents, stresses, and notations were not consistently recorded and were characterized by idiosyncratic handwritten features introduced to the texts by sighted copyists. But these differences across texts probably did not pose significant problems to readers in the understanding and interpretation of specific styles.

Composing the Correct Tunes of Heike

The print edition of Chiichi's *Correct Tunes of Heike* cited in many scholarly works today is based on the manuscripts of the Ozaki household—Chiichi's host in Nagoya and family through his daughter's marriage. The original work, by some standards, would likely have consisted of forty book volumes, with contents that substantively coincided with contemporary *Heike* texts, albeit in a different format.[94] According to Komoda's survey of adapted copies of texts written with musical notations, almost all of those texts were produced as handwritten manuscripts, with the exception of *Short Tunes of Heike Recitations*[95] (which became available in print by around 1800).[96] Chiichi had composed his text as a professional manuscript intended primarily for professional musicians but also distributed it among amateurs and aficionados.

Chiichi's text would hardly have qualified as a secret manuscript. The main *Heike* characters and episodes were generally well known to audiences as they were adapted by different genres. In imagining Chiichi's performances, I do not preclude the possibility that Chiichi, as well as instructors in musical lineages, continued to verbally impart to advanced students or disciples some intricate techniques of performance and style that were not recorded in manuals. Lineages were defined by texts and also by personalities and relationships. What was imparted (or not) within a lineage and what was shared (or not) with people unaffiliated with it depended on such factors as the level of trust between a master and his disciple and between them and the horizontal networks of their peers.

Through the proliferation of print culture, commercial markets were awash with vernacular manuals, commentaries, and guidebooks about music and the performing arts.[97] *Heike* texts such as Chiichi's *Correct Tunes of Heike* of the Tokugawa period were passed down through handwritten practices, which may have been for practical reasons; musical notations of texts varied from lineage to lineage, and from person to person, and had to be manually inscribed. Woodblock printing would have been expedient, but it did not suit *Heike* musicians' needs for handwritten notes. Also, on commercial grounds, the dwindling fan base of *Heike* music did not make large-scale printing of all manuscripts lucrative or even necessary. Yet, even a manuscript-based tradition would not have been impervious to the widespread growth of print culture, as previously discussed. The inexhaustible array of published sources whetted the growing public appetite for knowledge of any kind and satiated consum-

152 · BLIND IN EARLY MODERN JAPAN

ers' desires for self-guided learning that bypassed professional lineages and formal tracks of training.

A seasoned blind musician like Chiichi who performed *Heike* music would have developed a keen ear for different lineages' musical sounds and styles. For such a blind musician, writing a *Heike* text was less about helping him remember verses than it was about communicating certain interpretations of verses to his audiences. Chiichi's text, like other *Heike* texts, was not a verbatim transcription of an actual performance: it was a template that encoded his choices. These choices, which were inflected by his personal preferences and his knowledge of the heritage of lineages, conveyed the essential qualities of an ideal performance—what a good performance would have sounded like. This insight expands on musicologist Hugh de Ferranti's observation that "different reciters of *Heike* stood in different relation to the written documents of the *Heike* tale-complex, and specifically the 'performance texts' produced among distinct schools of blind professionals."[98] In similar fashion, we can guess at sighted copyists' motives: how they were intent on transcribing musical notes and sequences that blind musicians would mostly have learned by rote and through practice, and how they were resolved to codify the inscriptions of sounds with a system of identifiable and meaningful written signs and to explain the technicalities of musical performances on their own terms.

Against this backdrop, Chiichi's *Correct Tunes of Heike*, dated 1776, was written to be seen, read, and performed as an open text by audiences, as were many *Heike* texts. This work stood as a record of an insider's perspectives on the genre. Through its association with Chiichi's name and reputation, it was imbued with the authority of an actual, professional, blind performer of the guild—even though this characterization would obscure the collaborative nature of textual composition. The core content presented the narrative through episodes running along various chronologies. The performances enhanced the logic of parallel spaces in the unfolding narrative structure. In this respect, the shifting focal points intensified tensions between timelines, imparting an accompanying sense of jarring temporal dissonance. The revolving cast of characters elevated the harmony and clash of storytelling perspectives and moved the plot along (forward and backward).

Chiichi retained formulaic lyrical patterns and incorporated essential *Heike* secret tunes to pay homage to the overarching generic traditions. In the Maeda lineage's performance tradition, the secret tunes were performed by a blind musician in the context of the entire narrative, which would have been recited continuously over thirty days in a formal cere-monial setting.[99] Even in the age of print culture, when secret tunes were recorded, perhaps what made those tunes special was how they were performed—using the technical skills and exquisite performance styles that only distinguished blind musicians were allowed to learn.

Chiichi's text was taught to students in a sequence that progressed in difficulty.[100] At the most basic level, a student memorized fifty verses of "Heike content."[101] The "Heike content" (thirty volumes), recomposed from the original tale, made up the core storytelling. Next in the train-ing were verses about imperial decrees, a subcategory of the "transmit-ted content,"[102] and another one hundred verses of "Heike content." Students who demonstrated promise in their training could be taught the rest of the "transmitted content." At that stage some verses were "The Rebuilding of the Great Pagoda," "Mount Kōya," "Genbō," "The Seinan Detached Palace," and "The Moving of the Capital to Fukuhara."[103] The highest level of training was reserved only for exceptionally promising students—they were likely students who had strong connections to Chi-ichi or who excelled in their performances. They were taught "The Ini-tiates' Chapter," "Lesser Secret Tunes," and "Greater Secret Tunes."[104] Those secret tunes were said to have been passed down within the Maeda lineage long ago before Chiichi's time.[105]

The musicality, inflections, and tones encoded in Chiichi's *Correct Tunes of Heike* were not uncommon by the standards of existing musical notation. The moods and styles of narration ranged from the types befit-ting selfless love, sacrifice, and courage to those that plumbed the depths of despair and to still others that enveloped the excesses of violence.[106] The musical notations (which were written next to where the respective melody was played) were taken from preexisting sources that combined linear strokes and *kana* and *kanji* characters of the Japanese scripts. Much has been made of the significant variations in notational styles within the Maeda lineage (see figure 5.2)—whether they represented local and regional differences and how they represented musical sounds.[107] To reiterate my earlier point, a comparison of musical notations in the texts would say a lot about the individual choices of the sighted contribu-tors to these texts and the collaboration with blind musicians—choices that did not always strictly adhere to the written conventions of either lineage by the eighteenth and nineteenth centuries. In particular, the analysis suggests the sharing of written texts among sighted purveyors of the cosmopolitan literary cultures of Edo, Kyoto, and Nagoya.[108] The eclectic concurrent use of linear strokes and characters, for example,

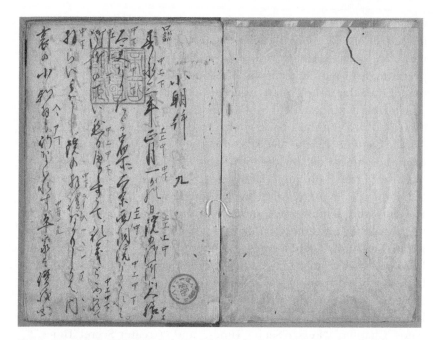

Fig. 5.2. Image of a *Heike* text linked to the Maeda lineage (*Maeda-ryū fushitsuki Heike monogatari*; likely from the late nineteenth century). This text (with verses from "Kochōhai") shows the notational style of the Maeda lineage with predominantly *kanji* notations written next to vertical verse lines. The mix of linear strokes and *kana* and *kanji* notations is not uncommon. Neither Hatano nor Maeda texts exclusively used one style of notation. National Diet Library Digital Collections.

has similarly been noted in the work of a blind musician in Edo named Toyokawa—this edition is commonly referred to as the "Toyokawa copy." The Edo-based handwritten texts are adduced as evidence of the concurrent circulation of Chiichi's text in the literary scene and as evidence of a marked shift toward modified notations among some sighted copyists of Edo.[109]

Sighted musicians could freely discuss *Heike* contents with blind musicians and form supportive relationships. In other genres—*koto* and *shamisen* music, for example—sighted and blind musicians would also have engaged one another in textual and musical studies, perhaps even to a greater extent as those genres were more popular than *Heike*. Sighted literati like Okamura Gensen in Edo produced their own *Heike* texts. Gensen was known for having written *The Musical Notations of Heike*.[110] A disciple of the Sōhen lineage of tea ceremony expert practitioners, he was originally trained as a physician. His interest in *Heike* texts and music harked back to the aesthetic training of his predecessors.[111] His work was supposedly completed in 1731, with an epilogue dated the third month of 1737, and represented the Sōhen lineage's understanding of *Heike* performance.[112] In the course of drafting the text, Gensen regularly convened with the guild's blind musicians. His network was centered on skilled, literate blind musicians such as Toyoda, Yamada, and Takaoka—these three musicians, and perhaps others, held the highest rank of *kengyō*. Some blind musicians also appeared to have supported him in an earlier *Heike* editorial project. Technical details about melodic arrangements and melodic refrains distinguished Gensen's interpretations of style from Chiichi's version.[113] Nonetheless, from what is known, both texts share the vocabulary and stylistic grammar of the genre.

In this micro-universe of intersecting codes and references, *Heike* texts were read differently, and their performances were also reimagined differently. By tracing these various circulation routes, it becomes clear that blind professionals themselves were entangled in the dense web of social and literary connections with sighted participants. More closely linked to Chiichi's *Correct Tunes of Heike* in light of similar structural arrangements and substantive overlapping contents was *Recitations of Heike*,[114] an oeuvre by Nagoya-based *haikai* poet Yokoi Yayū.[115] Also, Oka Masatake, an Edo-based sighted enthusiast of the genre, composed the manual *A Record of Questions and Answers about Heikyoku*[116] in 1820 together with a blind musician named Hoshino, who was one of Chiichi's students.[117] Masatake also tried to reconstruct the original content of Chiichi's *Correct Tunes of Heike*.[118]

The Nagoya-based copyists of Chiichi's *Correct Tunes of Heike* were scholarly, aesthetically cultured, sighted men. While we do not know how many sighted people were involved in writing the verses, or in writing the musical notations, one copyist we know of was Niwa Keichū, a samurai student. Another copyist was Neo-Confucian scholar of botany and natural history Matsudaira Kunzan. An active scholar in the Nagoya intellectual circuit who, not unlike other scholars in this regard, maintained a recreational interest in *Heike*, Kunzan prepared the text of the introduction perhaps sometime in 1776, several months ahead of Keichū's preface.[119] Both texts were appended to Chiichi's work together with an epilogue by Chimura Moronari, Kunzan's sighted student and fellow enthusiast. The finished work was disseminated in Edo. Through his sighted students and proxies, Toyokawa (the blind musician in Edo who produced the "Toyokawa copy" mentioned earlier) adapted Chiichi's text.[120] As the "Toyokawa copy" passed through different hands, it was critically examined by sighted audiences in Edo to recreate more familiar musical styles.

Conclusion

Being blind could mean being enabled by disabled identity for a career in music, and for those musicians, other enabling factors could make a difference between an exceptional career and an ordinary career. Guild membership and a person's connections and interactions with other people were enabling factors in the lives and careers of blind musicians like Chiichi.

Chiichi's career depended on the guild, which had a stake in the political regime of the Tokugawa period as a status institution—by creating, demarcating, and indexing blindness as disability (see chapters 3 and 4). While the guild had no charitable or moral mission to rescue all its members from poverty—in fact, it oppressed those who were most vulnerable and physically dependent—it did support guild members' rights to collect alms and also maintained an infrastructure of vocational training, which promised prospects in employable professions.

In the unforgiving environment that penalized lowly status and favored blindness among other kinds of impairment, guild membership was a stepping stone to a career. As the parallel between the careers of Chiichi and Hokiichi highlights, the guild became the most important platform to launch a blind person's career through the connections that it enabled. The same system, however, bound guild members to repay the favor to the guild.

Chiichi's situation would likely have been a familiar one among professional blind musicians. He could have chosen to broaden his repertoire and be known for composing and performing new and popular genres—the logical choice of most blind musicians, such as Kuzuhara. Instead, Chiichi chose to concentrate on *Heike* and forge a traditional career, even though that genre's clientele had shrunk greatly over the seventeenth century. The gamble was ultimately rewarding, because in the end, it thrust him into the limelight.

The approach adopted in this study illustrates that Chiichi crafted a role for himself by being associated with like-minded sighted and blind peers. (The same can be said of Hokiichi, who accomplished a lot in scholarship.) We have to think beyond our existing scholarly conventions of *Heike*—binaries that trace "recited texts" and "read texts"—that are aimed at taxonomic efficiency but do not adequately capture the complex stories of the people behind these texts. If Chiichi offered the literary blueprint for *Correct Tunes of Heike*, then his sighted intermediaries in textual composition and compilation were no less significant in transforming his vision into reality.

The context of eighteenth-century print culture is important for understanding why texts were essential and how sighted audiences became involved in writing texts for a genre that blind musicians like Chiichi knew very well. Once in the possession of the right sighted purveyors, *Heike* texts were turned into objects of intense scrutiny. With the growing stability of the written mode, the transmission of tunes was focused on written cues, to the benefit of sighted readers. Texts passed as convenient sources of recreational self-learning for sighted amateurs who did not wish to spend too much time or money on any form of professional training.

Oftentimes, those sighted individuals were outsiders with no previous or direct ties to blind musicians or the guild. However, in their various capacities linked to blind musicians, they rendered essential services—not so much (or if at all) as professional performers during the Tokugawa period but more as partners, collaborators, and editorial assistants in the textual aspects of *Heike*. They copied texts, scrupulously inserted musical notations into the interstices of knowledge, and shared draft copies through their networks. These were practices that, seen as a whole, had expanded and intensified after the late medieval period. It is unclear how well Chiichi knew, or if he even knew, Yayū and Gensen, two of the sighted literati mentioned in this chapter who wrote *Heike* texts. The fact remains that many musicians would not have encountered one another in person in their lifetimes, but they were linked through textual studies.

By the late nineteenth century, blind musicians of *Heike* almost completely disappeared from the scene. The dismantling of the guild in 1871 under the Meiji regime permanently displaced blind musicians who had relied on the guild to train in *Heike*. Blind musicians, particularly guild members, were left without institutional support (see the epilogue). In a stark reversal of roles, professional sighted musicians replaced blind musicians in the role of studying and performing *Heike* music. The situation with blind priests in Kyūshū (see chapter 4) was not too different. Sighted musicians, according to de Ferranti, inherited and adapted the repertoire and musical styles of blind priests, essentially resuscitating those blind musicians' fading lyrical traditions in modern Japan.[121]

Musical lineages of sighted musicians in the Meiji period such as the Nagoya lineage and the Tsugaru lineage performed a diverse repertoire of music, which included *Heike* music.[122] The Maeda-Hatano lineage differentiation of *Heike* ceased to be of direct relevance to sighted lineages. As sighted musicians defined their own distinctive standards, they interpreted *Heike* based on their modified readings of texts such as Chiichi's *Correct Tunes of Heike.*

CHAPTER 6

Healing by Touch

Blind Acupuncturists and Masseurs

———— ❧ ————

The Tale of Flowering Fortunes,[1] an eleventh-century Japanese literary text from the Heian period, recounts an episode in which imperial court minister and nobleman Fujiwara no Nobunaga suffers from such excruciating pain that he is reduced to tears.[2] To relieve his pain, he orders a therapy known as *haratori*[3] (abdominal massage) to be performed on him. Abdominal massage is also mentioned in *The Pillow Book*,[4] another literary text about the imperial court of that same period.[5] In both texts, abdominal massage appears to be a type of massage given by low-ranking court women (presumably midwives). These are some of the earliest mentions of massage being performed on people.

Massage was introduced to Japan in the eighth century (or possibly earlier) through contacts with China and Korea.[6] Along with massage, acupuncture was a prominent specialty. Specialists in acupuncture and massage were regularly appointed to posts in the imperial court's Bureau of Medicine and attended to the court nobility.[7] A ninth-century source[8] describes how massage was performed to relax the body's joints and expel "winds"[9]; when combined with acupuncture, it was said to dissipate blood stagnation.[10]

Over the following centuries in Japan, it seems that only sighted people were associated with the professions of massage and acupuncture. Blind acupuncturists or masseurs are not mentioned at all in the early literature. But in the Tokugawa period, they not only emerged onto the medical scene but were everywhere in society. How did that shift happen, and why did blind people find work as acupuncturists and masseurs?

This chapter provides some answers by examining aspects of the social and medical contexts of the Tokugawa period that changed the livelihoods of blind people—aspects that expanded the possibilities of what it meant to be blind and to work in new professions. Medical lineages, popular medical culture, and the Kyoto guild occupy important roles in this historical narrative, so this chapter builds on earlier discussions of these subjects in chapters 1 through 3. The guild, which traditionally trained blind male musicians in *Heike* music starting in the thirteenth or fourteenth century, greatly expanded its membership in the seventeenth century by embracing early blind pioneers who practiced medicine and became famous as acupuncturists—one of those blind acupuncturists was Sugiyama Wa'ichi. In light of their accomplishments, blind acupuncturists promoted acupuncture as a fitting, lucrative profession for blind people. Wa'ichi's efforts to build an institutional foundation for acupuncture through the guild and to start his own medical lineage had a profound impact on the teaching of Japanese acupuncture, giving new impetus to the professional work of blind acupuncturists.

Like acupuncture, massage was a medical therapy, but blind people did not find their way into the profession until after blind acupuncturists had already achieved tremendous success. A factor that particularly encouraged the boom in massage was the growing cultural value that Tokugawa Japanese placed on cultivating good health[11] (Chinese: *yangsheng*; Japanese: *yōjō*; health cultivation). Hence, this chapter's discussion of massage also explores health cultivation: how it had roots in Chinese philosophy, how it was popularized starting in the eighteenth century, and how, in this popular context of health cultivation, massage was promoted as a therapy to improve anyone's bodily circulation of blood and *ki* (Chinese: *qi*; Japanese: *ki*; breath or vital energy).

As the demand for masseurs grew, blind masseurs entered the field and created a niche profession. Blind people became so widely associated with massage that blind masseurs were featured in popular literature. Massage was such a commonplace profession that even blind people who did not join the guild could obtain training through other means. All things considered, the guild's support for vocational training in acupuncture and massage, the social organization of medical knowledge through lineages, and an emerging medical culture centered on new ways of caring for the body converged as social and medical developments that were instrumental in enabling the work of blind people.

Blind Pioneers of Acupuncture: Who Were They?

THE SHOGUNATE'S MEDICAL HIERARCHY

The shogunate's medical organization provides some context that will help us understand the early reputation of blind acupuncturists. A hierarchy of physicians attended to the shogun and his aides. The posts were not created all at once, but as the bureaucracy burgeoned in strength over the seventeenth century, it became imperative to delineate roles for physicians. In or around 1683, the medical hierarchy was formalized, with the physician to shogun Tokugawa Tsunayoshi at the top of it.

Narinobu (or Roan) of the Nakarai clan and Manase Gensaku[12] of the Imaōji clan and his son Chikakiyo were several of the earliest physicians mentioned in *The Veritable Records of the Tokugawa Shoguns*, the official history of the Tokugawa shoguns.[13] In the first month of 1623, for example, these physicians were given privileged access to the inner chambers of the shogun's residence.[14] The Nakarai and Imaōji clans were forerunners of the hereditary office of shogunate physician.[15] Due to his proximity to the shogun, a shogunate physician was also known as a personal physician-in-waiting. Physicians broadened their coverage and duties to serve domain lords and samurai vassals.[16]

Over successive shoguns' rule, from the third shogun Tokugawa Iemitsu in the mid-seventeenth century to Yoshimune in the early eighteenth century, the medical hierarchy acquired complex layers.[17] To meet the rising demand for a range of medical specialties, the pool of physicians serving the shogunate was diversified; specialists such as shogunate acupuncturists, shogunate ophthalmologists, and shogunate pediatricians became prominent fixtures. By the early eighteenth century, the shogunate employed a whole array of physicians poised to perform their duties, a system that ensured the self-sufficiency of medical services for the shogunate's ranks of officials. The shogunate's tight command structure placed physicians in office under the rule of the Council of Junior Elders.[18]

For centuries after acupuncture was integrated into Japanese mainstream medicine, sighted men dominated the field. We do not know for sure how the earliest blind acupuncturists of the Tokugawa period were trained in acupuncture, but it is likely that they trained with medical lineages of the late medieval period—as the example of Sugiyama Wa'ichi (whom I will discuss shortly) tells us. It also is likely that they formed connections with the shogunate and leveraged them to secure positions in the shogunate's medical hierarchy. For example, Yamakawa Jōkan, about whom little is known, enjoyed the prestige of being called upon to administer acupuncture to shogun Tokugawa Iemitsu in the early seventeenth century.[19] Early blind acupuncturists' successful careers with the shogunate strengthened the general perception that blind acupuncturists were as skillful as sighted acupuncturists and could rely on their sense of touch to make up for impaired vision.

There were practical reasons why blind people were not trained in other medical specialties. For example, ophthalmology demanded delicate skills that depended on sight to a greater extent than acupuncture did. In ophthalmology, the diagnosis of eye conditions would have required a good degree of sight for recognizing and distinguishing colors and symptoms (see chapter 1). In an actual clinical procedure, treatments that involved the use of needles (needling techniques) would also have required an ophthalmologist to use good sight to observe the progress of an operation, anticipate outcomes, and adjust methods.

SUGIYAMA WA'ICHI AND HIS DISCIPLES

A well-known blind acupuncturist in his time was Sugiyama Wa'ichi—perhaps the blind acupuncturist we know the most about from the Tokugawa period. The collection *Biographies of Eminent Physicians in the Imperial Land*[20] by Asada Sōhaku, a nineteenth-century shogunate physician, is one of several early sources of information about Wa'ichi's life. It tells us that Wa'ichi learned acupuncture from a blind acupuncturist named Yamase Taku'ichi, who was a disciple of the late medieval Irie medical lineage and had studied under a sighted master named Irie Yoshiaki.[21] Wa'ichi also sought direct instruction from Yoshiaki's descendant Toyoaki (also of the Irie lineage) and assimilated his masters' knowledge into his own teachings. It is possible that Wa'ichi started his training in acupuncture after he joined the guild, but it is not clear when he became a guild member or in what other fields he was trained as a guild member. In 1680, Wa'ichi, who was in his forties, was granted an audience with shogun Tokugawa Ietsuna for the first time, probably because he had earned a good reputation as an acupuncturist.[22] Through the meeting, he was introduced to the shogun's networks and elevated his profile in the shogunate. What we do know from *The Veritable Records of the Tokugawa Shoguns* is that Wa'ichi's chief sponsor was shogun Tokugawa Tsunayoshi, who generously awarded him stipends from 1685 through 1692.[23] What we also know from that source is that Wa'ichi reached the pinnacle of his career in 1692 when he became the guild's top leader (*sōkengyō*)—this suggests that prior to the promotion, he had held the top rank of *kengyō* for years.[24]

Prominent blind acupuncturists such as Wa'ichi were committed to the guild. Of particular significance is the acupuncture training that the guild offered, the foundation of which was laid down by Wa'ichi's predecessors. But Wa'ichi had a bigger vision for the guild than what his predecessors probably had in mind. According to Sōhaku's account, Wa'ichi established his school of acupuncture.[25] Information about the exact layout of the original school, which is thought to have been set up for the guild at his residence in Edo, is lacking; institutional records about the school and other training schools that he had supposedly founded are also elusive.[26] At his school, Wa'ichi's styles of acupuncture and content of teaching were inaugurated as the Sugiyama lineage. Wa'ichi concentrated his attention on training blind students of the guild but did not codify his criteria for the selection of students—disciples had more direct relationships with their masters than students did, as chapter 5 explained. It seems that Wa'ichi accepted sighted students, but it is less clear whether he did that regularly. One student (a sighted man) whom he taught was Kurimoto (Sansetsu) Toshiyuki, who was familiar to local elites and the shogunate. Formerly a physician to Ōkubo Tadatomo, lord of Odawara domain (in Kanagawa prefecture today), Toshiyuki was promoted to become shogunate physician in 1693.[27]

Two top guild members, Mishima Yasu'ichi and Shimaura (or Wada) Ekiichi, carried on Wa'ichi's work. We may not have much information about their early lives, but there is some information about their profiles. In 1691, Yasu'ichi, who was a preeminent acupuncturist, was ordered to serve the shogun's close aides.[28] Based in Edo, he rose through the hierarchy of the guild and, sometime in 1693, took over Wa'ichi's role in overseeing the guild's instruction of acupuncture.[29] After Wa'ichi's demise, he assumed leadership of the guild. No less important was Yasu'ichi's successor, Ekiichi. Born into the Wada clan of samurai vassals of Yonezawa domain (in Yamagata prefecture today), Ekiichi became a guild member and was trained in acupuncture under Yasu'ichi; over time, in 1709, after consecutive promotions and with his base in Edo, he succeeded Yasu'ichi as the guild's top leader.[30] This Edo-based office was later reestablished as a permanent proxy to represent the Kyoto guild (see the discussion of the guild's hierarchy in chapter 3).

SUGIYAMA WA'ICHI'S MEDICAL LINEAGE

The Sugiyama lineage, or Wa'ichi's lineage, is notable for being a lineage that cultivated blind acupuncturists. Wa'ichi developed his styles of acupuncture in the seventeenth century within the overarching framework of medical lineages in Japan and in a milieu influenced by Chinese medical thought and practices.[31] To summarize the discussion of medical lineages from chapter 1, Japanese medical scholars had historically synthesized their approaches to Chinese medicine to develop Japanese medicine (also called Sino-Japanese medicine). The transmission of theoretical and practical knowledge from master to disciple within lineages was justified, systematized, and standardized by the early Tokugawa period—some of the knowledge was transmitted primarily by oral teachings. Lineages provided the social and intellectual frameworks of instruction in medicine. They transmitted and taught ideas that formed the germ of intellectual learning. The intellectual foundations of the Sugiyama lineage attest to the fact that Japanese acupuncture developed from Chinese acupuncture.[32]

If the means allowed, a blind or sighted person seeking rigorous training in acupuncture so as to gain credibility in the profession could choose to start a career with a lineage. By the eighteenth century, educational facilities that had evolved from the lineage-based system had sprouted up across Japan; Igakkan (the elite shogunate-sponsored medical school), domain-sponsored schools, and privately owned academies are well-known examples.[33] Wa'ichi's lineage and school of acupuncture were among the early institutions that propagated intellectual learning defined by lineage-based knowledge. Even in the nineteenth century, it was not uncommon for some medical lineages, such as the Ikeda lineage of smallpox medicine at the shogunate medical school, to try to preserve a balance between open instruction and secret knowledge.[34] As Federico Marcon explains, private academies that prioritized secret teachings manipulated the nature of secrecy to advertise their ownership and control of knowledge.[35] While it is likely that Wa'ichi relied on verbal methods of instruction, his followers derived their authority by attributing to him the authorship of *The Three Treatises of Sugiyama*,[36] named for the three basic texts that recorded Wa'ichi's teachings. The production of texts is a sign that Wa'ichi's lineage accepted sighted disciples and trusted the most qualified ones to transmit knowledge in writing and in print. (See the discussion in chapter 5 of collaboration between blind masters and sighted students in *Heike* music.)

Wa'ichi was known for the advanced acupuncture technique of needling with a guide tube—a technique still used today that features a slender, hollow tube through which a needle is inserted into an acu-point (or acupuncture point). His technique was said to be closely related to the technique of needling with a hammer tool[37] by the Mubun lineage,[38] a lineage of sighted acupuncturists that probably dated back to the sixteenth century. Both the Mubun and Sugiyama lineages, as well as later medical scholars, understood that the abdomen enveloped the totality of life and that physical health depended on the constant flow and circulation of *ki* and blood.[39] For example, arguments by the Sugiyama lineage about medical examination and diagnosis through abdominal palpation[40] were articulated in its early medical treatises.[41] The logic of abdominal palpation suggests that a good physician with a discerning sense of touch could uncover the secrets of diseases by palpating sites around the abdomen. The Mubun lineage insisted that ancient acupuncturists had been averse to the risks of agitating the abdomen and endangering the patient's life. But, with the hammering method, the Mubun lineage argued, an acupuncturist could safely tap an acupuncture needle with a hammer at any targeted spot on the abdomen. In technical applications, Wa'ichi's pairing of a needle and a guide tube was an improvement in efficiency. It is reasonable to imagine that a blind acupuncturist could use Wa'ichi's technique to perform acupuncture without relying on sight. Perception through a keen sense of touch was a skill that blind acupuncturists honed through long periods of practice.

The Shinden or "true transmission" lineage, a lineage that emerged early in the eighteenth century, expanded the audience of Wa'ichi's teachings beyond the guild. The Shinden lineage fits the description of a sub-lineage, an aspect of the history of medical lineages discussed in chapter 1, because it descended from and closely identified with the parent (Sugiyama) lineage. Overlaps between the two lineages point to common understandings of medical traditions in a broader epistemic context in which Japanese medical lineages organized knowledge. However, the Shinden lineage shifted its focus to train sighted disciples, likely in response to demands from sighted persons interested in studying Wa'ichi's acupuncture styles to become professional acupuncturists. It appears that in Ekiichi's lifetime, his clan (the Wada clan) transformed Wa'ichi's original school of acupuncture into a platform for inaugurating the new Shinden lineage, which grew into a hereditary lineage dominated by the Wada clan and gradually cut off ties with the guild. To preserve the records of that lineage, Ekiichi's sighted son Naohide, a shogunate physician, compiled and edited medical texts.[42] Generations later, Masanaga of the Wada clan sought to restore the former teachings of his predecessors.[43] As proof of his high stature, he had connections with shogunate physician Sōhaku, the author of medical biographies of eminent physicians who was mentioned earlier in this chapter. As Sōhaku recounted in his medical case histories, both he and Masanaga were involved in treating a high-profile foreigner named Léon Roches, a French government official posted to Yokohama who near the end of Tokugawa rule was a linchpin in the shogunate's policies to normalize relations with France.[44]

Historical records analyzed by Japanese historians of medicine Ōura Hiromasa and Ichikawa Yuri allow us to reconstruct the formal acupuncture training process of the Shinden lineage. From start to finish, instruction emphasized reading and reciting texts—tasks that were suited for the abilities of sighted people.[45] A potential disciple was required to sign a contract of agreement[46] to confirm that he had been selected and accepted by a master. Rote memorization was the primary method of learning for any disciple. The disciple had to take lessons and learn to flawlessly recite the main texts of the lineage (this was called line recitation[47]). His master corrected mistakes in the recitation. The disciple also had to demonstrate an accurate grasp of the semantics of core teachings. If he misunderstood any of the teachings, he was given a chance to restudy the main texts and copy excerpts. Simultaneously, under the close supervision of his master, the disciple had to master clinical techniques. In the final stage, when he exhibited full proficiency in theory and practice, he was examined by the head of the lineage. Once the disciple satisfactorily passed the examination, he earned his qualification as an acupuncturist—by that time, he was said to have reached the ultimate level of "divine needle."[48] Certain disciples were selected to master the lineage's secret needling techniques.

In light of Wa'ichi's reputation and contributions to the guild, we can imagine that in the centuries following his death, the guild continued to focus on teaching acupuncture to guild members according to the requirements of Wa'ichi's Sugiyama lineage. Guild members underwent training to learn content that was probably quite similar to that taught to sighted acupuncturists of the Shinden lineage, and distinguished disciples were additionally taught exclusive content. The steps would not have been too different from those outlined in the Shinden lineage's training, but we can assume that the training of a blind acupuncturist emphasized verbal instruction. Clinical training would also have been integral to his training. In general, a guild member training in massage would have received some basic training in acupuncture, and for a trainee concentrating on acupuncture, massage would still have been included in his training. This seems to be consistent with Wakuda Tetsuji's suggestion that a blind person in his basic training spent three years learning massage and another three years learning acupuncture.[49]

The intertwining of acupuncture and massage in professional work was common during the Tokugawa period, but the following section on massage will suggest that blind people had practical reasons to focus only on learning massage. Nonetheless, anecdotes about blind masseurs in Japan reported in the foreign press in the late nineteenth century support the view that even after the Tokugawa period, many blind people continued to be trained in both acupuncture and massage (see figure 6.1). As quoted in the *New-York Tribune* in 1891, "The art of shampooing [massage] as practised by the Japanese blind takes nine years to learn. The pupil for the first three years practises on his master; then he spends three years acquiring the art of acupuncture; and for the remaining three years he is on probation, his master receiving half his earnings."[50] The period of training would likely have varied according to factors such as a person's aptitude.

ASHIHARA HIDETOSHI: A BLIND ACUPUNCTURIST
IN THE LATE TOKUGAWA PERIOD

While general training would have sufficed for most blind acupuncturists, a privileged minority leveraged the connections formed through the guild's networks. The guild was useful through the nineteenth century in enabling some guild members to gain privileges to advance their careers. Ashihara Hidetoshi from the Kiso clan of samurai vassals was one such guild member. Born in Edo in 1797, Hidetoshi boasted the exceptional profile of someone who charted a course from humble beginnings in the guild to a position of influence.[51] At the age of six or seven, he became blind after he contracted measles, a disease that medical scholars at that time believed had "poison" that could cause blindness (see chapters 1 and 2). He entered the guild as an unranked disciple of a blind senior named Kishimura and acquired skills in acupuncture. As a fledgling acupuncturist in his early teens, he attended to the Sanada clan (samurai lord) of Matsushiro domain (in Nagano prefecture today), who resided at the domain domicile in Edo.[52] Hidetoshi's early career with the guild

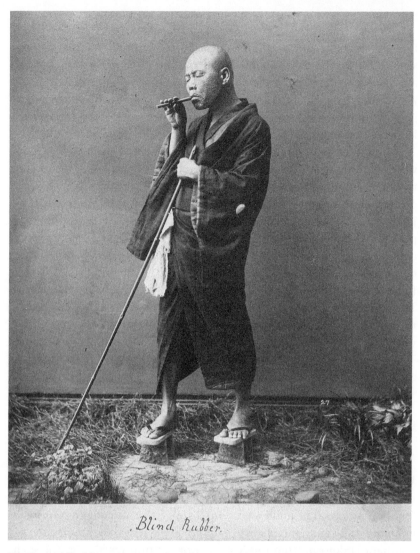

.Blind Rubber.

Fig. 6.1. "A blind Japanese masseur with a pipe in his mouth and a long pole in his hand." A photograph likely from the late nineteenth century shows a "blind rubber" (blind masseur) of the Meiji period with recognizable characteristics of blind masseurs from the Tokugawa period: as seen here, his head is shaven, and he walks with a staff and blows a whistle. Foreigners who visited Japan during the Meiji period were impressed with blind masseurs or, as they were also called, blind shampooers—because massage was called shampooing. American geographer Frank Carpenter published a vivid account of his encounter with massage at a hotel in Tokyo. "I am very tired, and I have just heard the whistle of the blind shampooer on the streets outside my hotel. I have clapped my hands, called a servant, and ordered a shampoo. . . . He [the blind shampooer] now begins to pass his hands over my body. He first seeks out two spots at my shoulders, and into these his thumbs go, it seems to me, almost to the joints. The places he touches are evidently nerve centers; for, as he gouges them, my whole frame quivers" (Carpenter, 1888–89, 216). From the Wellcome Collection.

was boosted when he acquired the basic rank of *zatō* at age seventeen through that clan's financial sponsorship.

In the decades following his promotion, Hidetoshi continued to climb up the guild's hierarchy and used his relationships to access the inner circles of the shogunate. He traveled to provide acupuncture services to samurai officials, including members of the collateral clans (descendent clans) of the shogun.[53] He also treated shogun Ienari, who was plagued with severe ailments that were believed to be caused by "winds." In return for treating him, the shogunate conferred a title on Hidetoshi, and he received generous rewards of rice stipends—privileges usually reserved for political elites. After the shogun's demise in 1841, Hidetoshi retired but stayed on as a physician in a lower office.

His success, however, was far from typical. Most blind acupuncturists who were not associated with the shogunate, with the networks of vassals, or with elite guild members had little access to opportunities beyond their regular, immediate circles.

Cultivating Health with Massage and Masseurs

THE CHINESE ORIGIN OF HEALTH CULTIVATION

As mentioned at the beginning of this chapter, the Tokugawa Japanese context of *yōjō* (health cultivation or nourishment) gave massage an essential role in maintaining health. Health cultivation did not develop overnight in Tokugawa society. A survey of its history tells us that it had deep roots in Chinese medical and cultural thought and practices. This would explain why Japanese medical literature even in the Tokugawa period shares a common vocabulary with Chinese medical literature on massage and its various functions.

The Chinese philosophy of health cultivation was intertwined with ancient Daoist goals of prolonging life.[54] It was founded on the principal tenet of cultivation at the physical, mental, and spiritual (and metaphysical) levels—for example, through the interplay of healing exercises of the breath and mind to experience the unity of the body as a dense, microcosmic universe. Ancient Chinese medical scholars thought of massage as a routine of stretching and massage exercises that could be performed in solitude to benefit a person's health.[55]

Daoist influences did not completely disappear during the historical periods that followed. Through the late medieval period of Sino-Japanese medicine in Japan, in the fifteenth and sixteenth centuries, discourses of health cultivation were still heavily interlaced with Daoist language. For example, in the sixteenth-century medical text *Transmitted Notes*,[56] which is attributed to Manase Dōsan, a highly respected medical scholar of the prominent Manase-Imaōji clan of the imperial court, the section "Immortal techniques of constant health cultivation" draws upon the Chinese Daoist text *Treatise on Immortals*.[57] It emphasizes the consumption of medicines and outlines prescriptive formulas to treat certain disorders, poor appetite and fatigue, and aches of the head and waist.[58]

Even as late as the nineteenth century in Tokugawa Japan, some writers cleverly employed the original Daoist meanings to appeal to the public's fascination with longevity and immortality. One author, Tanaka Utarō (perhaps a pseudonym), published the treatise *Formulas of Denshi's Health Cultivation*.[59] In it, by reviving the Daoist context, he magnified the literal meaning of the idiom "not growing old and living a long life"[60] to promote regimens such as techniques of breathing, stretching, and massage.[61]

MASSAGE AND HEALTH CULTIVATION

To understand why blind masseurs became popular, it is important to first understand how massage became popular in the context of health cultivation and, in particular, how people understood and promoted massage as a therapy with uses in everyday life. Massage was different from acupuncture in important respects. A good acupuncturist had to have intimate knowledge of the body's anatomy, conduits, and acu-points (including prohibited sites for certain medical conditions and seasons). While such knowledge also enhanced the training in massage, acupuncture was more exacting because it involved special technical competence with needles. Yet, it was because massage could be performed with a person's bare hands, and without the same level of expertise as acupuncture, that massage became such a commonplace practice in health cultivation. The relative ease with which blind people could pick up skills in massage enabled them to focus on training as masseurs and also enabled them to find work as masseurs. But it was also for this reason—that massage required less technical skills and expertise than acupuncture—that massage was not regarded in mainstream medicine as having the prestige and rigor of acupuncture.

The widespread public interest in health cultivation and in massage was linked to increased literacy in Tokugawa society. As chapter 2 discussed, by the eighteenth century, print culture had become a powerful element of popular culture, so integral to popular literature, consumer culture, and popular medical culture that readers and consumers were enabled by easy access to information and an array of choices of how to obtain it. Printed books covered a variety of subjects, and many of them were intended for the general reading public.[62] By some estimates, at least forty-one titles of books with health cultivation as the main subject were in print from the mid-1600s to the 1800s.[63] Well-read audiences were important consumers and proponents of health cultivation—and this phenomenon was not limited to urban areas.

It does not come as a surprise, then, that village leaders or provincial elites in the eighteenth century, Richard Rubinger explains, were avid readers and collectors of books.[64] For instance, in Daigatsuka village (in the Osaka area), a rice wine merchant named Kawachiya Kashō took heed of health cultivation both as a business model and as a personal health model, coupling good work ethics with healthy lifestyles and good habits of the mind.[65] Kashō argued that invaluable precepts had to be observed for a person to stay in good health. Taking a preventive and preemptive approach to health was critical—this was the essence of health cultivation.[66] By his reasoning, each day spent living purposefully was worth more than gold.

Health cultivation starting in the early eighteenth century was emphasized in popular medical culture because of its practical health benefits. For example, Shigehisa Kuriyama highlights that health cultivation animated the popular imagination about massage and labor. Stagnations were taboo: stagnated *ki* in the body was a manifestation of a lack of physical exertion, an aversion to hard work, and a predilection to delight in material excesses.[67] Abdominal massage, a specific type of massage around the abdomen, was believed to disperse *ki* that had slowed to a halt and congealed under the deleterious influences of "winds," poor diet, and emotions.[68]

Personal health acquired social and even economic significance. Popular perceptions of the health benefits of massage translated into ideas about good economic outcomes: massage was conducive to an individual's wellness because it stimulated movements of vital essences around the body. People who enjoyed good health were more likely to be able to labor beyond their prime years to support themselves and their families. Abdominal massage and abdominal palpation, thus, can be seen as logical outgrowths of the growing and deepening association of personal health with productive labor.

The metaphor of health cultivation as an ordering of the larger
social body found resonance in popular thought through works by Neo-
Confucian scholars.[69] Nishikawa Joken's *A Bagful of Miscellaneous Knowledge for Townspeople*[70] tells us that drinking alcohol with abandon led to
unruly and disruptive behaviors.[71] Self-indulgence, he warned, could
cause the breakdown of order in society. In the same vein, *A Useful Guide
on Health Cultivation and Food in Everyday Living*[72] by Tatsuno Ryōboku
can be understood as a work about the precepts of self-restraint and pru-
dence. Ryōboku asserted that people could attune their bodies through
physical labor and stave off diseases.[73] He made the analogy that flowing
water does not stagnate and the hinges of constantly swinging doors do
not rot. Quite literally, because he thought that massage kept the body
in perpetual motion, it was an antidote and an alternative to medicines
to cure inactivity and unproductivity.

By far the most influential and enthusiastic Japanese advocate of
health cultivation in the eighteenth century was Kaibara Ekiken, whose
treatise *Lessons on Cultivating Health*[74] (1713) was one of the most highly
regarded works published at the peak of public discourses of health cultivation. Ekiken discussed health as a style of self-cultivation and, ultimately, as a profoundly moral enterprise. He equated health cultivation
with moral cultivation, ascribing to the body symbolic meanings that continued to be appropriated later—for example, during the Meiji period,
health cultivation influenced notions and categories of public health.[75]

Ekiken understood the body to be an irreplaceable gift from one's
parents and the heavens and earth, implicated in complex social relationships and moral obligations. Nourishing health and leading a long
and productive life, he argued, were essentially acts of filial piety and
ways of repaying one's parents and the heavens and earth.[76] Instead of
going into the abstract metaphysics of health, Ekiken prioritized concrete actions. His key to good health can be summarized by the ideas
of moderation and thrift. By his standards, doing things in moderation,
from diet to sex, underpinned success in everything.[77]

Ekiken recommended massage and acupuncture for health cultivation. In fact, according to him, massage could be practiced daily and
surpassed acupuncture in its practical applications. There were manifold
benefits of observing a daily schedule of massage: *ki* flowed smoothly,
food was digested and did not stagnate in the body, and pain in the legs
and feet was relieved. Ekiken's instructions consisted of detailed steps
that anyone could follow.[78] He approved of acupuncture but instructed
that the conditions had to be ideal.[79] He considered acupuncture effi-

cacious in treating ailments related to stagnation in the abdomen and afflictions such as stubborn pains in the arms and legs, maintaining that it produced greater results than medicines and moxibustion under the same conditions.

Japanese medical literature about health cultivation from the eighteenth century onward devoted significant attention to using massage to improve the health of women and children. Popular instructional manuals on massage recommended different styles of massage for women and children. For example, *A Guide on Massage*[80] (by Tachibana Shunki and Fujibayashi Ryōhaku, dated 1799) advocates the therapeutic uses of abdominal massage.[81] The text says that children had delicate constitutions and that even if they were found to be in good health, massage could prevent the buildup and stagnation of breast milk and food and also could protect children from constipation and from debilitating illnesses, such as measles, smallpox, and epilepsy. To care for a pregnant woman and to ensure a safe and smooth childbirth, a masseur was advised to focus on performing massage in such a way as to safely shift the fetus, stimulate the flow of blood and *ki* around the abdomen, and encourage appetite and food consumption.

A blind masseur's visual impairment was his advantage: he was free to apply his skills on women's bodies without reproach and without fear of violating decency and modesty.

BLIND MASSEURS AND THE GUILD

In every aspect of popular medical culture, massage was recommended for everyone, and people were encouraged to include massage in their everyday routines. As interest in massage grew, so too did opportunities for people who wanted to become masseurs. Perhaps because blind people were thought to excel in jobs that involved tactile skills, such as music and acupuncture, they were enabled by this popular perception to find work in massage.

Even though blind masseurs were in such great demand that massage became the most common profession (even the default profession) among blind people, we have less information about the profiles of blind masseurs than what we have about blind acupuncturists. This comparative lack of sources could be because massage was less prestigious than acupuncture, as mentioned earlier, and also because blind people who worked as masseurs were generally poor and were less known than blind

174 · BLIND IN EARLY MODERN JAPAN

acupuncturists for professional accomplishments. Acupuncture had a head start as a profession among blind people, and because of this, we know more about blind acupuncturists than we do about blind masseurs in the seventeenth century. Moreover, acupuncture, not massage, was the profession that launched early guild members such as Wa'ichi to fame, as it did also for later guild members such as Hidetoshi of the Kiso clan.

Wa'ichi's contributions to the guild and to acupuncture resulted in the training of guild members as acupuncturists. The guild probably developed a systematic way to teach massage to guild members starting in the late seventeenth century after Wa'ichi's Sugiyama lineage was inaugurated. Although blind masseurs should have gone through the proper route of acquiring medical knowledge and skills in both massage and acupuncture, many chose not to do this, so as to shorten their training. This was possible in part because massage was less complex than acupuncture and also in part because among books about health cultivation there were self-help books that either featured or focused on massage and acupuncture.

Thanks to instructional manuals on massage and acupuncture, which were widely circulated as printed texts, anyone wishing to learn about either profession would have found those texts useful. While there is no clear evidence to suggest if (or how) such manuals were used in professional instruction, self-instruction with texts could have replaced formal training. It is likely that blind people who trained on their own studied those texts with the help of sighted readers and practiced their skills to become masseurs.

In light of the growing popularity of massage starting in the early eighteenth century, blind people could employ their disabled identities to their advantage, and the popular perception about their tactile skills probably also enhanced that advantage: because they were blind, they were suitable to train as masseurs. For a blind man without ties to a lineage or to the guild, the path to become an acupuncturist or masseur could have involved less rigorous training. Accounts about filial children discussed in chapter 4 suggest that blind women tried to find work as masseuses to provide for their families. The shogunate did not object to blind women's participation in the profession, nor does it seem that blind women were banned from learning or practicing acupuncture and massage. But blind masseuses would surely have faced strong competition from blind masseurs, and it would have been more difficult still for blind women than for blind men to train in either profession because of gender discrimination. Blind women were also disadvantaged because they were not represented by the Kyoto guild and were excluded from opportunities.

In the competitive commercial markets, particularly from the early eighteenth century onward, massage was valued commercially. Blind masseurs were free to offer massage to anyone for a fee; they were hired and paid for their labor. Well-informed and well-to-do merchants would surely have been ideal clients. As proof, massage, as well as acupuncture, was mentioned in accounts about approaches to health and illness. References to kneading therapy,[82] Umihara Ryō points out, bespeak the varieties of massage that blind people were engaged to perform.[83]

Could sighted people find employment as masseurs? Likely so. An anecdote from the mid-nineteenth-century source *Stories of Medicine on the Road*,[84] a collection of entertaining stories compiled from hearsay, informs us that Hara Nan'yō was a sighted physician who was said to have practiced massage and acupuncture at his shop in Edo before becoming a physician of the domain lord of Mito domain (in Ibaraki prefecture today).[85] It is possible that there are many more stories out there of sighted people who found work as masseurs, especially in big cities, where job opportunities abounded. Because the guild only had authority over the blind status category, it could not stop sighted people from dabbling in massage for a living. But foreigners who were in Japan in the late nineteenth century were so impressed with blind masseurs that they remarked that blind people monopolized the profession of massage; this suggests a trend that had started in the Tokugawa period that favored the employment of blind masseurs over sighted masseurs.[86]

Evidence from historical records in the Tokugawa period, however, does not always give us clear answers about masseurs' identities. Sighted people interacted with blind people, and Yao Yazaemon's diary offers some perspectives on their complex interactions. Yazaemon was a wine merchant of Itami (near Osaka) who lived in the eighteenth century. He was no stranger to blind visitors and blind professionals because he periodically encountered them in his social circles. He found ways to stay healthy but suffered from frequent ailments, such as abdominal pains and headaches. In his diary, he reported being treated with moxibustion and acupuncture; at least twice, he specifically sought Kōhaku, who may have been a sighted acupuncturist of considerable repute, to perform acupuncture for his benefit.[87] Yazaemon knew a blind musician named Kaden who had been trained in music from the age of twelve, and Yazaemon greatly enjoyed Kaden's musical performances.[88] One time, Yazaemon hired a blind masseur named Ichi no San'uemon (it is unclear if this person was a guild member)—the same blind person to whom, it seems, he had given alms some years earlier.[89] At another time, Yazaemon hired a masseur named Yūsen to perform a massage of acupoints.[90] Yūsen's name, however, does not bear the usual "Jō-" prefix or "-ichi" suffix of the name of a guild member, so it is hard to tell if he was a sighted person, a blind masseur unaffiliated with the guild, or just a novice guild member without a rank.[91]

The shogunate had a vested interest in encouraging the professionalization of massage, particularly through the guild. The guild received support from the shogunate to recognize massage as a mainstay in the professional work that blind people could do for a living. Under status rule, by ensuring that blind people were employed, and employed in a popular profession like massage, the shogunate could count on blind people to provide for themselves and, at the same time, compel them to abide by the laws of the blind status category—working blind people, the shogunate declared, earned their blind status identities through the guild. But, no matter how hard the shogunate tried to strengthen the guild's authority, a blind person's ease of finding work in massage left the guild with the problem of dealing with blind people who should have joined the guild but did not, a problem that chapter 4 discussed.

In a decree of 1813, one of many examples from the eighteenth and nineteenth centuries, the shogunate demanded that all working blind professionals such as masseurs, acupuncturists, medical practitioners, lay religious performers, and musicians register as subjects of the guild.[92] That decree was a variation on earlier decrees and was intended to redefine the guild's scope of authority and to reiterate that the guild's mandate of authority was affirmed by the shogunate. Heads of towns and villages had to cooperate by keeping proper records about blind people and the names of their respective guild masters. Yet, if guild leaders had found out that a blind masseur was not a guild member, it would have been difficult to bar him from continuing his work. Being a nonmember, he had no legal obligation to the guild—his disabled identity was not tied to the guild. In fact, a local government would have considered it more expedient for a blind person to be working in an approved profession despite not having guild membership than to be relying on local charity.

BLIND MASSEURS IN POPULAR LITERATURE

Blind masseurs were literally everywhere by the eighteenth century. While it would be difficult to gather statistical information about them in every town or city, they were so common in the major cities of Edo and Osaka that, in fact, they were widely represented in print culture. In his kaleidoscopic, illustrated series on trades and professions, prolific woodblock print artist Katsushika Hokusai (1760–1849) portrayed blind masseurs. In one style of massage called "foot strength,"[93] a masseur stepped on his client's back and dug in his feet to apply pressure while performing massage with his feet.[94] In another style, a masseur used his hands and fingers to massage his client's shoulders and back.[95] On a regular day, a blind masseur would have walked in the streets, navigating his way with a wooden cane and blowing a small whistle to announce his arrival—this scene would have resonated with the vivid depictions of blind masseurs by foreigners in Japan in the late nineteenth century.[96]

Popular literature reminds us that although the employment options available to blind people were restricted by prevailing circumstances, a blind person had a good chance of being employed as a masseur. *Drops of Japanese Hop: Gossips from Here and There*,[97] a nineteenth-century collection of miscellaneous essays, narrates an account about a blind man named Mizuno Saga'ichi.[98] Saga'ichi considered becoming a musician but was unable to find anyone to teach him music. He abandoned his original plan and instead took up massage. He was said to have trained in the style of the Sugiyama lineage and made a living as a masseur. Though the account neglects to say how exactly he was instructed, or whether he was concurrently trained as an acupuncturist, it is clear that being a masseur was an expedient choice. This account would have reflected the choices of many blind people like Saga'ichi.

Stories in Tokugawa-period popular vernacular literature featured blind masseurs in incidental roles. In a late eighteenth-century popular work of the *kibyōshi* genre (literally, yellow-back book, a genre of illustrated comic and satirical works), such a character serves as a marker of someone's wealth and entitlement. *Dreams of Splendor of Master Flashy*,[99] a yellow-back book by the genre's pioneer, Koikawa Harumachi, tells the story of Kinbē, an unremarkable, provincial person but the perfect protagonist for this genre's comical setting. The story is told through a dream sequence—Roger Thomas discusses the playful use of "dream" in this genre.[100] As we are told, one day, on his way to Edo, Kinbē dozes off at a shop that sells millet cakes. He has a dream that is so vivid that he believes it is real. In this dream, he is an heir to a wealthy merchant. He revels in an extravagant, hedonistic lifestyle and splurges his wealth in the pleasure quarters of the Yoshiwara district of Edo, where he becomes enamored with a courtesan named Kageno. At one point in his dream, to flaunt his nouveau riche status, he hires a blind man named Go'ichi

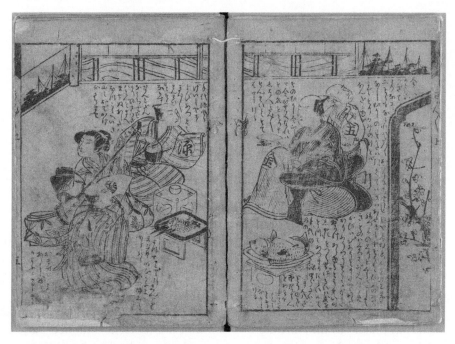

Fig. 6.2. Image of a blind masseur. In the right frame, Kinbē, marked by the character *kin* (a reference to Kinkin Sensei), appears to be receiving a back massage given by a blind masseur. From Koikawa Harumachi, *Dreams of Splendor of Master Flashy* (Japanese title: *Kinkin sensei eiga no yume*, 1775). National Diet Library Digital Collections.

(or Gu'ichi) and a personal assistant, Genshirō.[101] Although the blind man's role is not elaborated, an illustration from the book suggests that he is Kinbē's personal masseur (see figure 6.2). The plot is animated by a hilarious twist at the end. When Kinbē is finally roused from his slumber, he is immediately disabused of his fantasy of riches. In an instant, he is struck by the realization—which passes for a crude and ultimately farcical enlightenment—that life's fleeting splendor is over while he is waiting for a millet cake.[102]

Massage was also featured in at least one work by Jippensha Ikku, another writer who, like Harumachi, was known for writing irreverently humorous fiction. That work, *Travels along the Eastern Highway*[103] (colloquially translated as *Shank's Mare*), is infused with place names, dialects, and innuendoes that linguistically enliven the picaresque adventures of the two bungling, quarrelsome protagonists, Yajirobei (Yaji) and Kitahachi (Kita). Along their travels west of Edo, they stop at an inn in the town of Miya, where they are entertained by two blind female musicians and are treated to a massage by a blind masseur.[104] In an outrageous comedy, the sighted, able-bodied Yaji and Kita are unsympathetically abandoned to the unexpected instincts and whims of disabled characters. While giving a massage, the blind masseur plugs his fingers into Kita's ears and sings a nonsensical chorus. In this fleeting "deaf" instant, the masseur unashamedly belts out vulgarities and mocks Kita, who cannot hear any of the insults. Later that night, one of the blind musicians is rudely awakened from her slumber when Yaji creeps upon her and tries to take liberties with her. Assuming that the intruder is a thief, she reacts violently to his sexual advances. Her startled cries send him scurrying back to his room.

Time and again, for the rest of their escapades, Yaji and Kita are ensnared in blunders of their own doing (and undoing). The "narrative prosthetic" moments in the story, to use the term elaborated by disability studies scholars David Mitchell and Sharon Snyder, turn "disability into both a destabilizing sign of cultural prescriptions about the body *and* a deterministic vehicle of characterization for characters constructed as disabled."[105] Disability is playfully invoked in the narrative episode through two-dimensional blind characters—the blind masseur and the blind musicians—for the purpose of driving the plot to its absurd conclusion. The story succeeds by exploiting the comic potential of sensory impairment. But as it also turns out, much to the surprise of the two lead characters, the blind characters they encounter are not as vulnerable as they appear to be.

Instructional manuals are important sources in popular literature that not only present information about massage and acupuncture but also provide perspectives on popular opinions about blind masseurs and acupuncturists. These sources generally acknowledge the benefits of massage and acupuncture for health cultivation but also include pointed commentary on the skills of blind masseurs and acupuncturists. For example, the vernacular medical treatise *A Convenient Guide on Acupuncture*,[106] published in around 1735 by Hongō Masatoyo, claims to be a source that distilled the most essential truths about acupuncture from various sources.[107] It is critical of the existing state of inadequately trained lay physicians and blind acupuncturists, alleging that in their haste to practice professionally, many blind acupuncturists did not complete their training. Perhaps that was how the work was advertised to readers: as an introduction to the correct principles and techniques of acupuncture.

Another related perspective that blind masseurs were inadequately trained is echoed in many other popular instructional manuals. One of them is *A Guide for Self-Instruction in Massage*[108] (1793), which we consider to be a reproduction of the early eighteenth-century classic manual *Records of the Oral Teachings of Massage*[109] (1713). The text argues that massage was a real medical practice whose health benefits rivaled those of moxibustion and medical prescriptions but advises blind masseurs to undergo thorough vocational training so as to earn proper credentials.[110] Aspirants of shallow learning as well as aspirants without aptitude, the text adds, could not grasp the principles of massage.

A Guide on Massage by Shunki, discussed earlier, offers similar commentary. It says that masseurs were too eager to indulge the fancies of affluent clients that they neglected the historical roots of massage and discredited the profession by causing serious harm to their clients.[111] The influential treatise *An Illustrated Handbook on Massage*[112] (1827), which is attributed to Ōta Shinsai, remarks that many masseurs in society were blind and concurs with the general sentiment that blind masseurs were desperate to earn a living.[113] One important detail is mentioned in *A Guide on Massage*: deaf people also worked as masseurs. This reference to deaf people here suggests that consumers were open to employing deaf masseurs, and it is possible that throughout the Tokugawa period, it was common—or more common than we think—for disabled people with other kinds of impairment to become masseurs.[114]

Conclusion

Being blind could mean being enabled for work in the new niche professions of acupuncture and massage. The context for understanding this argument begins with the seventeenth century. Over that century, social and political developments carved out new professional niches for blind people. Perhaps by chance, blind people who trained in medicine early in the seventeenth century were also people with connections to the shogunate. Because they were recognized by the shogunate for their expertise in acupuncture, they leveraged their success to promote acupuncture as a profession for blind people.

In this regard, the guild, which had become the main institution in governing the blind status category, played a very important role. As the guild broadened its membership, it accepted new professions. Blind acupuncturists who had ties to the shogunate furthered their careers by earning power through the guild's hierarchy. Among them was Wa'ichi, a blind acupuncturist who rose to the apex of the medical profession and the guild in the late seventeenth century. Wa'ichi founded his school of acupuncture and medical lineage, the Sugiyama lineage, with the guild and focused on the vocational training of guild members. While training in acupuncture, guild members also learned massage—we understand that massage and acupuncture have significant overlaps because they both deal with ideas of enhancing the bodily circulation and flow of blood and *ki*. Yet, because the guild had an exclusively male membership, blind women lacked similar access to training in those professions.

Wa'ichi did not develop his ideas in a vacuum. Rather, the development of his medical lineage points to common intellectual frameworks in medical traditions in Japan. His reputation was so broadly associated with his acupuncture styles that sighted students were interested in learning acupuncture from him. To this end, the Shinden lineage, an eighteenth-century lineage that can be traced to Wa'ichi's successors, trained sighted acupuncturists.

By the eighteenth century, ideas of health cultivation that spread through popular medical culture emphasized good health for men, women, and children and stimulated interest in the therapeutic role of massage. Readers and consumers of print culture read books about health cultivation and hired masseurs, and this context in which massage became popular encouraged guild members to focus on massage. By asserting their disabled identities, blind people could even try to train in massage without joining the guild. Massage became the default profession of blind people and was so intertwined with blind masseurs that they were represented in popular literature. This fact that massage employed so many blind people that they dominated the profession certainly attracted the attention of foreign visitors to Japan in the late nineteenth century.

Epilogue

Onward to the Meiji Period

———— ·ᘐᐩ· ————

When we look back on the history of blind people in Tokugawa Japan, we will remember the Kyoto guild as a formidable political institution in that culture and period. As chapters 3 and 4 discussed, the guild influenced—both directly and indirectly—blind people's lives and livelihoods. For most guild members, the guild's most important role was to prepare them for careers in music and medicine or to give them broad access to alms. The guild's elites, who formed a minority, acquired more power and influence than the rest of the guild. As much as the guild enabled blind people's disabled identities, it also exploited vulnerable guild members and disabled them in social and economic ways. Just as significant is the fact that many blind people who did not join the guild for various reasons were not free from the guild's dictates to conform to its expectations.

In 1871, several years after the Meiji government came to power, the guild was dismantled.[1] Regarded as a remnant of the Tokugawa regime, the guild simply did not have a place in Meiji Japan's vision of a modern future. The government's repudiation of Tokugawa-era institutions, which included the abolition of domains, set Japan on the path of nation building.

The guild's demise signaled the end of an important chapter in the history of blind people.[2] More important, its demise had a profound impact on society. Guild members who had spent their savings on ranks were left with ranks that were rendered meaningless overnight. As government authorities took a tough stance against itinerant professions, the guild's blind musicians and religious performers no longer had recourse to justify their rights to alms from patrons. Blind people who received stipends from the guild and those who accessed charity through their domain governments were ever more dependent on their families and home communities for support.[3]

Blind lay priests and blind female musicians—the two main social groups of blind people against whom the guild discriminated, as discussed in chapter 4—were not immune to social and political reforms in Meiji society.[4] Blind priests were forced to reorganize their groups under a new form of temple administration, while blind female musicians tried to maintain their musical traditions in their kinship groups.

The Meiji regime's modernizing impulse that catalyzed the elimination of the guild also stimulated the gestation of modern medicine. Modern medicine was introduced in Meiji Japan through the university-based medical education that supplanted Tokugawa-period academies and the lineage-based system of learning. Traditional medical lineages, which were discussed in chapters 1 and 6, were denigrated as being outdated. They were excluded from the new university-based teaching model and declined in importance and influence.

Europeans such as German military physician Leopold Müller were welcomed by the Meiji government to professionalize Japanese medicine and align Japanese medical education with the standards in Europe.[5] German-Japanese medical exchanges became prominent, with the transfer of medical expertise from Germany to Japan through German physicians stationed in Japan as well as through Japanese students educated abroad in Europe. Ophthalmology was fundamentally transformed on the basis of Western medical thought and clinical methods, eclipsing the Tokugawa-period models of Sino-Japanese and Dutch-method medicine, which chapter 1 discussed. As networks of medical training colleges and hospitals expanded across Japan from the late nineteenth century onward, ophthalmology was more widely taught to medical students, producing a critical mass of Japanese ophthalmologists with the expertise to engage in research.

The Tokugawa period's culture of health cultivation, which chapter 6 discussed, gave way in the Meiji period to a national culture that interpreted physical, mental, and intellectual fitness through a different framework. While the traditional term for health cultivation (*yōjō*) remained in use in Meiji society, the Japanese term that gained currency was *eisei* (hygiene).[6] The Meiji state's preoccupation with public sanitation and public health, which were studied as aspects of hygiene, reflected the national, and also ideological, turn toward biological, medical formulations of health. Able-bodiedness was a concrete expression of biological health and, by extension, the symbolic health of the national body writ large.[7]

In the new context of health in which the Meiji state regarded personal health as a reflection of collective health, the goals of ophthalmology and hygiene converged in significant ways. Standards for testing vision were developed in the military to evaluate conscripts' visual acuity.[8] As schools and compulsory education for children were introduced,[9] a specific branch of hygiene called school hygiene[10] studied the relationship between the school environment and students' psychological and physical health, including vision.[11]

In that same context, the Meiji state identified highly communicable diseases, such as smallpox, measles, syphilis, and trachoma (which were discussed in chapters 1 and 2), as threats to public health. The national approach to public health expanded vaccinations against smallpox.[12] Eye clinics played a major role in these national public health campaigns. In fact, trachoma was so politicized as a stigma of underdeveloped societies that its eradication was viewed as a political measure of Japanese society's progress vis-à-vis Western societies.[13]

In light of the Meiji state's coordinated, national efforts to strengthen medical education and improve public health, we can imagine that people suffering from any kind of visual impairment could choose from, as well as benefit from, a wide array of medical treatments.[14] We can also imagine that people in Meiji society were open to trying different kinds of cure for their eye conditions. What was new in Meiji society, however, was the prevalence of a rhetoric of cure that suited the national agenda— the agenda that elevated Western medicine and promoted Western cures as modern cures, as opposed to native, popular cures.[15]

Another area of change was education. Education of disabled students, which was inaugurated in major Japanese cities, was a notable feature of Meiji education that was in sharp contrast to the Tokugawa period. The first school for blind and deaf students was the Kyoto Deaf-Mute Institution (Kyoto Mōain), established in 1878 to fulfill the Ministry of Education's plan for "schools for handicapped people" (*haijin gakkō*).[16] Schools that were founded in close succession in 1879 and 1880 included the Tokyo Institution for Blind Education (Tokyo Kunmōin), which was the predecessor of the Tokyo School for the Blind and Deaf-

Mute (Tokyo Mōagakkō), and the Osaka Model School for the Blind and Deaf-Mute (Osaka Mohan Mōagakkō).[17] Early experimental forms of braille were developed with tactile Japanese characters; the braille template that was developed by Ishikawa Kuraji was approved for use in classrooms in 1890.[18] Those schools underwent institutional reorganization in the early twentieth century to form separate schools for blind students and for deaf students.[19]

As education of blind students was a novel idea in the Meiji period, it is likely that the vast majority of Japan's blind population did not have access to education. What did not change during the Meiji period, and even thereafter, was that blind people worked in the niche professions of music, acupuncture, and massage—professions that the guild in the Tokugawa period had enabled and supported. The popularity of those professions in the Tokugawa period, discussed in chapters 5 and 6, explains why schools in Meiji society prepared blind students for similar careers. For example, at the Tokyo School for the Blind and Deaf-Mute, the general ordinary track underscored the study of academic subjects, while through the vocational track, blind students were taught music, acupuncture, massage, and moxibustion.[20] Musical training in the latter track focused on *koto* music, which was popularly performed by blind musicians during the Tokugawa period. It is likely that many blind people without the means to go to school learned vocational skills on their own.

To break with the preceding Tokugawa-period practices of medical lineages and academies in medical learning, the Meiji state developed a system to license acupuncturists and masseurs. Sighted people were recognized in those professions, and anyone, including blind people, seeking to practice professionally was required to earn accreditation. The Ministry of the Interior issued directives in 1911 (which were revised in 1920) that gave the superintendent general of the government police the power to approve the licensing of acupuncturists and masseurs.[21] Cities and prefectures approached the regulation of acupuncturists and masseurs differently within a broadly defined national framework that devolved authority to local bureaucratic apparatuses to conduct licensing and checks.[22]

For those blind students with some means, education gave them opportunities to become leaders. Blind graduates of schools could aspire to become teachers, while sighted trainees could also train to become teachers in blind education.[23] Exceptional blind students even attended universities. One of the most prominent blind activists was Iwahashi

Takeo, who was born in the late Meiji period in 1898. He briefly attended the Osaka Municipal (City) School for the Blind and later graduated from Kwansei Gakuin University.[24] Throughout his career as an activist, he was an advocate for blind people's rights to welfare and education, and through his friendship with blind-deaf American activist Helen Keller he played a crucial role in introducing transnational disability activism to Japan in the years shortly before World War II.[25]

This epilogue does not, of course, offer a comprehensive view of the developments in Meiji society. Rather, it traces in broad strokes those developments that continue the discussion of Tokugawa society. In the Meiji period, blindness was still studied and treated as an array of disabling conditions, and in medicine, ophthalmology was redefined through the interpretive, authoritative perspectives of Western medical education and hygiene.

As the social, cultural, and political contours of Meiji Japan's history show, in Tokugawa Japan's transition to the Meiji period, not all developments were contiguous; some breaks were more disruptive than others. Old institutions were displaced and removed. Lives that were sustained by those institutions were even upended. Yet, as new institutions took root, some remnants of old lives persisted and found new ways to survive. Blind people did not relinquish their agency on the historical stage of Meiji society.

Certainly, tracing Japan's historical narrative from Tokugawa society to Meiji society appears to confirm the current linear, teleological narrative of modern history: that as societies marched inexorably toward progress, lives became better because of advances in areas such as science, medicine, technology, and education. Yet, instead of searching for evidence that fits a teleological narrative, it is more important for us to conclude that Tokugawa society developed in important ways: that the ways blindness—or, more generally, visual impairment—was socialized, politicized, and medicalized in the Tokugawa period made Tokugawa society different from Meiji society, not less modern than Meiji society.

When we peer into the histories of blindness and blind people in Tokugawa society, we realize that those histories are unique because they were shaped by particular conditions in Tokugawa society: its intellectual frameworks, popular thought and culture, laws, political ideologies and rhetoric, and social and political values and practices.

In Tokugawa society, the lives of blind people—how they were supported, how they chose to live, and how their lives were disabled and enabled—were torn by tensions between enablement and exploitation in a social and political system unlike any seen in other societies, and that constructed unique experiences of disability. Blindness was the most remarkable disability of Tokugawa society in ways that were not equivalent or even comparable in the Meiji period.

Examining Tokugawa society in its own right lets us make sense of disability and the social, political, medical, and cultural contexts in which we understand the complex answer of what it meant to be blind in that period: that being blind was about being disabled and that it was also about being enabled in ways that we can only interpret and appreciate through those same contexts.

More broadly, this approach allows us to understand Tokugawa society through the perspectives of disability history. This analysis offers a starting point for future discussions of how we can narrate and connect a nation's history through studies of disability in different periods. Perhaps we can envision a future of greater interdisciplinary scholarship in which new disability histories blossom in new writings about national histories.

Notes

Preface

1. Wortley, "Yellow Brick Roads," August 22, 2020.
2. Choe, "Blind Masseurs in South Korea Worry about the Loss of Status," September 17, 2008. South Korea, as well as China, hires blind people as masseurs.
3. Sean O'Reilly, personal email communication, October 10, 2020. I thank Sean O'Reilly for reminding me of the memorable scenes of massage and music in the movies.

Introduction

1. Japanese title: *Heike monogatari*. *Heikyoku* or *Heike* music is the lyrical performance of the tale.
2. Japanese title: *Gunsho ruijū*.
3. *Shōgai*: [障害]; *shikaku shōgai* (visual impairment): [視覚障害]. *Shōgai* is sometimes written as [障がい] to avoid using the second *kanji* character, which can mean "harm" or "detriment." See also Stevens, *Disability in Japan*, 47–57. Expressions used today such as *me ga/no mienai hito* (a person who cannot see) and *me ga/no fujiyū na hito* (literally, a person with an inconvenience with the eyes) describe a visually impaired person's lack of sight (or diminished ability to see).
4. "Shōgaisha kihonhō" (E-Gov Japan).
5. Inasaka, *Sanba kokoroe*, image 79; Hirahara, *Ganka kanmei*, image 14. Meiji-period authors used *shōgai* for its literal meaning of "obstruction," "damage," or "impediment" in the medical context—hence, it could refer to "impairment." For example, it appears in texts on obstetrics and gynecology to refer to "obstruction" in birth. It also means "impairment" of vision in some texts on ophthalmology. *Shōgai* was not a standard word in the Tokugawa period.
6. Japanese term: *kanpō igaku* (Sino-Japanese medicine). Elman, "Rethinking the Sino-Japanese Medical Classics," 1–18; Trambaiolo, "Ancient Texts and New Medical Ideas in Eighteenth-Century Japan," 81–104.
7. Berry, *Japan in Print*, 209.

189

8. Gordon, *A Modern History of Japan*, 11–21; Hall, "The *Bakuhan* System," 150–69.

9. Japanese: *daimyō* (or daimyo in Anglicized spelling).

10. This system is known as *mibunseido* or *mibunsei*.

11. Howell, *Geographies of Identity in Nineteenth-Century Japan*, 21.

12. Howell, *Geographies of Identity in Nineteenth-Century Japan*, 33–34 and 45.

13. This is a streamlined picture of the status system. See also Groemer, "The Creation of the Edo Outcaste Order," 264. I use the word "outcast" to refer to the outcast status of the Tokugawa period instead of "outcaste," which Groemer and other scholars have used to separate the medieval and early modern outcast identities.

14. Ehlers, *Give and Take*, 5–6.

15. Howell, *Geographies of Identity in Nineteenth-Century Japan*, 22. I share Howell's reasons for avoiding the conventional language of the Confucian hierarchical ordering of status. Social organizations, as Howell points out, were dynamically composed, and among commoners, for example, there were various occupations and intersecting status identities.

16. Japanese characters: [当道座] (*tōdōza*).

17. Howell, *Geographies of Identity in Nineteenth-Century Japan*, 40.

18. Katō Yasuaki's book *Nihon mōjin shakaishi kenkyū*, to date, offers the most comprehensive book-length study of the guild. See also Groemer, "The Guild of the Blind in Tokugawa Japan," 349–80.

19. Groemer, *Goze*, xvii.

20. Nakamura, *Deaf in Japan*, 12. As Nakamura notes, "The diverse identities created by the product of a physical impairment, social institutions, family, history, and individuality all contradict an essentialized, unitary, and mandatory nature to deaf existence."

21. Yamada, *Tsūshi: Nihon no shōgaisha*, 168–80; Pennington, *Casualties of History*, 216–17. The Law on the Welfare of People with Physical Disabilities (*Shintai shōgaisha fukushi hō*) of 1949 was enacted in 1950. The original law identified the categories of visual and hearing impairment, linguistic impairment, physical impairment (due to severed limbs or the impaired functions of limbs), and impairment of the central nervous system.

22. The Japanese word *rai* is often translated as "leprosy." This translation preserves the historical meaning of the original Japanese word. (The current standard translation is "Hansen's disease.")

23. Suzuki, "Kinsei raibyōkan no keisei to tenkai," 96–100; Burns, *Kingdom of the Sick*, 47–73.

24. Yokota, "Monoyoshi kō," 13–27. The Japanese word *raisha* refers to people with leprosy. The word "leper" is used only to show the direct link to the word for leprosy.

25. Groemer, *Street Performers and Society in Urban Japan*, 56.

26. Howell, *Geographies of Identity in Nineteenth-Century Japan*, 33–34 and 45.

27. De Ferranti, *The Last Biwa Singer*; Kinda'ichi, *Heikyoku kō*; Komoda, *Heike no ongaku*.

28. See Rapp and Ginsburg, "Enabling Disability," 552. Rapp and Ginsburg eloquently discuss kinship in the lives and stories of people with disabilities and their families to create more inclusive practices in society. Here, I interpret how disability was enabled in a different kind of historical context, with a focus on disability history, not anthropology.

29. Batten, "From Segregation to Civil Rights," 399.

30. Section 4: "Disability Defined and Rules of Construction," ADA Amendments Act of 2008.

31. Heyer, *Rights Enabled*, 126–28 and 165–66.

32. Heyer, *Rights Enabled*, 146.

33. Stevens, *Disability in Japan*, 64.

34. Otake, "New Law Bans Bias against People with Disabilities, but Shortcomings Exist, Say Experts," May 2, 2016.

35. Nielsen, *A Disability History of the United States*, 54–56.

36. Weygand, *The Blind in French Society from the Middle Ages to the Century of Louis Braille*, 175–77.

37. Curran, "Diderot's Revisionism," 75–93; Paulson, *Enlightenment, Romanticism, and the Blind in France*, 39–71. In France and England, philosophers such as Denis Diderot and John Locke were heavily invested in philosophical investigations of blindness to test theories about sensory deprivation. The Molyneux problem, discussed by Locke, was a thought experiment. It focused on solving in empirical terms whether a person born blind, if he had gained sight, could recognize physical shapes that he had only learned conceptually.

38. Weygand, *The Blind in French Society from the Middle Ages to the Century of Louis Braille*, 87–109.

39. Husson, *Reflections*, 8–9. For more about the medieval origins of the Quinze-Vingts, see Weygand, *The Blind in French Society from the Middle Ages to the Century of Louis Braille*, 11–23.

40. Weygand, "Blind Love," 224–25.

41. Freeberg, *The Education of Laura Bridgman*, 7–28.

42. Burch and Rembis, "Re-Membering the Past," 5–6.

43. Burch and Rembis, "Re-Membering the Past," 3.

44. Nielsen, *The Life of Anna Ott*, 6.

45. DasGupta, "Medicalization," 120.

46. Nielsen, *A Disability History of the United States*, 86. Nielsen explains that the American Civil War (1861–65) precipitated large-scale systemic changes in pensions for disability that had been in place after the Revolutionary War, and medical diagnoses were increasingly invoked to certify disabled veterans for disability pensions.

47. Linker, "On the Borderland of Medical and Disability History," 519–20.

48. Shakespeare, "The Social Model of Disability," 216–17.

49. Shakespeare, "The Social Model of Disability," 217–18.

50. Couser, "Illness," 105–107.

51. Horn and Frohne, "On the Fluidity of 'Disability' in Medieval and Early Modern Societies," 18. As Klaus-Peter Horn and Bianca Frohne write about the premodern European context, "Even though the term 'disability' was not used by medieval and early modern authors, this concept may be helpful to understand aspects of corporeal 'difference' in pre-modern societies."

52. Scalenghe, *Disability in the Ottoman Arab World*, 10. Scalenghe supports "a social constructionist approach that employs the 'social model' of disability." She adds that "disability is the systemic societal response to perceived impairments."

53. Metzler, *A Social History of Disability in the Middle Ages*, 4.

54. Scalenghe, *Disability in the Ottoman Arab World*, 79.

55. Scalenghe, *Disability in the Ottoman Arab World*, 79.

56. Siebers, "Returning the Social to the Social Model," 47.
57. Siebers, "Returning the Social to the Social Model," 47.
58. Siebers, "Returning the Social to the Social Model," 47.
59. Wheatley, *Stumbling Blocks before the Blind*, 6.
60. Wheatley, *Stumbling Blocks before the Blind*, 13–14.
61. Kudlick, "Social History of Medicine and Disability History," 119; Kudlick, "Comment: On the Borderland of Medical and Disability History," 549.
62. Waldschmidt, "Disability Goes Cultural," 24–25.
63. Snyder and Mitchell, *Cultural Locations of Disability*, 7.
64. Hughes and Paterson, "The Social Model of Disability and the Disappearing Body," 329. Hughes and Paterson criticize the social model because "the definition of impairment proposed by the social model of disability recapitulates the biomedical 'faulty machine' model of the body" that is "a pre-social, inert, physical object, as discrete, palpable and separate from the self."
65. Hughes and Paterson, "Disability Studies and Phenomenology," 603. Sociological approaches to impairment have challenged the assumed stability of impairment as an unchanging biological and medical fact.
66. Bolt, *The Metanarrative of Blindness*, 17–22.
67. Kim, *Curative Violence*, 11–17.
68. Kim, *Curative Violence*, 15.
69. Kim, *Curative Violence*, 14.

Chapter 1

1. Japanese: *zō* (organs, or depots) and *fu* (viscera, or palaces).
2. *Huang Di Nei Jing Su Wen*, vol. 1, 17–18.
3. Chinese title: *Huangdi neijing*; Japanese title: *Kōtei daikyō/daikei*.
4. Japanese: *kanpō yaku*.
5. Japanese: *sanshō*, or "triple burner."
6. *Kōtei daikyō/daikei somon*, image 23; *Huang Di Nei Jing Su Wen*, vol. 1, 106.
7. *Kōtei daikyō/daikei somon*, image 20; *Huang Di Nei Jing Su Wen*, vol. 1, 91.
8. *Huang Di Nei Jing Ling Shu*, 255.
9. Kuriyama, *The Expressiveness of the Body and the Divergence of Greek and Chinese Medicine*, 168.
10. *Kōtei daikyō/daikei somon*, image 43; *Huang Di Nei Jing Su Wen*, vol. 1, 190.
11. *Huang Di Nei Jing Ling Shu*, 191.
12. Kuriyama, *The Expressiveness of the Body and the Divergence of Greek and Chinese Medicine*, 161–62.
13. *Huang Di Nei Jing Su Wen*, vol. 1, 168.
14. Japanese title: *Ishinpō*.
15. Japanese: Ten'yakuryō.
16. Triplett, "Using the Golden Needle," 543–45.
17. Kogawa, *Kōhon Nihon ganka gakushi*, 49–53.
18. Japanese title: *Owari meisho zue*.
19. Japanese name: Yakushi Nyorai (Sanskrit: Bhaiṣajyaguru).
20. Yamada, "Hōraiji to Mikawa Owari no Yakushi shinkō," 79–96.
21. Suzuki, *Medicine Master Buddha*, 16–24.
22. Shinmura, *Nihon iryōshi*, 106–7.
23. Mishima, *The History of Ophthalmology in Japan*, 134–35. Mishima suggests that

the Myōgen'in parent lineage was systematized through the textual transmission of a scroll that only highly qualified disciples were allowed to receive.

24. *Owari meisho zue* (chūkan), 223–28. Myōgen'in was said to be a temple affiliated with the Japanese Tendai Buddhist sect.

25. Tanihara, "Hyōshi no kaisetsu," 978–79.

26. Japanese title: *Majima Myōgen'in megusuri*. The preface suggests the author to be someone named Toyoshima Hōkyō Rōgetsusai.

27. *Majima Myōgen'in megusuri*, images 11–13.

28. The temple was Kōenji. In the text, the temple Kōenji is periodically mentioned with the *kanji* characters reversed (Enkōji), suggesting some confusion about the name.

29. Kornicki, "Manuscript, not Print," 34.

30. Japanese: *hidensho*.

31. Japanese title: *Ganryō tōun hiroku*. The text is attributed to Majima Daikōbō (a Majima sub-lineage leader). Comparisons with other Chinese and Japanese texts suggest that the text was copied from different sources.

32. *Ganryō tōun hiroku*, image 15. Some phrases are "shinchi kuden," "hari o mochiyu kuden," and "kuden ari."

33. Umihara, "Kinsei ganka'i no mibun sonritsu to gakutō," 20–21. Secret texts still retained some value for the lineage that asserted ownership of them, even though a text could be circulated to any extent upon the discretion of the actual owner.

34. Chinese title: *Yinhai jingwei*; Japanese title: *Ginkai seibi*. Mishima, *The History of Ophthalmology in Japan*, 102.

35. Kovacs and Unschuld, *Essential Subtleties on the Silver Sea*, 53–54. This ophthalmological treatise is sometimes attributed to the famous Chinese physician Sun Simiao, whose life spanned much of the seventh century. But as Kovacs and Unschuld highlight, it is more likely a Ming-dynasty work because of its medical references to the Song-Jin-Yuan dynasties.

36. Chinese: *wu lun*; Japanese: *gorin*.

37. Chinese: *ba kuo*; Japanese: *hakkaku*.

38. Kovacs and Unschuld, *Essential Subtleties on the Silver Sea*, 44–45 and 58–59. I follow Kovacs and Unschuld in using the translations "five spheres" and "eight boundaries." See also Mishima, *The History of Ophthalmology in Japan*, 101. Mishima suggests that the idea of "eight boundaries" (or enclosures) had Chinese origin, traced to a medical text of the Yuan dynasty.

39. *Ganryō tōun hiroku*, image 11.

40. *Ganryō tōun hiroku*, image 12. Among the viscera, the *sanshō* was replaced by the *meimon* (gate of life) conduit.

41. *Suwa shishi* (chūkan), 734–35; *Ganmoku taizen*, images 8–10. In the treatise *Ganmoku taizen*, the lineage of Takeuchi Shinpachi (the Takeuchi lineage), known for its activities in and around Shinshū (in the Shinano area) in the early Tokugawa period, reiterated the same concept for understanding the eyes' interdependent relationships with the organs and viscera.

42. Chinese: *feng*. Chinese and Japanese medical texts, in general, mention that "winds" caused diseases.

43. Kuriyama, *The Expressiveness of the Body and the Divergence of Greek and Chinese Medicine*, 234.

44. *Kōtei daikyō/daikei somon*, images 55 and 83; *Huang Di Nei Jing Su Wen*, vol. 1, 269 and 359 (Zhang Jiebin's commentary).

45. *Kōtei daikyō/daikei somon*, image 157.
46. *Kōtei daikyō/daikei somon*, image 158.
47. *Huang Di Nei Jing Ling Shu*, 672.
48. Trambaiolo, "Epidemics and Epistemology in Early Modern Japan," 162.
49. Kovacs and Unschuld, *Essential Subtleties on the Silver Sea*, 173–74. Chinese: *tianxing chiyan*; Japanese: *tenkō sekigan*. As the Japanese and Chinese references appear similar, I use the translation "epidemic red eyes."
50. Japanese: *maku*.
51. Japanese: *doniku*.
52. Japanese: *yami me*.
53. *Ganryō tōun hiroku*, image 13.
54. Japanese: *yonjū hachi gan*.
55. Kovacs and Unschuld, *Essential Subtleties on the Silver Sea*, 174. As Kovacs and Unschuld explain, the five-day period of recovery mentioned in the Chinese source was calculated based on Chinese divisions of seasonal periods.
56. Kovacs and Unschuld, *Essential Subtleties on the Silver Sea*, 170–73.
57. Kovacs and Unschuld, *Essential Subtleties on the Silver Sea*, 236–37.
58. Inoue, *Ganbyō torahōmu ron*, 10–13 (images 25–26); Inoue, *Kingan torahōmu ryōyōhō*, 98–105 (images 55–58).
59. Inoue, *Kingan torahōmu ryōyōhō*, 72–76 (images 42–44).
60. Japanese: *kasumi* (blurred or blurry); Japanese: *daku* (*nigoru*), literally, "cloudy" or "muddy."
61. See also *Ganryō tōun hiroku*, image 25. Names of foreign substances imported from (and through) China were written with the *kanji* notation "tō" or "kara" (a reference to China). The Majima lineage could have studied the more contemporary Chinese, Ming-dynasty *Bencao gangmu* (*Encyclopedia of Materia Medica*) by Li Shizhen. However, it is not clear how extensively the Majima lineage appropriated the pharmacological knowledge of *Bencao gangmu* because it drew heavily upon traditional formularies of Majima medicines.
62. *Ganryō tōun hiroku*, image 24.
63. *Ganryō tōun hiroku*, image 25.
64. Chinese: *qing mang* [清盲]; Japanese: *seimō*.
65. Chinese: *qing mang* [青盲] (a homonym of [清盲] in modern Chinese; Japanese: *seimō*). See also Deshpande, "Indian Influences on Early Chinese Ophthalmology," 308–16. Here, I follow Deshpande's translation of *qing mang* [青盲] as "glaucous blindness," as the symptoms were quite characteristic of glaucoma.
66. Japanese: *akishii* (clear blindness). *Ishinpō*, images 277–78. For a full translation of the entry in *Ishinpō*, see Triplett, "Using the Golden Needle," 545–47.
67. Chinese: *fu yi*.
68. *Ishinpō*, image 279.
69. *Ishinpō*, image 280.
70. Deshpande, "Ophthalmic Surgery," 378.
71. Japanese: *naishō* or *sokohi* (internal obstruction); *uwahi* or *gaishō* (external obstruction).
72. Japanese title: *Byōmei ikai*. *Byōmei ikai*, vol. 3, image 69.
73. Chinese: *nei zhang* (internal obstruction); *wai zhang* (external obstruction). Deshpande, "Indian Influences on Early Chinese Ophthalmology," 318–19. See also Zhang and Unschuld, *Dictionary of the Ben Cao Gang Mu*, vol. 1, 353–54. Zhang and

Unschuld translate *nei zhang* as "internal screen" and *wai zhang* as "external screen"; the related term *zhang yi* is translated as "obstructive shade."

74. *Ganryō tōun hiroku*, images 47–48; *Majima-ryū megusuri hisho*, image 5.

75. For an overview of the "obstructive" conditions described in the Majima texts, see Mishima, *The History of Ophthalmology in Japan*, 117.

76. Japanese title: *Majima-ryū ganmoku hidensho*.

77. *Majima-ryū ganmoku hidensho*, image 9.

78. *Ganryō tōun hiroku*, image 14.

79. *Ganryō tōun hiroku*, images 14–15 and 33.

80. *Ganmoku taizen*, images 37 and 69.

81. Jannetta, "Diseases of the Early Modern Period in Japan," 386.

82. Jannetta, *The Vaccinators*, 132–49 and 160–80.

83. Trambaiolo, "Vaccination and the Politics of Medical Knowledge in Nineteenth-Century Japan," 431–35. As Trambaiolo points out, the shogunate favored Sino-Japanese medicine and proponents of Sino-Japanese medicine.

84. Japanese: *doku*.

85. Aoki, *Edo jidai no igaku*, 82–83. Yoshimasu Tōdō favored the concrete formularies and therapies of *Shanghanlun* (*Treatise on Cold Damage*; Japanese: *Shōkanron*) of the late Han dynasty of China. For a discussion of Tōdō's ideas of drugs with "poison," see Trambaiolo, "Writing, Authority and Practice in Tokugawa Japan," 90.

86. Japanese title: *Idan*.

87. *Idan*, images 23–24.

88. One example is *hōsō no me* [疱瘡之目]. *Ganmoku taizen*, image 54; *Ganryō tōun hiroku*, image 20.

89. Japanese title: (*Zoku*) *Tōka ben'yō*.

90. (*Zoku*) *Tōka ben'yō*, images 109–10.

91. Japanese title: *Ikeda sensei chitō kuketsu*. It was written by Saitō (Jun) Kōan.

92. *Ikeda sensei chitō kuketsu*, image 39.

93. Japanese: *ryōkaku. Gardenia jasminoides* (*kuchinashi*); Forsythia (*rengyō*).

94. Japanese title: *Kōkei saikyūhō*.

95. The shogunate medical school was the Igakkan. Machi, "Igakkan no gakumon keisei (1)," 354–60.

96. *Kōkei saikyūhō*, images 177–78.

97. Japanese: *suisen no ne*.

98. Japanese: *rokujō*.

99. Japanese: *tsuki me*.

100. *Kōkei saikyūhō*, images 178–79.

101. *Mannō* ointment (an ointment for universal use) could be added.

102. Japanese: Nagasaki *bugyō*.

103. Jannetta, *The Vaccinators*, 3. I follow Jannetta's translations of *rangaku* and *ranpō* and use Dutch learning for *rangaku* and Dutch-method medicine for *ranpō* throughout this chapter.

104. Japanese: *jitsugaku* (practical learning).

105. Marcon, "Inventorying Nature," 203.

106. Jannetta, *The Vaccinators*, 96.

107. Dutch title: *Ontleedkundigen tafelen*. Tan, "The Brain in Text and in Image," 94–95; Low, "Medical Representations of the Body in Japan," 350–52. Kulmus's work, upon publication, was criticized by European scholars for lacking in scholarly value.

108. Japanese title: *Kaitai shinsho.*
109. Johnson, *Western Influences on Japanese Art,* 49–59.
110. For a discussion of the different approaches to Tokugawa medicine, see Trambaiolo, "Native and Foreign in Tokugawa Medicine," 299–324.
111. Jansen, "Rangaku and Westernization," 541–53.
112. Elman, "Sinophiles and Sinophobes in Tokugawa Japan," 115–16.
113. For an example of this common narrative, see Screech, *The Lens within the Heart,* 166–70.
114. Aoki, *Edo jidai no igaku,* 147–48.
115. Japanese title: *Ganka shinsho.*
116. Latin title: *Doctrina de morbis oculorum.*
117. *Ganka shinsho,* vol. 1, images 13–16.
118. *Ganka shinsho,* vol. 1, image 6.
119. *Ganka shinsho,* vol. 1, image 7.
120. Japanese title: *Ganka kinnō.*
121. Japanese: *shinkei* (nerve, or more literally, spirit conduits); *shōshieki* (vitreous humor).
122. *Ganka kinnō,* vol. 1, image 18. See also *Kaitai shinsho,* vol. 2, image 15; *Kaitai shinsho, jozu,* image 24.
123. *Ganka kinnō,* vol. 1, images 19 and 22.
124. Japanese: *suishōeki. Ganka kinnō,* vol. 1, image 18.
125. *Ganka kinnō,* vol. 3, images 19–20.
126. *Dassairoku,* images 4–5 and 10–11.
127. Japanese: *gankyū gan.*
128. *Byōmei ikai.*
129. *Byōmei ikai,* vol. 5, image 36.
130. This disease was known as *kohatsu.*
131. *Ganka shinsho,* vol. 2, image 23; *Ganka shinsho,* vol. 3, images 21–22.
132. Japanese: *taidoku. Ganka kinnō,* vol. 3, images 24–26; Thompson, *Vietnamese Traditional Medicine,* 19–20. This theory was likely postulated in the Song dynasty in China and had become influential in Tokugawa Japan. It considered "fetal poison," thought to be "poison" latent in the human body from birth, to be a cause of smallpox.
133. Shinmura, *Kodai iryō kanninsei no kenkyū,* 384–88. The medical use of leeches was an ancient technique discussed in medical texts of China and Japan and had been an accepted practice.
134. Shinmura, *Nihon iryōshi,* 164.
135. Rubinger, *Private Academies of the Tokugawa Period,* 107–11.
136. Ban, *Tekijuku o meguru hitobito,* 88–125.
137. For a discussion of *rangaku* networks, see Jackson, *Network of Knowledge,* 82–85.
138. Aoki, *Zaison rangaku no kenkyū,* 45–78.
139. Endō, "Iinuma-juku to sono monjin no dōkō," 77–78.
140. Rubinger, *Private Academies of the Tokugawa Period,* 115–17.
141. Rubinger, *Private Academies of the Tokugawa Period,* 117–18; Frumer, *Making Time,* 119–20 and 143–44. Siebold was accused of possessing and smuggling maps of Japan, considered to be a treasonous act that violated the shogunate's harsh isolationist and censorship policies.
142. Miyazaki, "Shīboruto no sandō tengan'yaku," 469–73.
143. Japanese name: *hashiridokoro.*

144. Japanese title: *Shīboruto kenpōroku.* For more about calomel, see image 9.

145. Japanese title: *Yakuhin ōshuroku.* The publication date is suggested to be 1886, but before then handwritten copies could have been circulated.

146. *Yakuhin ōshuroku,* image 7.

147. *Yakuhin ōshuroku,* image 8.

148. *Yakuhin ōshuroku,* image 13.

149. Trambaiolo, "Antisyphilitic Mercury Drugs in Early Modern China and Japan," 1010–13; Suzuki, "Edo jidai no igakusho ni miru baidokukan ni tsuite," 44–48.

150. Japanese title: *Kubai yōhō.*

151. *Kubai yōhō,* images 66–67.

152. *Shīboruto kenpōroku,* image 9.

153. Dormandy, *Opium,* 45–61. The name Laudanum, maybe from the word "laud," was linked to Paracelsus (or his disciple), a sixteenth-century Swiss physician and alchemist. After falling into disuse, the name was revived by Thomas Sydenham, a seventeenth-century English physician.

154. *Shīboruto kenpōroku,* image 10.

155. *Shīboruto kenpōroku,* image 19.

156. *Shīboruto kenpōroku,* image 8.

157. *Shīboruto kenpōroku,* image 19. A mixture without opium could be prepared by mixing mercury, rose honey, and gum Arabic in water.

Chapter 2

1. Recent studies of Greco-Roman antiquity and early modern England discuss how popular medicines and popular medical knowledge are not unproblematic categories. See, for example, Harris, "Popular Medicine in the Classical World," 1–21; Curth, *English Almanacs, Astrology, and Popular Medicine,* 1–8.

2. Hur, *Prayer and Play in Late Tokugawa Japan*; Hardacre, *Religion and Society in Nineteenth-Century Japan*; Nenzi, *Excursions of Identity.*

3. I interpret "folk" broadly and do not force a distinction between folk beliefs and popular beliefs.

4. Japanese title: *Kyūmin myōyaku* (or *Kyūmin myōyakushū*). The work was reissued with an updated preface as *Zōho kyūmin myōyaku* (*Expanded and Updated Edition: Miraculous Medicines for Saving the Populace,* 1806) and had a lot in common with *Shomin myōyakuhō* (*Prescriptions of Miraculous Medicines for Various Peoples*).

5. *Kyūmin myōyaku,* images 4–5. See also Suzuki Eiichi, "Mito-han no igaku to iryō," 160.

6. Japanese: *shomin.*

7. Japanese: *haijin.*

8. Japanese title: *Fukyū ruihō.*

9. Aoki, *Edo jidai no igaku,* 58–59.

10. Chinese title: *Bencao gangmu. Chuanxin youi fang* (*Traditional Reliable and Easy Prescriptions*) is another Chinese medical text that was cited.

11. *Kyūmin myōyaku,* image 39.

12. Japanese: *suzume no ogoke.*

13. *Shomin myōyakuhō,* images 65–66.

14. *Fukyū ruihō,* vol. 1, images 60 and 70–71.

15. Japanese: *ōdan.*

16. Japanese: *keifun; haraya.*

17. Japanese: *tori-me* (bird eyes).

18. Japanese: *shiokara* (a fermented fish meat paste).

19. Japanese: *yatsume unagi.*

20. *Shomin myōyakuhō,* image 66.

21. *Shomin myōyakuhō,* image 67; *Kyūmin myōyaku,* image 40.

22. Japanese: *shuppan bunka.* Kornicki, "Manuscript, Not Print," 23–52.

23. Rubinger, *Popular Literacy in Early Modern Japan,* 87–90.

24. Japanese title: *Rakuchū rakugai baiyaku chōhōki.*

25. *Rakuchū rakugai baiyaku chōhōki,* 181–85.

26. Japanese title: *Zoku Edo sunago onko meisekishi* (or, in short, *Zoku Edo sunago*). A sequel to *Edo sunago.*

27. *Zoku Edo sunago,* vol. 1, images 3–5. The title (*Zoku Edo sunago*) refers to the artisanal technique of blowing gold and silver dust. The work can be read as a sequel to Fujita Toshibē's gazetteer *Edo kanoko*—in the context of fashion and textiles, *kanoko* is a *shibori* technique of using fabric dyes. Senryō gathered new information about what he had seen and heard (mostly about temples and shrines) in the years after his own compilation of *Edo sunago.* Another important text is *Yōshū fushi,* a late seventeenth-century gazetteer written by scholar and essayist Kurokawa Dōyū about the surrounding area of Yamashiro.

28. *Zoku Edo sunago,* vol. 5, image 9.

29. Japanese: *megusuri.*

30. *Zoku Edo sunago,* vol. 5, images 14–15.

31. Japanese: *goreikō.*

32. Japanese: *kumokiri.*

33. *Zenkōji hitori annai,* image 34.

34. Japanese: *gedokuen.*

35. Williams, *The Other Side of Zen,* 87–97.

36. Japanese: *hangontan.*

37. *Toyama baiyaku gyōshi* (*jōkan*), 8–9 (image 22). Some ingredients were said to be bear gall, *Saussurea costus* (thistle) from China (*tōmokkō*), arsenic sulfide (orpiment or realgar; *keikan yūō*), Chinese skullcap (*tōōgon*), musk, cloves, frankincense (*gyoku nyūkō*), and buckwheat flour.

38. *Toyama kenshi: shiryō-hen,* vol. 5, 957–58 and 1013–14. Myōkokuji (a temple) of the Nichiren sect tried to claim the genealogy of the pill.

39. *Toyama kenshi: tsūshi-hen,* vol. 4, 17–37. See also Shinmura, *Nihon iryōshi,* 132.

40. *Toyama kenshi: shiryō-hen,* vol. 5, 973–74 and 990–91.

41. Japanese: *meisho zue.*

42. *Owari meisho zue* (*chūkan*), 229–30.

43. Japanese: *manbyō kintaien.*

44. Japanese title: *Edo meisho zue. Edo meisho zue,* vol. 1, image 39; vol. 14, image 22.

45. In that vision, he received the pill from Nyojō Zenshi (who was possibly Mokusu Nyojō of the early seventeenth century of the temple Kōfukuji in Nagasaki).

46. Japanese: *hōshintan.*

47. Japanese title: *Yamato meisho zue.*

48. *Yamato meisho zue,* vol. 3, images 6–7.

49. Japanese: *mankintan.*

50. *Ise sangū meisho zue,* images 28–30.

51. Japanese title: *Ise sangū meisho zue.*

52. Japanese title: *Sakaemasu megane no toku*; Japanese: *megane-ya* (optician). The work was illustrated with the collaboration of Kitao Masayoshi.

53. For more about this work, see Screech, *The Lens within the Heart*, 181–83. Screech translates this title as *Great Wealth Made through the Virtue of Glasses*.

54. Japanese: *oshi*. Ambros, *Emplacing a Pilgrimage*, 85.

55. Nenzi, *Excursions of Identity*, 142–43; Nenzi, "To Ise at All Costs," 76–81.

56. Josephson, "An Empowered World," 121.

57. Hardacre, *Shintō and the State*, 9–15.

58. Japanese title: *Edo shinbutsu gankake chōhōki*.

59. *Edo shinbutsu gankake chōhōki*, 87–90.

60. Japanese: *shōichii*.

61. Japanese title: *Miya tera gankake chōhōki*.

62. *Miya tera gankake chōhōki*, 348.

63. Japanese: *kusuriburo*.

64. Butler, "'Washing off the Dust': Baths and Bathing in Late Medieval Japan," 2–7.

65. Nenzi, *Excursions of Identity*, 184; Vaporis, *Breaking Barriers*, 240–41.

66. Japanese title: *Shūi miyako meisho zue*.

67. *Shūi miyako meisho zue*, vol. 3, Yōkokuji (*yo* section), 55.

68. Japanese name: Senju Kannon.

69. Japanese: *yōryūsui*.

70. Japanese: *tokukosui*.

71. *Shūi miyako meisho zue*, vol. 2, Raigōin (*ra* section), 24.

72. Rotermund, "Demonic Affliction or Contagious Disease," 374–82.

73. Rotermund, "Illness Illustrated," 278. Japanese medical scholars and physicians such as Kazuki Gyūzan thought that measles was caused by "poison." (See also the discussion of smallpox in chapter 1.)

74. Hardacre, *Religion and Society in Nineteenth-Century Japan*, xv–xxi, 1–34, and 130–49.

75. Japanese title: *Shinpen Sagami no kuni fudokikō*.

76. *Shinpen Sagami no kuni fudokikō, jō no kan*, 840.

77. Japanese: *azukigayu*.

78. *Hashika karuku suru hō*, by Utagawa.

79. Aoki, *Zaison rangaku no kenkyū*, 95–100.

80. Hur, *Death and Social Order in Tokugawa Japan*, 49; Rowley, *An Imperial Concubine's Tale*, 25–28.

81. *Dai Nihon kinsei shiryō, Hosokawa-ke shiryō*, vol. 8, docs. 1842 and 1843, 16–17.

82. *Menkō shūroku* (*kan-20*), vol. 3, 77–78; *Dai Nihon kinsei shiryō, Hosokawa-ke shiryō*, vol. 8, docs. 1824 and 1828, 3–4 and 6–7.

83. Japanese political appointment: *rōjū*.

84. Japanese political appointment: *tairō*.

85. *Menkō shūroku* (*kan-20*), vol. 3, 79. For a brief biography of Doi Toshikatsu, see Tanihara, "Hosokawa Tadaoki to Edo jidai shoki no ganka," 678.

86. *Dai Nihon kinsei shiryō, Hosokawa-ke shiryō*, vol. 8, docs. 1847–49, 20–21.

87. *Suzuki Heikurō: Kōshi nikki*, vol. 4, 8–9.

88. For more about Yashichi's medical history, see Nagata, "Kinsei kōki ni okeru kanja no ishi sentaku," 325–26 and 333–34.

89. *Suzuki Heikurō: Kōshi nikki*, vol. 4, 18–22.

90. Japanese title: *Nansō Satomi hakkenden*.

91. *Kyokutei Bakin nikki*, vol. 4, 357–59.

92. Japanese: *rōgan*. Bakin also mentions "weak eyes" (*suigan*).

93. Japanese: *kasumi*.

94. *Kyokutei Bakin nikki*, vol. 4, 360–67.

95. *Kyokutei Bakin nikki*, vol. 4, 242 (21st day). See also Young, "Family Matters," 108–23. Young discusses the role of religious prayers for Bakin and his family when they had ailments.

96. *Kyokutei Bakin nikki*, vol. 4, 460 (17th day) and 477–78 (9th day).

97. Japanese: *shōsaiko*.

98. See, for example, *Kyokutei Bakin nikki*, vol. 4, 414 (21st day) and 417 (26th day).

99. *Kyokutei Bakin nikki*, vol. 4, 394 (15th day), 399 (24th day), 415 (22nd day), 417 (26th day), 427 (17th day), and 534 (26th day). For a list of the medicines' properties, see Young, "Family Matters," 103–6.

100. Japanese: *kiō*.

101. Japanese: *kurogan* or *kokugan*.

102. *Kyokutei Bakin nikki*, vol. 4, 411 (16th day), 413–14 (20th day), and 430 (23rd day).

103. *Kyokutei Bakin nikki*, vol. 4, 434 (2nd day).

104. *Kyokutei Bakin nikki*, vol. 4, 425 (13th day).

105. *Kyokutei Bakin nikki*, vol. 4, 426 (14th day).

106. *Kyokutei Bakin nikki*, vol. 4, 502 (15th day).

107. *Kyokutei Bakin nikki*, vol. 4, 445–46 (22nd day). During one visit, he prescribed an enhanced "energy-revitalizing" (*kakki*) decoction and adjusted his prescriptions.

108. *Kyokutei Bakin nikki*, vol. 4, 454–61 (9th day–18th day).

109. Japanese: *gorei*.

110. Omichi had a brief episode of worm-induced attacks and took bear gall to subdue the symptoms. (In the Sino-Japanese medical context, worm disease had roots in Daoist medical thought and should not be understood as parasitic worm infection.) The family received gifts of food and medicines from friends. Omichi was recommended a special plant called *mōgyūjimyō* (hairy-cow-calf sprout), which was apparently good for healing from diarrhea.

111. *Kyokutei Bakin nikki*, vol. 4, 461 (19th day).

112. Chadani, "Kaisetsu: Kadoya Yōan nikki no sekai," 523–26.

113. For some examples, see *Kadoya Yōan nikki: ge*, 249 (15th day), 261 (21st day), 322 (23rd day), 326 (19th day), 335 (24th day), 353 (2nd day), and 357 (17th day). I will refer to this source simply as *nikki* in the notes that follow.

114. *nikki: ge*, 71 (15th day), 116 (27th day), and 117 (15th day), and 199 (13th day and 15th day); *nikki: jō*, 87 (7th day). To get an idea of the distances, traveling along a westerly route from Shinjō to Sakata, located near the coast of the Sea of Japan, took him over a day. A trip to Yōan's home base from Kubota would have taken someone at least two days, and about a day from Shinjō to the same destination.

115. *nikki: ge*, 52 (13th day), 309 (8th day), and 320 (4th day).

116. *nikki: ge*, 54 (6th day and 7th day) and 102 (26th day). On one trip, Yōan traveled to the village of Nozoki to see Takahashi Yasujirō, who had been struggling with poor health for a long time, and returned home with gifts, given to him as tokens of gratitude. At another time, Yōan received an inquiry from the administrative office, which was asking a question perhaps on behalf of a superintendent about some medicines.

117. *nikki: jō,* 491 (23rd day); *nikki: ge,* 338 (13th day).

118. *nikki: ge,* 346 (12th day and 13th day) and 347 (28th day).

119. *nikki: jō,* 80 (25th day) and 515 (26th day); *nikki: ge,* 248, 251, and 265.

120. *nikki: jō,* 310 (14th day), 358 (11th day), 498 (28th day) and 579 (5th day); *nikki: ge,* 191 (18th day).

121. *nikki: jō,* 87 (4th day).

122. *nikki: ge,* 195 (4th day), 197 (26th day), and 199 (16th day).

123. *nikki: jō,* 290 (22nd day).

124. *nikki: ge,* 363 (22nd day).

125. *nikki: jō,* 530 (27th day and 29th day) and 531 (3rd day and 4th day).

126. *nikki: ge,* 396–98.

127. *nikki: ge,* 115 (11th day) and 511 (11th day).

128. *nikki: ge,* 117 (10th day), 120 (18th day), 140 (12th day), and 265 (8th day).

129. *nikki: ge,* 196 (9th day).

130. *nikki: ge,* 264 (23rd day).

131. *nikki: ge,* 95 (25th day), 264 (24th day and 26th day), and 308 (21st day and 22nd day).

132. *nikki: jō,* 566 (8th day).

133. *nikki: jō,* 182 (9th day).

134. *nikki: ge,* 242 (11th day). It seems that by the start of 1859, he did not have money to purchase goods from Osaka and pay the Shibata intermediary.

135. Japanese title: *Ika jinmeiroku.*

136. Vaporis, *Tour of Duty,* 12–14. The alternate attendance system was akin to an institutionalized arrangement of keeping daimyo families and vassals as hostages subject to the will and whims of the shogun.

137. *Ika jinmeiroku,* vol. 1, images 4–5.

138. Japanese: *hondō.*

139. *Ranpō* (Dutch-method medicine) constituted a marginal category in the listings. For a comparison of registers, see Umihara, "Edo no rangakusha," 97–105.

140. *Ika jinmeiroku,* vol. 1, image 28.

141. *Ika jinmeiroku,* vol. 2, image 24.

142. *Ika jinmeiroku,* vol. 2, image 31.

143. *Kinsei kanpō chiken senshū,* vol. 10, 54–56.

144. Japanese: *gekan.*

145. The Ancient Formulas medicine was promoted by medical scholars and physicians. One of them was Yoshimasu Tōdō (mentioned in chapter 1). Odai Yōdō was a proponent of Tōdō's medical thought.

146. *Kinsei kanpō chiken senshū,* vol. 11, 175–76.

Chapter 3

1. See figure I.1 in the introduction. Katsushika Hokusai used *akimekura* to gloss the word for "internal obstruction" (a reference to cataracts). To find other references mentioned in this paragraph, see vol. 4 of *Kinmō zui,* image 20.

2. *Kosha* and *mōjin* have the same meaning.

3. *Kinmō zui* glosses *goze* as *kojo.*

4. Howell, *Geographies of Identity in Nineteenth-Century Japan,* 21–22.

5. In the same way, we may not know who was visually impaired but not so visually impaired as to want to be identified as a blind person. Hence it is prudent to

think of "blind people" as those identified or self-identified as such in Tokugawa-era historical sources—I explain this reasoning in the introduction.

6. In most contexts, I refer to the Kyoto guild quite simply as the guild. On a small scale, when I discuss guild branches of the Kyoto guild, I call them local guilds or local guild groups because of their local-level configurations.

7. The tale was recorded in many variant copies. Chapter 5 will discuss the significance of one particular text in the late Tokugawa period.

8. *Heike* music was thought to have been performed to appease spirits; blind musicians were thought to be able to cross the liminal junction between the realms of the living and the dead.

9. *Nihon kodai chūsei jinmei jiten*, 1–2; Hyōdō, *Heike monogatari no rekishi to geinō*, 8–18.

10. Japanese title: *Kanmon nikki*.

11. *Kanmon nikki*, vol. 1, 168–69, 171, 210, 243–44. *Kanmon nikki* recorded events from 1416 to 1448. It is clear some *biwa hōshi* were in high demand. For example, in the years of Ōei 24 (1417) and 25 (1418), we can tell that Chin'ichi *kengyō* was invited at least eight times to perform music.

12. Japanese title: *Tsurezuregusa*.

13. Keene, *Essays in Idleness*, 186.

14. Japanese title: *Konjaku monogatarishū*.

15. *Konjaku monogatarishū*, vol. 16, 1061–63 (images 1151–53).

16. Ishii, "Sekkyō-bushi," 292–94; *Sekisemimaru jinja monjo*, 42; Hyōdō, *Heike monogatari no rekishi to geinō*, 111–12. According to the medieval records of Sekisemimaru shrine (now in Ōtsu city), Semimaru was born the fourth son of the Heian emperor Daigo and was honored as Sekikiyomizu Semimaru no Miya.

17. "Semimaru," in *Twenty Plays of the Nō Theatre*, 103–12.

18. *Dai Chikamatsu zenshū: kaisetsu chūshaku*, vol. 5, 143–44 (images 82–83); Matisoff, "Nō as Transformed by Chikamatsu," 206; Matisoff, *The Legend of Semimaru*, 145–46.

19. Japanese title: *Tōdō yōshū*.

20. For more about the genre of *kawara makimono*, see Wakita, *Kawara makimono no sekai*, i–iv. Socially discriminated groups produced works about their origins.

21. *Tōdō yōshū*, 539–41.

22. For more about the religious functions of stone stupas, see Plutschow, "The Placatory Nature of *The Tale of the Heike*," 75–77.

23. The rite was called *suzumi no tō* (cooling rite, perhaps a reference to a cooling respite from the summer heat). *Tōdō yōshū*, 540 and 568.

24. *Tōdōza heike biwa shiryō: Okumura-ke zō, Koshikimoku*, 65 and 72; *Tōdōza heike biwa shiryō: Okumura-ke zō, Shinshikimoku*, 80. For more about the ritual, see *Enpekiken ki*, 103–4; Hayami, *Shokoku zue nenchū gyōji taisei*, 166–67.

25. For a study of Myōon Benzaiten and the guild, see Fritsch, *Japans blinde Sänger*.

26. *Tōdōza heike biwa shiryō: Okumura-ke zō, Tōdō ryakki*, 147; *Tōdō ryakki, Mōjin shoshorui*, vol. 3, images 15–16; Suzuki, "Shiryō shōkai Tōdō ryakki," 35–46. Several versions of *Tōdō ryakki* have been studied to some extent.

27. Japanese title: *Hannyashingyō*.

28. *Nagoya shishi, fūzoku hen*, vol. 6, 386–87 (image 226); *Konrin tsukumo no chiri*, 24; Komoda, *Heike no ongaku*, 110.

29. Japanese title: *Awaji no kuni fūzoku toijōkotae*.

30. *Awaji no kuni fūzoku toijōkotae*, 785. The centerpiece of the worship was a scroll bearing the image of Myōon Benzaiten.

31. *Chishinshū*, 111–12.

32. Sub-grades were called *kizami.*

33. [惣検校]

34. [職検校]

35. Katō, *Nihon mōjin shakaishi kenkyū*, 180–81 and 213–15; *Tōdōza heike biwa shiryō: Okumura-ke zō, Tōdō daikiroku*, 8; Ubukata, "Okumura-ke monjo kaisetsu," 402. The analysis presents information from Katō's chart and from *Tōdō daikiroku* (*The Great Records of the Guild*), a late eighteenth-century manuscript from the Okumura clan's archives.

36. [惣録]

37. [検校]

38. [十老]

39. [別当]

40. [勾当]

41. [座頭]

42. [衆分]

43. [紫分]

44. [無官]

45. [初心]

46. [打掛]

47. I use the term "national" cautiously to mean countrywide, because it is difficult to speak of a nation or nation-state prior to the Meiji period.

48. *The History of Japan Together with a Description of the Kingdom of Siam, 1690–92*, by Kaempfer, vol. 2, book 3, 55–56.

49. Japanese: *kankin* or *zatōgane.*

50. Japanese title: *Mugura no shizuku: shoka zatsudan.*

51. *Mugura no shizuku: shoka zatsudan*, 274. Approximate values: 1 *ryō* (gold) = 4 *bu* = 4,000 *mon* (copper currency unit); 1 *monme* (a currency unit, usually used for counting silver; approximately 3.75 grams) = 10 *fun*; 1 *hiki* = 10 *mon.*

52. Chamberlain, *Things Japanese*, 277.

53. Japanese title: *Aizu fudoki.*

54. *Aizu fudoki fūzokuchō*, 272.

55. *Kenshōbo*, doc. 14, 504. Japanese: *hatō* or *ha no kami* (lineage or sect master, a position inherited from the medieval system of the guild's *Heike* musical sects).

56. *Koga-ke monjo*, vol. 4, 262–69 (doc. 1830), 274–75 (doc. 1835), and 404–12 (doc. 1868).

57. Howell, *Geographies of Identity in Nineteenth-Century Japan*, 46.

58. Howell, *Geographies of Identity in Nineteenth-Century Japan*, 46.

59. Howell, *Geographies of Identity in Nineteenth-Century Japan*, 48.

60. Howell, *Geographies of Identity in Nineteenth-Century Japan*, 48.

61. Howell, *Geographies of Identity in Nineteenth-Century Japan*, 34–35.

62. Ehlers, *Give and Take*, 6, 8, and 10.

63. Japanese: *Koshikimoku.*

64. *Koshikimoku*, 73–74.

65. Japanese: *Shinshikimoku.*

66. *Tōdōza heike biwa shiryō: Okumura-ke zō, Tōdō daikiroku*, 24. It is not clear how

the guild decided which expelled guild member could regain his rank, but in the example of a certain Shin'ichi *kengyō*, he was expelled and readmitted with his rank.

67. *Tōdōza heike biwa shiryō: Okumura-ke zō, Shinshikimoku*, 77–82; Katō, *Nihon mōjin shakaishi kenkyū*, 164; Groemer, "The Guild of the Blind in Tokugawa Japan," 359; *Tōkyō shishikō, shigai-hen*, vol. 11, 623.

68. Sometimes known as *haitōsho* or *haitō kaisho* (office of dividends).

69. *Kariya-machi shōya tomechō*, vol. 5, 733–35. As one example from 1789 shows, the local Kariya guild (in Nagoya) proposed to use the dwelling space of a sighted person named Shōshichi to succeed an earlier office headed by Seiya'ichi, a deceased guild member. Owning an autonomous office would have made the Kariya guild less dependent on the guild's office in Nagoya.

70. *Chishinshū*, 109–10. Some data from the eighteenth century yields a partial picture of the spread of local guild groups in one place and in the proximate area. In the late eighteenth century, five leaders or so appeared to be active in Hiroshima at one time, with thirty-six leaders in districts around Hiroshima overseeing approximately 1,200 blind people. Many of them were presumably guild members, but a significant proportion (about 366 of them) were blind women, who were nominally under the authority of local guild leaders.

71. Ogata, "Bakumatsu Higo ni okeru tōdōza," 6–7; Ogata, "Kinsei Higo ni okeru tōdōza no kakuritsu," 121–40; Ogata, "Zamoto kikiyaku senshutsu kara miru Kumamoto-han no tōdōza," 79–97.

72. Japanese: *bugyōsho* or *hanchō*. (See also footnote 71.)

73. Groemer, *Goze*, 16.

74. *Kenshōbo*, doc. 19, 507–8.

75. Namase, *Kinsei shōgaisha kankei shiryō shūsei*, 423–24.

76. Japanese title: *Seji kenbunroku*.

77. Teeuwen and Nakai, *Lust, Commerce, and Corruption*, 200–201.

78. *Shihō shiryō dai* 180 *gō* (*Tokugawa kinreikō, dai* 5 *shitsu*), 223–24 (images 117–18).

79. *Shihō shiryō dai* 180 *gō* (*Tokugawa kinreikō, dai* 5 *shitsu*), 224–25 (image 118).

80. Namase, *Kinsei shōgaisha kankei shiryō shūsei*, 417.

81. Japanese: *machi-bugyō*.

82. *Tokugawa kinreikō: goshū*, vol. 4, ed. Ishii, 303–6.

83. *Oshiokirei ruishū*, vol. 6, ed. Ishii, 516.

84. Japanese: *jisha-bugyō*.

85. The least severe was *keihō*, which banned exiled members from entering Edo and its environs. *Shihō shiryō dai* 180 *gō* (*Tokugawa kinreikō, dai* 5 *shitsu*), 234–36 (images 123–24).

86. *Ofuregaki Tenpō shūsei: ge*, doc. 6482, 833.

87. Japanese title: *Tōdōza haitōmotsu oboegaki*.

88. *Koga-ke monjo*, vol. 4, 723–25.

89. *Tokugawa jikki: dai 3-pen*, vol. 17 (1905 digital edition), 295 (image 153); *Tokugawa jikki: dai 3-pen*, vol. 18 (1905 digital edition), 327 (image 170).

90. Japanese title: *Tokugawa jikki*.

91. Shōji, *Aizu fudoki fūzokuchō*, 260 and 263.

92. See, for example, *Kaga-han shiryō*, 14-*hen*, 18 (image 13).

93. Botsman, *Punishment and Power in the Making of Modern Japan*, 50–58.

94. Groemer, "The Creation of the Edo Outcaste Order," 264–69.

95. Groemer, "The Creation of the Edo Outcaste Order," 281.

96. Groemer, "The Guild of the Blind in Tokugawa Japan," 351–55.

97. Howell, *Geographies of Identity in Nineteenth-Century Japan*, 29.

98. Howell, *Geographies of Identity in Nineteenth-Century Japan*, 34.

99. Ehlers, *Give and Take*, 25.

100. Ehlers, *Give and Take*, 86–105.

101. Ehlers, "Benevolence, Charity, and Duty," 56–57 and 69–73.

102. *Kaga-han shiryō, 4-hen*, 458 (image 233).

103. *Hanpōshū*, vol. 2, *Tottori-han*, doc. 27, 125.

104. Japanese: *Teiichi fuda.*

105. *Hanpōshū*, vol. 10, *Zoku Tottori-han*, doc. 44, 623.

106. *Hanpōshū*, vol. 2, *Tottori-han*, doc. 238, 278. Some of them were *komusō* (priests of the Fuke Buddhist sect) and *hachihiraki bōzu* (beggar priests traveling with alms bowls).

107. Japanese: *gotai fugu.*

108. *Hanpōshū*, vol. 2, *Tottori-han*, doc. 345, 426–27, and doc. 347, 428.

109. *Hanpōshū*, vol. 3, *Tokushima-han*, doc. 2718, 1048–49.

110. *Hanpōshū*, vol. 3, *Tokushima-han*, doc. 2733, 1052. In 1766, Tokushima domain authorities authorized blind people to travel up to ten *ri* (a unit of distance, approximately 2.44 miles or 3.92 kilometers per *ri*) in all four cardinal directions from their domiciles to seek alms from donors within this radius.

111. Groemer, *Goze to goze uta no kenkyū: shiryō-hen*, 121–22. See the example about Hagi domain (in Yamaguchi prefecture today) in 1728.

112. Japanese: *kōri-bugyō.*

113. *Hanpōshū*, vol. 1, *Okayama-han: ge*, doc. 314, 233–35.

114. He was a *kengyō.*

115. Roberts, *Mercantilism in a Japanese Domain*, 74.

116. *Kenshōbo*, docs. 7–9, 499–500.

117. In terms of cash, a *shubun* (*zatō*) could receive sixty *monme*. A *goze* received 25 *monme*, the least amount.

118. *Kenshōbo*, docs. 11 and 12, 501–2.

119. Smits, "Shaking Up Japan," 1046–47.

120. McClain, "Failed Expectations," 403–7.

121. *Kaga-han shiryō, 12-hen*, 309–11 (images 158–59).

122. Japanese: *ōjōya kaigiroku.*

123. For more about the *ōjōya* in Kurume domain, see Hibi, "Kurume-han ni okeru Kansei yonen zaikata showappu no shuhōgawari to ōjōya," 83–122.

124. Japanese: *ōjōya.*

125. *Kurume-han ōjōya kaigiroku*, vol. 5, 1–12.

126. *Kurume-han ōjōya kaigiroku*, vol. 5, 155.

127. *Kurume-han ōjōya kaigiroku*, vol. 5, 204.

128. Japanese: *moyaizutome nyūyōkin.*

129. *Kurume-han ōjōya kaigiroku*, vol. 5, 99.

130. *Kariya-machi shōya tomechō kaisetsu*, 36–38.

131. *Teihon Kaga-han hisabetsu buraku kankei shiryō shūsei*, 482–86.

Chapter 4

1. Japanese term: *goze.*

2. Japanese term: *mōsō.* I use the translation "blind priests."

3. *Shihō shiryō dai* 180 *gō* (*Tokugawa kinreikō, dai* 5 *shitsu*), 226 (image 119).

4. *Hanpōshū,* vol. 2, *Tottori-han,* doc. 338, 424–25. See also *Hanpōshū,* vol. 1, *Okayama-han: jō,* doc. 1359, 534–35.

5. *Shihō shiryō dai* 180 *gō* (*Tokugawa kinreikō, dai* 5 *shitsu*), 226–28 (images 119–20).

6. *Hanpōshū,* vol. 11, *Kurume-han,* doc. 249, 101.

7. Japanese: *rōjū.*

8. Sugano, "State Indoctrination of Filial Piety in Tokugawa Japan," 172. For other studies of the Kansei reforms and the impact, see Howell, "Hard Times in the Kantō," 349–71; Hur, *Prayer and Play in Late Tokugawa Japan,* 118–21. Despite the moralistic thrust of the Kansei reforms, the results were mixed. Hur's discussion of the religious site Sensōji in Edo during the Kansei period explains that the reforms did not succeed in curbing the cultural energies of the masses.

9. Japanese title: *Yoshino zōshi.*

10. He was part of Matsudaira Sadanobu's inner circle.

11. *Yoshino zōshi,* 458–59 and 497.

12. Japanese title: *Kōgiroku.*

13. Yamashita, *Edo jidai shomin kyōka seisaku no kenkyū,* 314–15.

14. Yonemoto, *The Problem of Women in Early Modern Japan,* 48–49.

15. *Kankoku kōgiroku* (*jōkan*), ed. Sugano, 132.

16. *Kankoku kōgiroku* (*chūkan*), ed. Sugano, 178–79.

17. For other stories, see *Kankoku kōgiroku* (*jōkan*), ed. Sugano, 87–88 and 143–44; Sugano, *Edo jidai no kōkōsha: Kōgiroku no sekai,* 72–73.

18. Japanese title: *Kiyū shōran.*

19. *Kiyū shōran,* vol. 3, 73–74.

20. Japanese title: *Sunkoku zasshi.*

21. *Sunkoku zasshi,* vol. 1, 241–42 (images 133–34); Sakuma, *Goze no minzoku,* 10–12.

22. Igarashi, *Goze,* 108–11. The northwestern parts of Japan around Niigata prefecture were home to generations of blind female musicians, whose entrenched networks and ties with local, sighted communities made them popular.

23. Ishii, "Sekkyō-bushi," 298–99.

24. Groemer, *Goze,* 3; Groemer, "Who Benefits?," 350–52.

25. Groemer, "Female Shamans in Eastern Japan during the Edo Period," 29; Kawamura, "A Female Shaman's Mind and Body, and Possession," 257–62.

26. Knecht, "Japanese Shamanism," 680; Kawamura, "A Female Shaman's Mind and Body, and Possession," 262–63.

27. Koida, *Hotoke to onna no Muromachi,* 84–86; *Onna chōhōki taisei,* image 66. In the early eighteenth century, *Onna chōhōki* (*A Convenient Guide for Women*), as well as other moralistic treatises, rehashed prescriptive arguments about gender roles.

28. Japanese title: *Soga monogatari.*

29. Japanese title: *Ochiboshū.*

30. *Ochiboshū,* 124–26 (images 441–42).

31. *Wagakoromo,* 331.

32. Itasaka, "The Woman Reader as Symbol," 104–5; Kornicki, "Women, Education, and Literacy," 12–14.

33. *Edo machibure shūsei,* vol. 14, doc. 13977, 390. One account focuses on a blind woman named Masue of Asakusa in Edo. Masue became blind after an episode of

smallpox at age forty-five. It seems that she worked as an acupuncturist. But we do not know how or where she was trained to become one. See also *Kankoku kōgiroku* (*jōkan*), ed. Sugano, 143–44; Sugano, *Edo jidai no kōkōsha*, 72–73. Sayo (a different person, not to be confused with Sayo from Fukagawa discussed earlier in the text), mentioned in an account from *Kōgiroku*, had a blind daughter. She wanted her daughter to pick up skills in massage and acupuncture, but there is no detail about how her daughter was to be trained.

34. *Edo machibure shūsei*, vol. 14, doc. 13819, 268–69.

35. *Goze shikimoku*, 249.

36. Japanese: *ichirō*.

37. Japanese: *chūrō*.

38. *Kenshōbo*, doc. 23, 509.

39. Japanese: *gogunka yakusho*.

40. *Kenshōbo*, doc. 38, 532.

41. Japanese title: *Ukiyo no arisama*.

42. *Ukiyo no arisama* (*kan no kyū jō: go*), 147 (image 159).

43. Yamada, "Matsushiro hanryō no mōjin," 179–240.

44. *Echigo goze nikki*, by Saitō, 22–28.

45. *Echigo goze nikki*, by Saitō, 29–30.

46. *Echigo goze nikki*, by Saitō, 46–51.

47. *Echigo goze nikki*, by Saitō, 51.

48. *Echigo goze nikki*, by Saitō, 63–66.

49. *Echigo goze nikki*, by Saitō, 68.

50. Umeda, "Kinsei Nara no mōsō soshiki." Some *mōsō* (blind priests) in Nara were allied with the home temple Kōfukuji.

51. Japanese: *mōsō*.

52. Nakano, "Mōsō to biwagaku," 12–14.

53. Nagai, *Nikkan mōsō no shakaishi*, 30–31; Nishioka, "Jishin mōsō no shakumon," 158–59.

54. Japanese title: *Jishinkyō*. Hoshino, "Mōsō no shoji kyōten," 69–84. It is hard to establish the origin of *Jishinkyō*.

55. *Mōsō biwa*, 124–27.

56. Japanese: *kuzure* music.

57. Japanese: *kama-barai*.

58. Japanese: *gokoku jōju* (success of the five grains).

59. *Kuzure* music varied across the Kyūshū region and developed from oral traditions.

60. Nagai, *Nikkan mōsō no shakaishi*, 32–37. The logic of classification was sometimes obscure and would defy easy generalization.

61. *Koga-ke monjo*, vol. 4, 382–83; *Fukuoka kenshi: bunka shiryō hen*, vol. 2, 64.

62. They were banned from playing the *Tsukushi-goto* (a type of *koto*).

63. Japanese title: *Tōdō daikiroku*.

64. *Tōdōza heike biwa shiryō: Okumura-ke zō, Tōdō daikiroku*, 9.

65. *Fukuoka kenshi: bunka shiryō hen*, vol. 2, 531–33; Chikuma, "Kōrasan shinkō no denpa," 33–50.

66. *Fukuoka kenshi: bunka shiryō hen*, vol. 2, 75–76. A *kogashira* was installed as a minor head of a *mōsō* group. The *furekogashira* was a minor head quite similar to the *kogashira*, and they reported to the *sōkogashira*, who was ranked above them in the hierarchy as the group leader.

67. *Fukuoka kenshi: bunka shiryō hen*, vol. 2, 79 and 91–95. The records suggest the transfer of leadership authority from Shōkai to Ukai.
68. *Fukuoka kenshi: bunka shiryō hen*, vol. 2, 95–96.
69. Narita, *Mōsō no denshō*, 46–48.
70. *Fukuoka kenshi: bunka shiryō hen*, vol. 2, 97–98. 1 *hiki* = 10 *mon*.
71. *Fukuoka kenshi: bunka shiryō hen*, vol. 2, 148.
72. *Fukuoka kenshi: bunka shiryō hen*, vol. 2, 43–46.
73. *Hanpōshū*, vol. 7, *Kumamoto-han*, docs. 532 and 533, 324–25; Miyano, "Kinsei kōki Shōren'in ni yoru mōsō shihai jittai," 17–40; Nagai, "Chikuzen Chikugo no mōsō shūdan to sono shūhen," 263–68.
74. Japanese: *monzeki*.
75. Terao, "Kinsei jiin no kashitsuke ni tsuite," 132.
76. *Kumomi-ke monjo*, 15–16.
77. *Hanpōshū*, vol. 1, *Okayama-han: jō*, docs. 1361 and 1362, 535–36; *Hanpōshū*, vol. 11, *Kurume-han*, doc. 2305, 803.
78. *Ofuregaki Tenpō shūsei: ge*, doc. 5511, 429.
79. Miyachi, "Hizen mōsō kō," 17–31.
80. *Fukuoka kenshi: bunka shiryō hen*, vol. 2, 65–69.
81. *Fukuoka kenshi: bunka shiryō hen*, 157–58.
82. *Ofuregaki Tenpō shūsei: ge*, doc. 5512, 429–30.
83. *Fukuoka kenshi: bunka shiryō hen*, vol. 2, 288.
84. *Fukuoka kenshi: bunka shiryō hen*, vol. 2, 283–84 and 289.

Chapter 5

1. *Tokugawa jikki: dai ichihen*, vol. 38 (1975 print edition), 659. As retired shogun, Tokugawa Ieyasu delighted in hosting entertainers at his residence. On one particular day, in 1614, they gathered to put on a show for him. Present among them were blind male musicians (*biwa hōshi*) of *Heike. Heike* music is also often referred to as *heikyoku*.
2. Rowden, *The Songs of Blind Folk*, 11.
3. Itō, *Ningyō jōruri no doramatsurugī*, 357–65; Saya, *Heike monogatari kara jōruri e*, 143–72; McCullough, *The Tale of the Heike*, 9.
4. We refer to these musical scores as *heikyoku fuhon*. They can also be considered "recited texts" (*katari-kei* or *katari-bon*)—see the section on musical lineages.
5. Komoda, "The Musical Narrative of *The Tale of the Heike*," 89; Tokita, *Japanese Singers of Tales*, 64. A verse or *ku* can be broken down into discrete music-text units called *dan*.
6. Komoda, "The Musical Narrative of *The Tale of the Heike*," 84; Komoda, *Heike no ongaku: tōdō no dentō*, 240–42; Tateyama, *Heike ongakushi*, 823–24.
7. *Tokitsugu kyō ki*, 537 (image 529); Muroki, "Jōrurihime monogatari," 16–17.
8. Japanese title: *Oku no hosomichi*.
9. *The Narrow Road to the Deep North and Other Travel Sketches*, 114.
10. Flavin, review of Johnson's *The Koto*, 131–32.
11. Flavin, "Sōkyoku-jiuta," 172–74.
12. Arisawa, "Ryūha," 101–4. These blind musicians held the rank of *kengyō*.
13. Japanese title: *Kiyū shōran*.
14. *Kiyū shōran*, vol. 11, 6.
15. Japanese title: *Yoshiwara zatsuwa*.
16. *Yoshiwara zatsuwa, Enseki jisshu*, vol. 3, 71 (image 42).

17. *Kaga-han shiryō, dai 13-hen*, vol. 13, 537 (image 272).

18. Japanese: *zahō no shikimoku.*

19. *Kenshōbo*, doc. 20, 508.

20. *Yao Yazaemon nikki*, 293.

21. *Tokugawa kinreikō zenshū*, vol. 5, 131; Katō, *Nihon mōjin shakaishi kenkyū*, 124–25.

22. For an example of a micro-historical approach, see Roberts, "Shipwrecks and Flotsam," 83–122.

23. De Ferranti, "Transmission and Textuality in the Narrative Traditions of Blind Biwa Players," 133. To employ Hugh de Ferranti's metaphor of "residual textuality," Chiichi's *Correct Tunes of Heike* maintained the durability of a written score to distinctly encode his interpretive choices within the permutations of a larger narrative to influence the desired performance contents and styles.

24. For additional works about print culture in Tokugawa Japan, see Clements, *A Cultural History of Translation in Early Modern Japan*, 21–24; Groemer, "Edo's 'Tin Pan Alley,'" 1–36.

25. I translate the Japanese term *hikyoku* as "secret tunes."

26. Yamada, "Rethinking *Iemoto*," 29–32; Corbett, *Cultivating Femininity*, 29. Yamada traces the origin of the term *iemoto* and argues for a flexible bottom-up view that focuses on individual agency within the *iemoto* system. Corbett examines texts on tea culture in the *iemoto* system.

27. Atsumi, "Ogino kengyō den: hoi," 183–230; Komoda, *Heike no ongaku*, 57–60; Ozaki, "Ogino kengyō to Heike mabushi no kōkeisha," 49–58.

28. Ozaki, "Ogino kengyō to Heike mabushi no kōkeisha," 51–54.

29. Ozaki, *Heike chūkō no so*, 10–12.

30. Tanizaki held the rank of *kengyō.*

31. *Heike mabushi*, vol. 1, 5–6. The Ozaki edition of the *Heike mabushi* is the source for my discussion. See also Ozaki, *Heike chūkō no so*, 102–3.

32. *Heike mabushi*, vol. 1, 6. The temples mentioned were Myōhōin, Shōren'in, and Shōgoin; and the imperial regent houses were Kan'in, Kujō, and Nijō.

33. Platt, *Burning and Building*, 42–45.

34. Komoda, *Heike no ongaku*, 53–54; *Tōdōza heike biwa shiryō: Okumura-ke zō, Sandai no seki*, 172–76.

35. Atsumi, *Gunki monogatari to setsuwa*, 340 and 363–64.

36. Komoda, *Heike no ongaku*, 54–55; Atsumi, *Gunki monogatari to setsuwa*, 371–75; *Tōdōza heike biwa shiryō: Okumura-ke zō, Sandai no seki*, 176.

37. *Heike monogatari* (*Zōho kokugo kokubungaku kenkyūshi taisei*, vol. 9), 438.

38. Ozaki, "Ogino kengyō to Heike mabushi no kōkeisha," 55–56.

39. Ozaki, *Heike chūkō no so*, 65; Atsumi, "Kaidai," 45–46.

40. Ozaki, *Heike chūkō no so*, 94–95.

41. *Tōdōza heike biwa shiryō: Okumura-ke zō, Koshikimoku*, 66–67.

42. Katō, *Nihon mōjin shakaishi kenkyū*, 215.

43. Komoda, *Heike no ongaku*, 47–48; *Omote bikae*, image 59; *Chishinshū*, 110; Katō, *Nihon mōjin shakaishi kenkyū*, 218.

44. *Tōdō shinshikimoku*, 529 and 535; Katō, *Nihon mōjin shakaishi kenkyū*, 210–11.

45. *Chishinshū*, 113.

46. Komoda, *Heike no ongaku*, 62–65; Tateyama, *Heike ongakushi*, 352. Fujii held the rank of *kōtō*. As pointed out by Komoda, Fujii *kōtō* belonged to a group of *sōkyoku* pioneers in Nagoya with *Fuji* [藤] in their names.

47. Komoda, *Heike no ongaku*, 64–65; Atsumi, "Ogino kengyō den: hoi," 219–20. Fujita held the rank of *kōtō*.

48. *Konrin tsukumo no chiri*, 75; Komoda, *Heike no ongaku*, 64; Tateyama, *Heike ongakushi*, 354.

49. *Heike mabushi*, vol. 1, 6; Atsumi, "Kaidai," 5. Chiichi could have introduced his criteria for selecting disciples whom he deemed worthy of being taught the secret tunes.

50. Komoda, "The Musical Narrative of *The Tale of the Heike*," 99.

51. Japanese title: *Tokugawa jikki*.

52. *Tokugawa jikki, dai 3-pen* (1907 digital edition), 259 (image 133), 295 (image 151), 327 (image 167), 369 (image 188), 594 (image 301), 632 (image 320), and 711 (image 359).

53. *Koga-ke monjo*, vol. 4, 353 and 382–86.

54. These musicians were Namikawa, Saitō, Inuzuka, and Ibaraki—all achieved the rank of *kengyō*. See *Tokugawa jikki, dai 3-pen* (1907 digital edition), 708–9 (image 358).

55. *Kuzuhara kōtō nikki*, 347–51; Saiki, *Kokiroku no kenkyū (ge)*, 298–303.

56. Matsuno was a *kōtō* and was later awarded the rank of *kengyō*.

57. For some examples, see *Kuzuhara kōtō nikki*, 46–75 (Tenpō years 3–7; 1832–36).

58. Some of the famous tunes from his repertoire were "Kumo no ue" (On Top of Clouds), "Shiki no yuki" (Snow of the Four Seasons), "Sato no akira" (Dawn at the Hometown), "Setsugekka" (Snow Moon Flowers), "Yaegasumi" (Multilayered Afterglow/Mist), and "Chikubushima."

59. For some examples, see *Kuzuhara kōtō nikki*, 177 (Kōka 4; 1847) and 190–91 (Kaei 3; 1850).

60. Japanese title: *Gunsho ruijū*.

61. Japanese title: *Onkodō Hanawa sensei den*.

62. *Gunsho ruijū, dai 19 shū*, 383–87 (images 198–200). See also Ueda, "Hanawa Hokinoichi to kokugaku," 29–55; Saitō, "Onkodō Hanawa sensei den ni tsuite," 111–38.

63. This was the *ritsuryō* code.

64. *Gunsho ruijū, dai 19 shū*, 386 (image 200) and 389 (image 201). This Chinese medical text was discussed in chapter 1.

65. Japanese: Wagaku kōdansho.

66. *Gunsho ruijū, dai 19 shū*, 394–97 (images 204–6).

67. *Gunsho ruijū, dai 19 shū*, 392–93 (image 203).

68. *Gunsho ruijū, dai 19 shū*, 392 (image 203), 395 (image 204), and 396 (image 205).

69. Japanese title: *Hanawa zen sōkengyō nenpu*.

70. *Gunsho ruijū, dai 19 shū*, 404–7 (images 209–10).

71. Japanese: *katari-kei* or *katari-bon*.

72. Japanese: *yomi-kei* or *yomi-bon*.

73. Butler, "The Textual Evolution of Heike Monogatari," 6 and 34. Butler, one of the earliest English-language scholars of *Heike*, espouses the view that *Heike* was written down before being adapted to suit different "read" and "recited" forms. The foundational texts of the two categories were completed during the Kamakura period.

74. Ichiko, *Heike monogatari kenkyū jiten*, 105 and 319; Atsumi, *Heike monogatari no kisoteki kenkyū*, 54; Yamashita, *Heike monogatari no seisei*, 7–12. Atsumi proposed renaming the *yomi-kei* as *zōho-kei* (supplemented texts), as texts from this category enriched the *katari-kei* by including references to written historical and literary sources. Yamashita's taxonomy of *tōdō-kei* (guild genealogy) for texts of the *katari-kei* and *hitōdō-kei* (non-guild genealogy) for the *yomi-kei* may more accurately reflect the role of the *katari-kei* in shaping recitative practices.

75. Oyler, *Swords, Oaths, and Prophetic Visions*, 18–19. In the same vein of "synchronic intertextuality" of medieval *Heike* texts, Chiichi participated in the contemporaneous textuality of *Heike*.

76. Tomikura, *Heike monogatari kenkyū*, 402–6 and 431–32; Yamashita, *Heike monogatari no seisei*, 102–7. Copies of the *Rufu-bon* were circulated starting in the early decades of the seventeenth century. See, for example, https://dl.ndl.go.jp/info:ndljp/pid/25 70057

77. *Tokugawa jikki: dai ichihen*, vol. 38 (1934 print edition), 622–30; *Sunpuki, Shiseki zassan*, vol. 2, 243–44.

78. Suzuki, "Tōdō no koshikimoku," 246–47. See the discussion of the guild's laws in chapter 3.

79. Japanese title: *Saikai yotekishū*.

80. *Saikai yotekishū*, 77–80.

81. Komoda, *Heike no ongaku*, 51–52; Tateyama, *Heike ongakushi*, 247–49, 269–71, and 280–81.

82. *Saikai yotekishū*, 5; Okumura, *Heikyoku fuhon no kenkyū*, 64; *Nagoya shishi: fūzoku-hen*, vol. 6, 96 (image 66).

83. Adriaansz, *Kumiuta and Danmono*, 10–12.

84. Japanese title: *Yatsuhashi kengyō kinkyokushō*.

85. *Yatsuhashi kengyō kinkyokushō jo*, images 37–40.

86. *Chikuzen meisho zue*, 210. This eminent temple was said to be founded before the sister temple in Hakata in Chikuzen province (in Fukuoka prefecture today).

87. Japanese title: *Sōkyoku taiishō*.

88. *Sōkyoku taiishō*, images 29–34.

89. The oldest lineages were supposedly inaugurated in Semimaru's time and blossomed centuries later during the Bunroku period (1592–96).

90. *Kiyū shōran*, vol. 11, 13 (image 29).

91. Another well-known blind musician was Kaga'ichi of Sesshū of the Yanagawa lineage.

92. *Yasumura kengyō busō gafushū*, image 41. Yasumura *kengyō*, who lived in Kyoto in the eighteenth century, likely compiled *Busō gafushū* (*A Collection of the Elegant Scores of the Koto*) to update the records of *Yatsuhashi kengyō kinkyokushō*.

93. Komoda, *Heike no ongaku*, 140–41; Ichiko, *Heike monogatari kenkyū jiten*, 463–64 and 555.

94. Forty volumes: *kan* or *satsu*. See also Hayashi, "Heike mabushi shoshi," 3–4. The original Ozaki manuscript seems to be missing the text of "The Greater Secret Tunes."

95. Japanese title: *Heigo shōkyoku*.

96. Komoda, "Heike mabushi no Edo denpa ni tsuite," 103.

97. See Fleming, "Restaging the Forty-Seven Rōnin," 392. By the late eighteenth century, as Fleming points out, the public could choose from many print materials on Japanese entertainment.

98. De Ferranti, "Transmission and Textuality in the Narrative Traditions of Blind Biwa Players," 149.

99. *Saikai yotekishū*, 89–90; Atsumi, "Kaidai," 16; Takahashi, *Heike monogatari Kaku'ichi-bon shinkō*, 200–201.

100. Kinda'ichi, *Heikyoku kō*, 18–19; Atsumi, "Kaidai," 16.

101. Japanese: *hira mono.*

102. Japanese: *yomi mono* (subcategory); *denju mono* (category of "transmitted content").

103. "Goku mono" (Five *ku*): "Daitō no konryū" (The Rebuilding of the Great Pagoda), "Kōya no maki" (Mount Kōya), "Genbō," "Seinan no rikyū" (The Seinan Detached Palace), and "Miyako utsuri" (The Moving of the Capital to Fukuhara). See Tyler, *The Tale of the Heike*, contents page. I mostly follow Tyler's English translations of chapter titles.

104. "Kanjō no maki" (The Initiates' Chapter), "Shōhiji" (Lesser Secret Tunes), and "Daihiji" (Greater Secret Tunes). See Komoda, *Heike no ongaku*, 142–43. Komoda highlights that *Heike mabushi* was probably the first *heikyoku* text with the "Greater Secret Tunes" listed under a specially designated title.

105. *Enpekiken ki*, 104; Takahashi, *Heike monogatari Kaku'ichi-bon shinkō*, 86–87; Ichiko, *Heike monogatari kenkyū jiten*, 65. "Engi no seidai" (The Saintly Reign of Emperor Daigo) and "Gion shōja" (The Jetavana Temple) made up the "Lesser Secret Tunes." "Engi no seidai" was traditionally incorporated into the longer *ku* of "Chōteki zoroe" (The Roster of Imperial Foes) in many adapted texts. The "Greater Secret Tunes" consisted of "Shūron" (a stand-alone *ku* adapted from "Mount Kōya"), "Tsurugi no maki" (The Sword), and "Kagami no maki" (The Mirror).

106. Kinda'ichi, *Heikyoku kō*, 18, 60, 63–72; Suzuki, *Heikyoku to Heike monogatari*, 10–12 and 82–83; Komoda, "The Musical Narrative of *The Tale of the Heike*," 84–87. In the range of melodic formulae, the *kudoki* was prevalent.

107. Komoda, *Heike no ongaku*, 182–83.

108. Suzuki, "Heikyoku fuhon toshite no tokushoku," 8–9.

109. For a brief introduction of the *Toyokawa-bon*, see Komoda, *Heike no ongaku*, 178–80; Ichiko, *Heike monogatari kenkyū jiten*, 421–22.

110. Japanese title: *Heike ginpu.*

111. Ozaki, "Ogino kengyō to Heike mabushi no kōkeisha," 55. For a brief biography of Okamura Gensen, see Nomura, *Sōhen-ryū*, 73.

112. *Heike ginpu*, 500–506. Though an abridgement of *Heike*, this work features *ku* that were arranged in the sequences common to the *Kaku'ichi-bon* and *Rufu-bon*.

113. Suzuki, "Koe no denshō, koe no kigōka," 1–19.

114. Japanese title: *Heigo.*

115. Komoda, *Heike no ongaku*, 150 and 173–75.

116. Japanese title: *Heikyoku mondōsho.*

117. Komoda, "Heike mabushi no Edo denpa ni tsuite," 104–5.

118. Komoda, "Kyōto Daigaku-zō *Heikyoku mabushi*," 31–32 and 48.

119. *Mugura no shizuku: shoka zatsudan*, 419. For more about Matsudaira Kunzan's place in Tokugawa scholarship on natural history, see Fukuoka, *The Premise of Fidelity*, 61–62.

120. Komoda, "Heike mabushi no Edo denpa ni tsuite," 103; Atsumi, "Ogino kengyō den: hoi," 94–115 and 162–63; Atsumi, *Yokoi Yayū jihitsu Heigo*, 3–4.

121. De Ferranti, "The Kyushu *Biwa* Traditions," 115–19.

122. Komoda, *Heike no ongaku*, 202–4 and 209–10; Komoda, "Nagoya heikyoku no

ryūha o megutte," 1 and 16–18. Among the sighted *heikyoku* musicians was Kusumi Taiso from the Kusumi clan of samurai vassals in Tsugaru. Taiso's teacher was Asaoka Chōsaiichi *kengyō*, who was taught by Nakamura *kengyō*—a student of Chiichi's lineage (mentioned earlier in this chapter as Ju'ichi). Through Taiso, *Heike mabushi* was transmitted within the Tsugaru-*kei* (Tsugaru lineage). In a parallel development, sighted male performers of *jiuta* and *sōkyoku* in Nagoya made up the Nagoya-*kei* (Nagoya lineage). Because of both lineages' emphasis on *jiuta* and *sōkyoku*, *heikyoku* was adapted to the performance styles and melodies of the dominant genres.

Chapter 6

1. Japanese title: *Eiga monogatari.* Watanabe, *Flowering Tales*, 1–20. Watanabe discusses this work's relationship with the *monogatari* genre.
2. *Eiga monogatari zenchūshaku*, vol. 7, 326–27.
3. Japanese verbal phrase: *hara nado toru*.
4. Japanese title: *Makura no sōshi*.
5. *Makura no sōshi*, 373.
6. See *Nihon shoki*, 97–98. The *Nihon shoki* (*The Chronicles of Japan*) contains scattered references to acupuncture.
7. Japanese: *hari-hakase, hari-shi*, or *hari-sei* (acupuncturists); Japanese: *anma-hakase, anma-shi*, or *anma-sei* (masseurs); Japanese: Ten'yakuryō (Bureau of Medicine). Shinmura, *Kodai iryō kanninsei no kenkyū*, 44–46. The Ten'yakuryō mirrored the precedent of Tang China, though on a reduced scale.
8. Japanese title: *Ryō no gige* (*Yōrōryō* or *Yōrō* codex).
9. See the discussion of "winds" in chapter 1.
10. *Ritsu, Ryō no gige*, 283.
11. Japanese: *yōjō* [養生].
12. Gensaku was Manase Dōsan's adopted son and heir; Dōsan was an early leader of the Latter Generations of medical scholars (*Goseiha*).
13. Japanese title: *Tokugawa jikki*.
14. *Tokugawa jikki: dai nihen*, vol. 39 (1976 print edition), 245; *Tokugawa jikki: dai ichihen*, 965 (image 490; 1907 digital edition); Nagao Eiichi Kyōju Taikan Kinen Ronbunshū Kankōkai, ed., *Shinkyū anmashi ronkō*, 8; Shinmura, *Nihon iryōshi*, 102–103.
15. Japanese: *okuishi* (also *gokinju, gokinjū ishi*, and *osoba ishi*).
16. *Tokugawa jikki: dai rokuhen*, vol. 43 (1976 print edition), 42; Nagao Eiichi Kyōju Taikan Kinen Ronbunshū Kankōkai, ed., *Shinkyū anmashi ronkō*, 10–11; Shinmura, *Nihon iryōshi*, 104–6.
17. Nagao Eiichi Kyōju Taikan Kinen Ronbunshū Kankōkai, ed., *Shinkyū anmashi ronkō*, 6.
18. Japanese: *Wakadoshiyori*.
19. *Tokugawa jikki: dai nihen*, vol. 39 (1976 print edition), 549 and 668.
20. Japanese title: *Kōkoku meii den*.
21. *Kōkoku meii den: jō*, 1851 (images 46–47); *Ryōchi no taigaishū* (*Shinkyū igaku tenseki taikei*, vol. 14), 4–5; Nagao Eiichi Kyōju Taikan Kinen Ronbunshū Kankōkai, ed., *Shinkyū anmashi ronkō*, 50.
22. *Tokugawa jikki, dai 3-pen*, 952 (image 480; 1907 digital edition). See also Katori, "Edoki no shinkyū anma to shikaku shōgaisha," 10. Katori suggests that a month before Wa'ichi's meeting with shogun Tokugawa Ietsuna, Wa'ichi and his

disciple Mitsu'ichi visited the residence of the Tottori domain lord in Edo, where Mitsu'ichi provided massage.

23. *Tokugawa jikki: dai gohen*, vol. 42 (1976 print edition), 334 and 553; *Tokugawa jikki: dai rokuhen*, vol. 43 (1976 print edition), 57 and 127; Katō, *Nihon mōjin shakaishi kenkyū*, 164.

24. *Tokugawa jikki: dai rokuhen*, vol. 43 (1976 print edition), 141. See the guild's hierarchy outlined in chapter 3.

25. Wa'ichi was said to have founded four schools in and around Edo and another forty-five schools across other regions.

26. Katō, *Nihon mōjin shakaishi kenkyū*, 531–32.

27. Katori, "Sugiyama kengyō Wa'ichi no deshitachi," 311–12; *Tokugawa jikki: dai rokuhen*, vol. 43 (1976 print edition), 156 and 162.

28. *Tokugawa jikki: dai rokuhen*, vol. 43 (1976 print edition), 115, 208, and 638.

29. Katori, "Sugiyama kengyō Wa'ichi no deshitachi," 305–9; Katori, "Mishima sōkengyō Yasu'ichi no shiryō to Tsuchiura no densetsu," 100–109; Ōura, Hanawa, and Ishino, "Sugiyama Shinden-ryū no keishōsha tachi," 70. Yasu'ichi likely lived at Wa'ichi's previous residence in Ogawa-*machi* (in today's Chiyoda-*ku* in Tokyo) instead of moving to Kyoto to supervise the guild's affairs.

30. Nagao Eiichi Kyōju Taikan Kinen Ronbunshū Kankōkai, ed., *Shinkyū anmashi ronkō*, 76–77; Ōura and Kosoto, "Sugiyama Kengyō Itoku Kenshōkaisho zō no 'Sugiyama shinden-ryū,'" 225–26.

31. Japanese: *ryū-ha* (or *gakutō*); Ōura, *Sugiyama Shinden-ryū rinshō shinan*, 243.

32. Vigouroux, "The Reception of the Circulation Channels Theory in Japan (1500–1800)," 121–23; Vigouroux, "Edo jidai ni okeru shinkyū igaku," 75. *The Deployment of the Fourteen Conduits* (Chinese: *Shisijing fahui*; Japanese: *Jūshikei hakki*), which was written in Yuan-dynasty China in the fourteenth century, was thought to have been annotated in Japan in the mid-seventeenth century and gained currency among acupuncturists as a foundational text about the theories of circulation.

33. Japanese: *hankō*; *shijuku*. Rubinger, *Private Academies of the Tokugawa Period*, 8–9. Rubinger argues that the term "school" should be interpreted broadly. See also Umihara, *Edo jidai no ishi shūgyō*, 26–33.

34. For a discussion of the Ikeda lineage, see Trambaiolo, "Writing, Authority and Practice in Tokugawa Medicine, 1650–1850," 144–78.

35. Marcon, *The Knowledge of Nature and the Nature of Knowledge in Early Modern Japan*, 182–83.

36. Japanese title: *Sugiyama sanbusho*.

37. Japanese: *uchibari*.

38. *Shinkyū chōhōki*, 17 and 46–47; Ono, *Kaisetsu Shinkyū chōhōki*, 5–7 and 46–50. This work on acupuncture will be introduced in this chapter's section on popular literature and blind masseurs.

39. *Idan*, 4 (image 11). Daidoji, "The Adaptation of the *Treatise on Cold Damage* in Eighteenth-Century Japan," 375 and 380–85. The abdomen was said to be where the "hundred diseases" arose.

40. Japanese: *fukushin*.

41. *Igaku setsuyōshū*, 8–11 (images 11–14); *Ryōchi no taigaishū*, 15 (image 21). In *Igaku setsuyōshū* (*A Collection of the Essentials of Medicine*), an entire section is devoted to methods of examining the abdomen. *Ryōchi no taigaishū* (*A Collection of the Outlines of Treatment*), another medical treatise of Wa'ichi's series, lists the categories of stagnation at the abdomen that could be diagnosed by palpation.

42. Ōura and Ichikawa, "Wada Masanaga no nokoshita *Sugiyama shinden-ryū* zenkan no kenshō," 337–38; Ōura, Hanawa, and Ishino, "'Sugiyama Shinden-ryū no keishōsha tachi," 70.

43. Ōura and Ichikawa, "Wada Masanaga no nokoshita *Sugiyama shinden-ryū* zenkan no kenshō," 341–42. Though it cannot be ascertained when or how long it took to edit and reorganize the contents, these handwritten copies were found to be in the possession of a blind disciple named Onozuka *kengyō* during the early Meiji years.

44. *Kissō shoei*, in *Asada Sōhaku*, vol. 6, 580–81; Ericson, "The Tokugawa Bakufu and Léon Roches," 34–36 and 229–31. The 1860s were tumultuous years in Japan as the Tokugawa regime was forced to open its borders to European powers.

45. Ōura and Ichikawa, "Wada Masanaga no nokoshita *Sugiyama shinden-ryū* zenkan no kenshō," 340–41.

46. Japanese: *shayaku*.

47. Japanese: *kudoku*.

48. Japanese: *shinshin*.

49. Wakuda, "Edoki no anma jutsu," 41. Wakuda suggests that the initial phase of training at the school of acupuncture of the guild was split evenly between acupuncture and massage for a total of six years.

50. "Condition of the Blind in Old Japan," Nov 29, 1891, 13.

51. Ōura, "Ashihara kengyō no ashiato," 52–54; Nagao Eiichi Kyōju Taikan Kinen Ronbunshū Kankōkai, ed., *Shinkyū anmashi ronkō*, 97–98.

52. Ōura, "Ashihara kengyō no ashiato," 64–67.

53. Ōura, "Ashihara kengyō no ashiato," 53, 66, and 71–73.

54. Takizawa, "Jūkyū seiki zenki yōjōron ni okeru ningen keiseikan no kōsatsu," 159. *Yangsheng* was roughly coterminous with *yangxing*.

55. Stanley-Baker, "'Indian Massage' from Sun Simiao's Prescriptions Worth a Thousand in Gold," 533–35. *Daoyin* exercises discussed in these early Chinese texts were mainly self-exercises or self-massage and developed under the influences of Indian traditions.

56. Japanese title: *Kirigami*.

57. Chinese title: *Xianjing*; Japanese title: *Sengyō*.

58. *Kirigami*, 44–45 (images 48–50).

59. Japanese title: *Denshi yōjōketsu*.

60. Japanese: *furo chōsei*.

61. *Denshi yōjōketsu*, images 2 and 14–15.

62. *Yōjō zokkaishū*, 4–9 (images 10–15). *Yōjō zokkaishū*, one of many printed illustrated manuals, provides instructions for massage.

63. Suzuki, "Edo jidai ni okeru yōjōsho no kenkyū," 413–15.

64. Rubinger, *Popular Literacy in Early Modern Japan*, 97–99.

65. Aoki, *Edo jidai no igaku*, 42–43.

66. *Kawachiya Kashō kyūki*, 49–50. By Kashō's estimation, a superior physician was someone who helped his patients by striving to prevent the onset of diseases so that even in times of illness, a patient quickly recovered from setbacks.

67. Kuriyama, "The Historical Origins of Katakori," 135–42. Stagnations: *henpeki/ kenpeki* and *katamari*.

68. Aoki, *Edo jidai no igaku*, 35–36.

69. Katafuchi, "Edo yōjōron e no michiyuki," 79–80.

70. Japanese title: *Chōnin bukuro*.

71. *Chōnin bukuro*, 124.

72. Japanese title: *Yōjō kanben nichiyō shokukagami.*

73. *Yōjō kanben nichiyō shokukagami,* images 7–9.

74. Japanese title: *Yōjōkun.*

75. Japanese: *eisei.* Takizawa, "Jūkyū seiki zenki yōjōron ni okeru ningen keiseikan no kōsatsu," 168.

76. *Yōjōkun,* vol. 1, images 4–5; Matsuda, *Yōjōkun,* 5.

77. *Yōjōkun,* vol. 2, images 40–41.

78. *Yōjōkun,* vol. 5, images 6–8; Matsuda, *Yōjōkun,* 116–19; Ōmachi, *Ekiken jikkun: ge,* 698–99 (image 53).

79. *Yōjōkun, kan 8,* vol. 8, images 40–41; Ōmachi, *Ekiken jikkun: ge,* 770–71 (image 89). According to Ekiken, acupuncture was forbidden when stagnation was absent or when a patient was gravely exhausted, starved and starving, parched from thirst, or devastated by shock. He warned about the age and constitution of a patient as factors not to be overlooked.

80. Japanese title: *Anma tebiki.*

81. *Gendaigo yaku anpuku shinjutsu anma tebiki zen,* 65–70 and 82–84.

82. Japanese: *momi chiryō.*

83. Umihara, *Kinsei iryō no shakaishi,* 50–51.

84. Japanese title: *Yūsō iwa.*

85. *Yūsō iwa,* 3–4 (image 5).

86. "New Field for the Blind," April 7, 1912, C5. According to this report, blind masseurs had gained a secure base in French society; there was a new institution in Paris for studying massage and training masseurs.

87. *Yao Yazaemon nikki,* 192, 216, and 254.

88. *Yao Yazaemon nikki,* 263.

89. *Yao Yazaemon nikki,* 225 and 289.

90. Japanese: *ana o ma [suru] sōrō.*

91. *Yao Yazaemon nikki,* 194; Umihara, *Kinsei iryō no shakaishi,* 30.

92. *Ofuregaki Tenpō shūsei: ge,* 432–33.

93. Japanese: *sokuryoku.*

94. *Hokusai manga,* vol. 1, image 9.

95. *Hokusai manga,* vol. 1, image 10.

96. Hasegawa, "Edo fūzoku ni anmashi no waza o egaita Katsushika Hokusai," 136.

97. Japanese title: *Mugura no shizuku: shoka zatsudan.*

98. *Mugura no shizuku,* 391.

99. Japanese title: *Kinkin sensei eiga no yume.* The word *kinkin* was a fashionable word for a flashy, ostentatious person at that time. Screech, *The Lens within the Heart,* 104. Screech translates this book title as *Master Moneypenny's Dreams of Glory.*

100. Thomas, "Approaches to Oneiric Texts and Imagery in Early Modern Japan," 60–63.

101. *Kinkin sensei eiga no yume,* 121–22 (images 69 and 70).

102. *Kinkin sensei eiga no yume,* 126 (image 72). See also *Shin Yoshiwara-chō sadamegaki, Enseki jisshu: dai 3,* 470 (image 242). There is some basis for imagining the association between massage and sensual indulgences. Massage was a medical therapy but it was probably also given for pleasure. Measures aimed at regulating safety in the pleasure quarters of Yoshiwara in Edo warned of pesky blind masseurs who waylaid customers and extorted high fees; when customers lost their belongings, these blind masseurs were accused of theft.

103. Japanese title: *Tōkaidōchū hizakurige.*
104. *Shank's Mare,* 157–64.
105. Mitchell and Snyder, *Narrative Prosthesis,* 50.
106. Japanese title: *Shinkyū chōhōki.*
107. *Shinkyū chōhōki,* 163.
108. Japanese title: *Anma hitorigeiko.*
109. Japanese title: *Dōin kuketsushō.*
110. *Anma hitorigeiko,* images 9–10; *Dōin kuketsushō,* images 7–9.
111. *Gendaigo yaku anpuku shinjutsu anma tebiki zen,* 7–9.
112. Japanese title: *Anpuku zukai.*
113. *Gendaigo yaku anpuku zukai,* 10.
114. *Anma tebiki,* images 2–3.

Epilogue

1. *Kuzuhara kōtō nikki,* 283. Kuzuhara *kōtō,* featured in chapter 5, recorded this news in his diary in an entry in the 12th month of 1871. We do not know, however, how he reacted to this news.
2. Katō, *Nihon mōjin shakaishi kenkyū,* 454–73.
3. Yamada, *Tsūshi: Nihon no shōgaisha,* 33–40. As Yamada's survey indicates, social welfare was reserved for the ambiguous category of the old, young, sick, and disabled (*rōyō haishitsu fuben no mono* and *byōsha*), including blind people and people with mental disabilities.
4. Katō, *Nihon mōjin shakaishi kenkyū,* 476–81; Groemer, *Goze to goze uta no kenkyū: shiryō hen,* 575–76.
5. Kim, *Doctors of Empire,* 16–53.
6. Rogaski, *Hygienic Modernity,* 136–64. "Eisei" literally means "guarding life"— the roots of Tokugawa Japanese health cultivation were also in Daoist thought.
7. Früstück, *Colonizing Sex,* 22–24. As Früstück explains, the national agenda was focused on the health of children and youths. It was informed by the political, socio-biological view of an organic living nation.
8. Hasegawa, *Rikugun senpei iji seiki,* 27–28 (images 18–19).
9. Platt, "Japanese Childhood, Modern Childhood," 970–75.
10. Japanese: *gakkō eisei.*
11. Inoue, *Ganka eiseigaku,* 53–55 (images 35–36) and 61–63 (images 39–40); Nakayama, "Posturing for Modernity," 364–72. Nakayama's study of Japanese school hygienist Mishima Michiyoshi tells a familiar story of Meiji government state agents intervening in education to carry out best practices for health as conceived by their formulations.
12. Jannetta, *The Vaccinators,* 178; Fukase, *Tennentō konzetsushi,* 278–81.
13. Inoue, *Kingan torahōmu ryōyōhō,* 72–76 (images 42–44). The discussion of trachoma was cast in racializing, nationalistic language, and it empowered the rhetoric of disease prevention in Japan's modernization.
14. Ding, "Iyaku iryō to Nichū rentai," 220–22. One famous eye medicine was medical entrepreneur Kishida Ginkō's eye medicine. It was not only sold all over Japan starting in the late nineteenth century but also exported overseas.
15. Figal, *Civilization and Monsters,* 92–96. Public health authorities looked upon popular medicines to treat trachoma as baseless, unenlightened, and even harmful to health, in contrast to evidence of the compelling logic and results of Western medicine.

16. Ogasawara, "Shichōkaku shōgaiji kyōiku no akebono ni okeru kigyōka fuiransoropī," 170–72; Tsukuba Daigaku Fuzoku Mōgakkō Dōsōkai Kōenkai, ed., *Mōa kyōiku bunrigo hyakunen*, 6.

17. *Short Account of the Tōkyō Blind and Dumb School*, 1–3; Ogasawara, "Shichōkaku shōgaiji kyōiku no akebono ni okeru kigyōka fuiransoropī," 166–70. The Tokyo School welcomed its first cohort of blind and deaf students in 1880.

18. *Short Account of the Tōkyō Blind and Dumb School*, 25–31; Tsukuba Daigaku Fuzoku Mōgakkō Dōsōkai Kōenkai, ed., *Mōa kyōiku bunrigo hyakunen*, 7–10. The Japanese braille system was refined in 1899 to accommodate characteristics of the Japanese language and was successfully readapted for more widespread use in print publications.

19. Tōkyō Mōgakkō, ed., *Tōkyō mōgakkō ichiran*, 23–24 (images 18–19). At the Tokyo School, the general length of primary education was six years; secondary education was four years.

20. *Short Account of the Tōkyō Blind and Dumb School*, 31–32; Yamada, *Tsūshi: Nihon no shōgaisha*, 76–77. In 1885, the vocational program was temporarily suspended.

21. Tōkyō Mōgakkō, ed., *Tōkyō mōgakkō ichiran*, 40–44 (images 27–29). Candidates for acupuncture and massage licensing were examined in subjects, such as the human anatomy.

22. Kurihara, *Hikari usure iku toki*, 15–23 and 35–65.

23. Yamada, *Tsūshi: Nihon no shōgaisha*, 77–79; Tōkyō Mōgakkō, ed., *Tōkyō mōgakkō ichiran*, 30–33 (images 22–23); Kurihara, *Taishō no Tōkyō mōgakkō*, 96.

24. Iwahashi, *Light from Darkness*, 40–48; Murota, "Iwahashi Takeo kenkyū oboegaki," 29–35; Honma, *Mōjin no shokugyōteki jiritsu e no ayumi*, 70–71.

25. "Helen Keller Hailed as Miracle in Japan: Royally Feted, She Expresses a Wish to Launch a Project to Aid Nation's Blind," April 16, 1937; Murota, "Iwahashi Takeo kenkyū oboegaki," 36–37. See also Nielsen, *The Radical Lives of Helen Keller*, 62.

Bibliography

~~~

The primary sources are arranged in three main sections: (1) digital sources and databases; (2) published sources; and (3) websites. For ease of reference, the primary sources are arranged in a title-first format, followed by relevant information.

All URLs were correct at the time of access, but may be subject to change by hosts.

Primary Sources

1. Digital Sources and Databases

+Adeac

Zenkōji hitori annai. (Shinshū chiiki shiryō archive) https://trc-adeac.trc.co.jp/Html
  /ImageView/2000515100/2000515100100020/011/?p=34

Aichi Prefectural Library

Denshi yōjōketsu. By Tanaka Utarō. 1826. [Kichō wahon digital library; item number:
  Wラ/490/タ]

Hathitrust Digital Library

Fukyū ruihō. Vol. 1. By Niwa Seihaku and Hayashi Ryōteki. 1729. https://babel.hathitr
  ust.org/cgi/pt?id=mdp.39015078134817&view=1up&seq=1
Kiyū shōran. Vol. 11. By Kitamura Nobuyo. *Zonsai sōsho.* Edited by Kondō Keizō. Tokyo:
  Kondō Keizō, 1887. https://babel.hathitrust.org/cgi/pt?id=keio.10811562441;vi
  ew=1up;seq=15
Konjaku monogatarishū. Kokushi taikei, vol. 16. Edited by Keizai Zasshisha. Tokyo: Keizai

Zasshisha, 1901. https://babel.hathitrust.org/cgi/pt?id=osu.32435025974916;vie
w=1up;seq=9

Sōkyoku taiishō (okusho). By Yamada Shōkoku. Kariganeya Ihē, 1811. https://babel.hat
hitrust.org/cgi/pt?id=keio.10811696553

Tokitsugu kyō ki. By Yamashina Tokitsugu. Edited by Hayakawa Junsaburō. Tokyo:
Kokusho Kankōkai, 1915. https://babel.hathitrust.org/cgi/pt?id=pst.000022214
911;view=1up;seq=529

Ukiyo no arisama. Kokushi sōsho, vol. 40. Edited by Yano Tarō. Tokyo: Kokushi
Kenkyūkai, 1917. https://babel.hathitrust.org/cgi/pt?id=mdp.39015082787543;
view=1up;seq=159

Yasumura kengyō busō gafushū. Likely by Yasumura *kengyō.* Included in *Sōkyoku taiishō
(okusho).* Kariganeya Ihē, 1811. https://babel.hathitrust.org/cgi/pt?id=keio.1081
1696553

Yatsuhashi kengyō kinkyokushō jo. Included in *Sōkyoku taiishō (okusho).* Kariganeya Ihē,
1811. https://babel.hathitrust.org/cgi/pt?id=keio.10811696553

Internet Archive

Light from Darkness. By Takeo Iwahashi. Tokyo: Christian Literature Society of Japan,
1932. https://archive.org/details/lightfromdarknes00take_0

Kyoto University Rare Materials Digital Archive:
Main Library, Fujikawa Collection

Anma hitorigeiko. By Hitogushi. 1793. https://rmda.kulib.kyoto-u.ac.jp/en/item/rb0
0000821

Anma tebiki. By Tachibana Shunki and Fujibayashi Ryōhaku. 1799/1835. https://rmda
.kulib.kyoto-u.ac.jp/en/item/rb00000442

Dassairoku. By Habu Genseki. Year unknown. https://rmda.kulib.kyoto-u.ac.jp/en/it
em/rb00004047

Dōin kuketsushō. By Miyawaki Chūsaku. 1713. https://rmda.kulib.kyoto-u.ac.jp/en/it
em/rb00000676

Ganmoku taizen. Author and year unknown. https://rmda.kulib.kyoto-u.ac.jp/en/it
em/rb00001783

Ganryō tōun hiroku. By Majima Daikōbō. Year unknown. https://rmda.kulib.kyoto
-u.ac.jp/en/item/rb00001803

Idan. By Yoshimasu Tōdō. 1812. https://rmda.kulib.kyoto-u.ac.jp/en/item/rb0000
0483

Igaku setsuyōshū. By Sugiyama Wa'ichi. 1887 (reprint). https://rmda.kulib.kyoto-u.ac
.jp/en/item/rb00000887

Ikeda sensei chitō kuketsu. By Kii Jakusan (Saitō Junkōan). Year unknown. https://rmda
.kulib.kyoto-u.ac.jp/en/item/rb00000960

Ishinpō. By Tanba Yasuyori. 1855 (reprint). https://rmda.kulib.kyoto-u.ac.jp/en/item
/rb00013365

Kirigami. By Manase Dōsan. 1649. https://rmda.kulib.kyoto-u.ac.jp/en/item/rb000
02008

Kōkei saikyūhō. By Taki Motoyori (and Taki Motoyasu). 1790. https://rmda.kulib.kyo
to-u.ac.jp/en/item/rb00002357

Kōtei daikyō/daikei somon. Author and year unknown. https://rmda.kulib.kyoto-u.ac.jp/en/item/rb00002408

Kubai yōhō. By Kō Ryōsai. 1838. https://rmda.kulib.kyoto-u.ac.jp/en/item/rb00002108

Kyūmin myōyaku. By Hozumi Hoan. 1693. https://rmda.kulib.kyoto-u.ac.jp/en/item/rb00001965

Majima Myōgen'in megusuri. By Hoshima Hōkyō Rōgetsu. Year unknown. https://rmda.kulib.kyoto-u.ac.jp/en/item/rb00005205

Majima-ryū ganmoku hidensho. Author and year unknown. https://rmda.kulib.kyoto-u.ac.jp/en/item/rb00005206

Majima-ryū megusuri hisho. Author unknown. 1712. https://rmda.kulib.kyoto-u.ac.jp/en/item/rb00005207

Ryōchi no taigaishū. By Sugiyama Wa'ichi. 1887 (reprint). https://rmda.kulib.kyoto-u.ac.jp/en/item/rb00005760

Shīboruto kenpōroku. By Inoue Yūki (Aritoki). Circa 1828. https://rmda.kulib.kyoto-u.ac.jp/en/item/rb00002839

Shomin myōyakuhō. Author unknown. Circa 1697. https://rmda.kulib.kyoto-u.ac.jp/en/item/rb00003368

Yakuhin ōshuroku. By Kō Ryōsai. 1886. https://rmda.kulib.kyoto-u.ac.jp/en/item/rb00005455

Yōjō kanben nichiyō shokukagami. By Tateno Ryōboku. Year unknown. https://rmda.kulib.kyoto-u.ac.jp/en/item/rb00005606

Yōjō zokkaishū. By Matsuo Dōeki. 1731. https://rmda.kulib.kyoto-u.ac.jp/en/item/rb00005617

(Zoku) Tōka ben'yō. By Ikeda Mukei. 1827. https://rmda.kulib.kyoto-u.ac.jp/en/item/rb00003474

National Diet Library Digital Collections

Dai Chikamatsu zenshū: kaisetsu chūshaku. Vol. 5. By Chikamatsu Monzaemon. Edited by Kitani Hōgin. Tokyo: Dai Chikamatsu Zenshū Kankōkai, 1923. http://dl.ndl.go.jp/info:ndljp/pid/969896

Ganka kanmei. Edited by Hirahara Motoyoshi. Tokyo: Hirahara Motoyoshi, 1893. https://dl.ndl.go.jp/info:ndljp/pid/836248

Gunsho ruijū, dai 19 shū. By Hanawa Hokiichi. Tokyo: Keizai Zasshisha, 1902. http://dl.ndl.go.jp/info:ndljp/pid/1879582

Heike monogatari (Rufu-bon). Author unknown. 1600. https://dl.ndl.go.jp/info:ndljp/pid/2570057

Hokusai manga. Vol. 1. By Katsushika Hokusai. Nagoya: Katano Tōshirō, 1878. https://dl.ndl.go.jp/info:ndljp/pid/851646

Kaga-han shiryō. 4-hen: http://dl.ndl.go.jp/info:ndljp/pid/1123775; 12-hen: http://dl.ndl.go.jp/info:ndljp/pid/1123980; 13-hen: http://dl.ndl.go.jp/info:ndljp/pid/1124011; 14-hen: http://dl.ndl.go.jp/info:ndljp/pid/1124027. Edited by Maeda-ke Henshūbu. Tokyo: Ishiguro Bunkichi, 1942.

Kinkin sensei eiga no yume. By Koikawa Harumachi. *Kinsei bungaku senshū.* Edited by Ehara Taizō. Tokyo: Meiji Shoin, 1939. http://dl.ndl.go.jp/info:ndljp/pid/1457605

Kinmō zui. Vol. 4. By Nakamura Tekisai. Yamagataya, 1666. https://dl.ndl.go.jp/info:ndljp/pid/2569343

Nagoya shishi. Vol. 6, *fūzoku-hen.* Edited by Nagoya Shiyakusho. Nagoya: Nagoya Shiyakusho, 1915. https://dl.ndl.go.jp/info:ndljp/pid/950890

Ochiboshū. By Daidōji Yūzan. *Shiseki shūran, dai* 10 *satsu.* Edited by Kondō Heijō. Tokyo: Kondō Shuppanbu, 1926. http://dl.ndl.go.jp/info:ndljp/pid/1920299

Omote bikae. Author and year unknown. http://dl.ndl.go.jp/info:ndljp/pid/253855 6/59

Onna chōhōki taisei. Vol. 4. By Kusada Sunbokushi. Osaka: Aburaya Heiemon, 1711. http://dl.ndl.go.jp/info:ndljp/pid/2543232

Sanba kokoroe. By Inasaka Sankichi. Kanazawa: Unkondō, 1886. https://dl.ndl.go.jp /info:ndljp/pid/836073

Shihō shiryō dai 180 *gō. Tokugawa kinreikō, dai* 5 *shitsu.* Edited by Shihōshō Chōsaka. Tokyo: Shihōshō Chōsaka, 1934. http://dl.ndl.go.jp/info:ndljp/pid/1449473

Shin Yoshiwara-chō sadamegaki. Enseki jisshu, dai 3. Edited by Iwamoto Kattōshi. Tokyo: Kokusho Kankōkai, 1907–8. http://dl.ndl.go.jp/info:ndljp/pid/991270/242

Sunkoku zasshi. Vol. 1. Edited by Abe Masanobu. Shizuoka: Yoshimi Shoten, 1912. https://dl.ndl.go.jp/info:ndljp/pid/765114

Tōdō ryakki. Mōjin shoshorui, vol. 3. Author and year unknown. https://dl.ndl.go.jp/in fo:ndljp/pid/2538554

Tokugawa jikki: dai ichihen. Edited by Keizai Zasshisha. Tokyo: Keizai Zasshisha, 1907. http://dl.ndl.go.jp/info:ndljp/pid/772965

Tokugawa jikki: dai 3-*pen. Zoku Kokushi taikei*, vols. 11, 17, and 18. Edited by Keizai Zasshisha. Tokyo: Keizai Zasshisha, 1905. http://dl.ndl.go.jp/info:ndljp/pid/991118; Tokyo: Keizai Zasshisha, 1907. http://dl.ndl.go.jp/info:ndljp/pid/772967

Yoshiwara zatsuwa. Enseki jisshu, vol. 3. Edited by Iwamoto Kattōshi. Tokyo: Kokusho Kankōkai, 1907–8. https://dl.ndl.go.jp/info:ndljp/pid/991270

Yūsō iwa. By Mori Yōchiku. 1864. http://dl.ndl.go.jp/info:ndljp/pid/2536610/5

National Institute of Japanese Literature Digital Collections

Kōkoku meii den: jō. By Asada Sōhaku. 1800s. (Call number: DIG-KNIK-20)

Nichibunken (International Research Center for Japanese Studies)

Hashika karuku suru hō. By Utagawa Fusatane. 1862. (Call number: YR/8/Ut; Folklore illustrations database)

Shūi miyako meisho zue. Vols. 2 and 3. By Akisato Ritō et al. 1787. (Illustrations of historic places in Kyoto database)

Waseda University Kotenseki Sōgō Database (Japanese and Chinese Classics)

Byōmei ikai. Vols. 3 and 5. By Ashigawa Keishū. Circa 1686. (Call number: ヤ09 00581)

Edo meisho zue. Vols. 1 and 14. By Saitō Gesshin et al. Year unknown. (Call number: 文 庫30 E0204)

Ganka kinnō. Vols. 1 and 3. By Honjō Fu'ichi. Circa 1830–36. (Call number: ヤ09 00725)

Ganka shinsho. Vols. 1, 2, and 3. By Sugita Ryūkei. Circa 1815–16. (Call number: ヤ09 00726)

Ika jinmeiroku. Vols. 1 and 2. By Shiratsuchi Ryūhō. 1820. (Call number: ヌ05 05784)

Ise sangū meisho zue. By Shitomi Kangetsu et al. 1797. (Call number: 文庫30 E0211)

Kaitai shinsho. Jozu and vol. 2. By Sugita Genpaku et al. 1774. (Call number: ﾔ03 01366)

Yamato meisho zue. Vol. 3. By Akisato Ritō et al. Circa 1791. (Call number: ﾉﾚ04 05326)

Yōjōkun. Vols. 1, 2, 5, and 8. By Kaibara Ekiken. 1834. (Call number: ﾔ09 00705)

Zoku Edo sunago onko meisekishi. Vols. 1–5. By Kikuoka Senryō. 1735. (Call number: ﾉﾚ 04 03228 0007)

2. Published Sources

Aizu fudoki fūzokuchō. Jōkyō fūzokuchō, vol. 2. Edited by Shōji Kichinosuke. Tokyo: Yoshikawa Kōbunkan, 1979.

Awaji no kuni fūzoku toijōkotae. Nihon shomin seikatsu shiryō shūsei, vol. 9. Edited by Takeuchi Toshimi, Harada Tomohiko, and Hirayama Toshijirō. Tokyo: San'ichi Shobō, 1969.

Chikuzen meisho zue. Edited by Kasuga Komonjo o Yomukai. Tokyo: Bunken Shuppan, 1985.

Chishinshū. Shinshū Hiroshima shishi, vol. 6, *shiryō-hen.* Edited by Hiroshima Shiyakusho. Hiroshima: Hiroshima Shiyakusho, 1959.

Chōnin bukuro. By Nishikawa Joken. *Nihon shisō taikei: kinsei chōnin shisō,* vol. 59. Edited by Nakamura Yukihiko. Tokyo: Iwanami Shoten, 1975.

Dai Nihon kinsei shiryō, Hosokawa-ke shiryō, vol. 8. Edited by Tōkyō Daigaku Shiryō Hensanjo. Tokyo: Tōkyō Daigaku Shuppankai, 1982.

Echigo goze nikki. By Saitō Shin'ichi. Tokyo: Kawade Shobō Shinsha, 1975.

Edo machibure shūsei. Vol. 14. Edited by Kinsei Shiryō Kenkyūkai. Tokyo: Hanawa Shobō, 2000.

Edo shinbutsu gankake chōhōki. Shōgyō chishi, vol. 2; *Chōhōki shiryō shūsei,* vol. 32. Edited by Nagatomo Chiyoji. Kyoto: Rinsen Shoten, 2007.

Eiga monogatari zenchūshaku. Vol. 7. Edited by Matsumura Hiroshi. Tokyo: Kadokawa Shoten, 1978.

Enpekiken ki. By Kurokawa Dōyū. *Nihon zuihitsu taisei: dai ikki,* vol. 10. Edited by Nihon Zuihitsu Taisei Henshūbu. Tokyo: Yoshikawa Kōbunkan, 1955.

Essays in Idleness: The Tsurezuregusa of Kenkō. By Yoshida Kenkō. Translated by Donald Keene. New York: Columbia University Press, 1998.

Fukuoka kenshi: bunka shiryō-hen. Vol. 2. Edited by Nishi Nihon Bunka Kyōkai. Fukuoka-shi: Nishi Nihon Bunka Kyōkai, 1993.

Gendaigo yaku anpuku shinjutsu anma tebiki zen. Translated and edited by Wakuda Tetsuji. Tokyo: Ōunkai Tenji Shuppanbu, 2010.

Gendaigo yaku anpuku zukai. Translated and edited by Wakuda Tetsuji. Tokyo: Ōunkai Tenji Shuppanbu, 2013.

Goze shikimoku. Nihon shomin seikatsu shiryō shūsei (minkan geinō, vol. 17). Edited by Tanigawa Ken'ichi. Tokyo: San'ichi Shobō, 1972.

Hanpōshū. Edited by Hanpō Kenkyūkai. Tokyo: Sōbunsha, 1959–73. Vol. 1: *Okayama-han (jō/ge,* 1959); vol. 2: *Tottori-han* (1961); vol. 3: *Tokushima-han* (1962); vol. 7: *Kumamoto-han* (1966); vol. 10: *Zoku Tottori-han* (1972); vol. 11: *Kurume-han* (1973).

Heike ginpu: Miyazaki Bunko Kinenkan zō Heike monogatari. Edited by Murakami Mitsunori and Suzuki Takatsune. Tokyo: Mizuki Shobō, 2007.

Heike mabushi. 2 vols. By Ogino Chiichi. Edited by Heike Mabushi Kankōkai. Kyoto: Daigakudō Shoten, 1974.

Heike monogatari. Zōho kokugo kokubungaku kenkyūshi taisei, vol. 9. Edited by Takagi Ichinosuke, Nagazumi Yasuaki, Ichiko Teiji, and Atsumi Kaoru. Tokyo: Sanseidō, 1977.

The History of Japan Together with a Description of the Kingdom of Siam, 1690–92. Vol. 2, book 3. By Engelbert Kaempfer. Glasgow: Robert MacLehose. For James MacLehose and Sons, 1919.

Huang Di Nei Jing Ling Shu. Translated by Paul U. Unschuld. Berkeley: University of California Press, 2016.

Huang Di Nei Jing Su Wen: An Annotated Translation of Huang Di's Inner Classic—Basic Questions. Vol. 1. Translated by Paul U. Unschuld, Hermann Tessenow, and Zheng Jinsheng. Berkeley: University of California Press, 2011.

Kadoya Yōan nikki (jō/ge). By Kadoya Yōan. *Kinsei shomin seikatsu shiryō: mikan nikki shūsei (dai 2-kan).* Edited by Chadani Jūroku and Matsuoka Sei. Tokyo: San'ichi Shobō, 1996–97.

Kankoku kōgiroku (jōkan; chūkan). Edited by Noriko Sugano. Tokyo: Tōkyōdō Shuppan, 1999.

Kanmon nikki. Vol. 1. By Gosukōin. *Zushoryō sōkan*, vol. 26. Edited by Kunaichō Shoryūbu. Tokyo: Kunaichō Shoryūbu, 2002.

Kariya-machi shōya tomechō. Vol. 5. Edited by Kariya-shi Kyōiku Iinkai. Kariya-shi: Aichi-ken Kariya-shi, 1979.

Kariya-machi shōya tomechō kaisetsu: dai 11 kan yori dai 20 kan made. Edited by Kariya-shi Kyōiku Iinkai. Kariya-shi: Aichi-ken Kariya-shi, 1988.

Kawachiya Kashō kyūki. By Kawachiya Kashō. Edited by Nomura Noboru and Yoshii Kitarō. Osaka: Seibundō Gakushū Shuppansha, 1955.

Kenshōbo. Tosa-han hōsei shiryō, vol. 5. Edited by Kōchi Kenritsu Toshokan. Kōchi-shi: Kōchi Kenritsu Toshokan, 1984–85.

Kinsei kanpō chiken senshū. Vols. 10 and 11. Edited by Yakazu Dōmei, Ōtsuka Yasuo, and Yasui Hiromichi. Tokyo: Meicho Shuppan, 1986.

Kinsei shōgaisha kankei shiryō shūsei. Edited by Namase Katsumi. Tokyo: Akashi Shoten, 1996.

Kissō shoei. In *Asada Sōhaku*, vol. 6. By Asada Sōhaku. *Kinsei kanpō igakusho shūsei*, vol. 100. Edited by Ōtsuka Keisetsu and Yakazu Dōmei. Tokyo: Meicho Shuppan, 1983.

Kiyū shōran. Vol. 3. By Kitamura Nobuyo. Edited by Nihon Zuihitsu Taisei Henshūbu. Tokyo: Yoshikawa Kōbunkan, 1979.

Koga-ke monjo. Vol. 4. Edited by Kokugakuin Daigaku Koga-ke Monjo Hensan Iinkai. Tokyo: Kokugakuin Daigaku, 1987.

Konrin tsukumo no chiri. Nagoya sōsho, vol. 7, *chiri-hen*. Edited by Nagoya-shi Kyōiku Iinkai. Nagoya: Nagoya-shi Kyōiku Iinkai, 1960.

Kumomi-ke monjo: Shimonoseki mōsō shiryō. Edited by Shimonoseki Shiritsu Chōfu Toshokan. Shimonoseki-shi: Shimonoseki Shiritsu Chōfu Toshokan, 1992.

Kurume-han ōjōya kaigiroku: kansei sannen—bunsei gonen. Vol. 5. Edited by Kyūshū Daigaku Kyūshū Bunkashi Kenkyūjo Shiryōshū Kankōkai. Fukuoka: Kyūshū Bunkashi Kenkyūjo Shiryōshū Kankōkai, 2001.

Kuzuhara kōtō nikki. By Kuzuhara kōtō. Edited by Ogura Toyofumi. Tokyo: Ryokuchisha, 1981.

Kyokutei Bakin nikki. Vol. 4. By Kyokutei Bakin. Edited by Shibata Mitsuhiko. Tokyo: Chūō Kōron Shinsha, 2009.

Lust, Commerce, and Corruption: An Account of What I Have Seen and Heard, by an Edo Samurai. Translated by Mark Teeuwen, Kate Wildman Nakai, Miyazaki Fumiko, Anne Walthall, and John Breen. Edited by Mark Teeuwen and Kate Wildman Nakai. New York: Columbia University Press, 2014.

Makura no sōshi. By Sei Shōnagon. *Nihon koten bungaku zenshū*, vol. 11. Edited by Matsuo Satoshi and Nagai Kazuko. Tokyo: Shōgakkan, 1974.

Menkō shūroku. Izumi sōsho, vol. 3. Edited by Hosokawa Morisada et al. Kumamoto-shi: Kyūko Shoin, 1989.

Miya tera gankake chōhōki. Shōgyō chishi, vol. 2; *Chōhōki shiryō shūsei*, vol. 32. Edited by Nagatomo Chiyoji. Kyoto: Rinsen Shoten, 2007.

Mōsō biwa. Nihon shomin seikatsu shiryō shūsei (minkan geinō, vol. 17). Edited by Tanigawa Ken'ichi. Tokyo: San'ichi Shobō, 1972.

Mugura no shizuku: shoka zatsudan. Nagoya sōsho sanpen, vol. 12. Edited by Nagoya-shi Hōsa Bunko. Nagoya-shi: Nagoya-shi Kyōiku Iinkai, 1981.

The Narrow Road to the Deep North and Other Travel Sketches. By Matsuo Bashō. Translated by Nobuyuki Yuasa. New York: Penguin Books, 1966.

Nihon kodai chūsei jinmei jiten. Edited by Hirano Kunio and Seno Seiichirō. Tokyo: Yoshikawa Kōbunkan, 2006.

Nihon shoki. Shinpen Nihon koten bungaku zenshū, vol. 3. Edited by Kojima Noriyuki, Naoki Kōjirō, Nishimiya Kazutami, Kuranaka Susumu, and Mōri Masamori. Tokyo: Shōgakkan, 1998.

Ofuregaki Tenpō shūsei (ge). Edited by Takayanagi Shinzō and Ishii Ryōsuke. Tokyo: Iwanami Shoten, 1977.

Oshiokirei ruishū. Vol. 6. Edited by Ishii Ryōsuke. Tokyo: Meicho Shuppan, 1971.

Owari meisho zue. By Okada Kei et al. Edited by Aichi-ken Kyōdo Shiryō Kankōkai. Nagoya: Aichi-ken Kyōdo Shiryō Kankōkai, 1973.

Rakuchū rakugai baiyaku chōhōki. Ihō yakuhō, vol. 4; *Chōhōki shiryō shūsei*, vol. 26. Edited by Nagatomo Chiyoji. Kyoto: Rinsen Shoten, 2006.

Ritsu, Ryō no gige. Edited by Kuroita Katsumi. Tokyo: Yoshikawa Kōbunkan, 2000.

Ryōchi no taigaishū. By Sugiyama Wa'ichi. *Shinkyū igaku tenseki taikei*, vol. 14. Edited by Nihon Koigaku Shiryō Sentā. Tokyo: Shuppan Kagaku Sōgō Kenkyūjo, 1978.

Saikai yotekishū. Edited by Tomikura Tokujirō. Tokyo: Koten Bunko, 1956.

Sekisemimaru jinja monjo. Kenkyū sōsho, vol. 46. Edited by Muroki Yatarō and Sakaguchi Hiroyuki. Osaka: Izumi Shoin, 1987.

Shank's Mare. By Jippensha Ikku. Translated by Thomas Satchell. Boston: Tuttle Publishing, 2001.

Shinkyū chōhōki. By Hongō Masatoyo. *Ihō yakuhō*, vol. 3; *Chōhōki shiryō shūsei*, vol. 25. Edited by Nagatomo Chiyoji. Kyoto: Rinsen Shoten, 2007.

Shinpen Sagami no kuni fudokikō. Edited by Senshūsha. Tokyo: Senshūsha, 1888.

Shokoku zue nenchū gyōji taisei. By Hayami Shungyōsai. *Kinsei fūzoku chishi sōsho*, vol. 15. Edited by Nakamori Hiroshi. Tokyo: Ryūkei Shosha, 1996.

Sunpuki. Shiseki zassan, vol. 2. Edited by Kokusho Kankōkai. Tokyo: Zoku Gunsho Ruijū Kanseikai, 1974.

Suwa shishi. Edited by Suwa Shishi Hensan Iinkai. Suwa-shi: Suwa Shiyakusho, 1988.

Suzuki Heikurō: Kōshi nikki. Vol. 4. By Suzuki Heikurō. Edited by Kōshi Nikki Kenkyūkai. Tachikawa: Tachikawa-shi Kyōiku Iinkai, 2014.

The Tale of the Heike. Translated by Helen Craig McCullough. Stanford: Stanford University Press, 1988.

The Tale of the Heike. Translated by Royall Tyler. New York: Viking, 2012.

Teihon Kaga-han hisabetsu buraku kankei shiryō shūsei. Edited by Tanaka Yoshio. Tokyo: Akashi Shoten, 1995.

Things Japanese, Being Notes on Various Subjects Connected with Japan for the Use of Travellers and Others. By Basil Hall Chamberlain. London: John Murray, Albemarle Street, 1898.

Tōdō shinshikimoku. Shintei zōho shiseki shūran, vol. 30. Edited by Tsunoda Bun'ei and Gorai Shigeru. Kyoto: Rinsen Shoten, 1967.

Tōdō yōshū. Shintei zōho shiseki shūran, vol. 30. Edited by Tsunoda Bun'ei and Gorai Shigeru. Kyoto: Rinsen Shoten, 1967.

Tōdōza heike biwa shiryō: Okumura-ke zō. Documents included: *Koshikimoku, Shinshikimoku, Tōdō daikiroku, Tōdō ryakki, Sandai no seki.* Edited by Atsumi Kaoru, Maeda Mineko, and Ubukata Takashige. Kyoto: Daigakudō Shoten, 1984.

Tokugawa jikki: dai ichihen. Shintei zōho kokushi taikei, vol. 38. Edited by Kokushi Taikei Henshūkai. Tokyo: Yoshikawa Kōbunkan, 1934; 1975.

Tokugawa jikki: dai nihen. Shintei zōho kokushi taikei, vol. 39. Edited by Kokushi Taikei Henshūkai. Tokyo: Yoshikawa Kōbunkan, 1976.

Tokugawa jikki: dai gohen. Shintei zōho kokushi taikei, vol. 42. Edited by Kokushi Taikei Henshūkai. Tokyo: Yoshikawa Kōbunkan, 1976.

Tokugawa jikki: dai rokuhen. Shintei zōho kokushi taikei, vol. 43. Edited by Kokushi Taikei Henshūkai. Tokyo: Yoshikawa Kōbunkan, 1976.

Tokugawa kinreikō: goshū. Vol. 4. Edited by Ishii Ryōsuke. Tokyo: Sōbunsha, 1960.

Tokugawa kinreikō zenshū. Vol. 5. Edited by Ishii Ryōsuke. Tokyo: Sōbunsha, 1959.

Tōkyō shishikō. Vol. 11, *shigai-hen.* Edited by Tōkyō Shiyakusho. Tokyo: Kyōdō Insatsu, 1931.

Toyama kenshi: shiryō-hen. Vol. 5, *Toyama-han, kinsei: ge.* Edited by Toyama-ken. Toyama-shi: Toyama-ken, 1974.

Toyama kenshi: tsūshi-hen. Vol. 4, *kinsei: ge.* Edited by Toyama-ken. Toyama-shi: Toyama-ken, 1983.

Wagakoromo. By Katō Ebi'an. *Nihon shomin seikatsu shiryō shūsei*, vol. 15, *toshi fūzoku.* Edited by Tanigawa Ken'ichi et al. Tokyo: San'ichi Shobō, 1971.

Yao Yazaemon nikki. By Yao Yazaemon. *Nihon toshi seikatsu shiryō shūsei*, vol. 10, *zaigō machi-hen.* Edited by Harada Tomohiko. Tokyo: Gakushū Kenkyūsha, 1981.

Yoshino zōshi. Zuihitsu hyakkaen, vol. 9. Edited by Mori Senzō et al. Tokyo: Chūō Kōronsha, 1981.

3. Websites

"Condition of the Blind in Old Japan." *New-York Tribune*, Nov. 29, 1891. ProQuest Historical Newspapers.

"Disability Defined and Rules of Construction." ADA Amendments Act of 2008, Sept. 25, 2008. https://www.eeoc.gov/laws/statutes/adaaa.cfm

"Helen Keller Hailed as Miracle in Japan: Royally Feted, She Expresses a Wish to Launch a Project to Aid Nation's Blind." *New York Times*, April 16, 1937. ProQuest Historical Newspapers.

"The Japanese at Play." By Frank Carpenter. *The Cosmopolitan* VI. New York: John Brisben Walker, November 1888–April 1889. Google Books.

"New Field for the Blind." *New York Times*, April 7, 1912. ProQuest Historical Newspapers.

"Shōgaisha kihonhō." E-Gov Japan. https://elaws.e-gov.go.jp/search/elawsSearch/elaws_search/lsg0500/detail?openerCode=1&lawId=345AC1000000084_20160401_425AC0000000065

Short Account of the Tōkyō Blind and Dumb School. Tokyo: Nomura Sōjūrō, 1903. Google Books.

Other Sources

Adriaansz, Willem. *Kumiuta and Danmono: Traditions of Japanese Koto Music.* Berkeley: University of California Press, 1973.

Ambros, Barbara. *Emplacing a Pilgrimage: The Ōyama Cult and Regional Religion in Early Modern Japan.* Cambridge, MA: Harvard University Asia Center, Harvard University Press, 2008.

Aoki Toshiyuki. *Edo jidai no igaku: meii tachi no 300 nen.* Tokyo: Yoshikawa Kōbunkan, 2012.

Aoki Toshiyuki. *Zaison rangaku no kenkyū.* Kyoto: Shibunkaku Shuppan, 1998.

Arisawa, Shino. "*Ryūha*: Construction of Musical Tradition in Contemporary Japan." *Japan Forum* 24, no. 1 (2012): 97–118.

Atsumi Kaoru. *Gunki monogatari to setsuwa.* Tokyo: Kasama Shoin, 1979.

Atsumi Kaoru. *Heike monogatari no kisoteki kenkyū.* Tokyo: Sanseidō, 1962.

Atsumi Kaoru. "Kaidai." In *Heike mabushi*, edited by Heike Mabushi Kankōkai, 2:5–52. Kyoto: Daigakudō Shoten, 1974.

Atsumi Kaoru. "Ogino kengyō den: hoi." In *Heike mabushi no kenkyū*, edited by Atsumi Kaoru and Okumura Mitsuo, 183–230. Kyoto: Daigakudō Shoten, 1980.

Atsumi Kaoru, ed. *Yokoi Yayū jihitsu Heigo.* Tokyo: Kadokawa Shoten, 1977.

Ban Tadayasu. *Tekijuku o meguru hitobito: rangaku no nagare.* Osaka: Sōgensha, 1981.

Berry, Mary Elizabeth. *Japan in Print: Information and Nation in the Early Modern Period.* Berkeley: University of California Press, 2006.

Bolt, David. *The Metanarrative of Blindness: A Re-reading of Twentieth-Century Anglophone Writing.* Ann Arbor: University of Michigan Press, 2014.

Botsman, Daniel. *Punishment and Power in the Making of Modern Japan.* Princeton: Princeton University Press, 2007.

Bulliet, Richard W., Pamela Kyle Crossley, Daniel R. Headrick, Steven W. Hirsch, Lyman L. Johnson, and David Northrup. *The Earth and Its Peoples: A Global History.* Vols. 1 and 2. Stamford, CT: Cengage Learning, 2015.

Burch, Susan, and Michael Rembis. "Re-Membering the Past: Reflections on Disability Histories." In *Disability Histories*, edited by Susan Burch and Michael Rembis, 1–13. Springfield: University of Illinois Press, 2014.

Burns, Susan L. *Kingdom of the Sick: A History of Leprosy and Japan.* Honolulu: University of Hawai'i Press, 2019.

Butler, Kenneth Dean. "The Textual Evolution of Heike Monogatari." *Harvard Journal of Asiatic Studies* 26 (1966): 5–51.

Butler, Lee. "'Washing off the Dust': Baths and Bathing in Late Medieval Japan." *Monumenta Nipponica* 60, no. 1 (2005): 1–41.

Chadani Jūroku. "Kaisetsu: Kadoya Yōan nikki no sekai." In *Kadoya Yōan nikki: ge, Kinsei shomin seikatsu shiryō: mikan nikki shūsei (dai 2-kan)*, edited by Chadani Jūroku and Matsuoka Sei, 523–43. Tokyo: San'ichi Shobō, 1997.

Chikuma Yasuyuki. "Kōrasan shinkō no denpa: Chikugo no kuni Mizuma Yamato Miike gun no yonsha o chūshin toshite." *Sangaku shugen*, no. 31 (March 2003): 33–50.

Choe, Sang-Hun. "Blind Masseurs in South Korea Worry about the Loss of Status." *New York Times*, September 17, 2008.

Clements, Rebekah. *A Cultural History of Translation in Early Modern Japan.* New York: Cambridge University Press, 2015.

Corbett, Rebecca. *Cultivating Femininity: Women and Tea Culture in Edo and Meiji Japan.* Honolulu: University of Hawai'i Press, 2018.

Couser, G. Thomas. "Illness." In *Keywords for Disability Studies*, edited by Rachel Adams, Benjamin Reiss, and David Serlin, 105–7. New York: New York University Press, 2015.

Curran, Andrew. "Diderot's Revisionism: Enlightenment and Blindness in the 'Lettres sur les aveugles.'" *Diderot Studies* 28 (2000): 75–93.

Curth, Louise Hill. *English Almanacs, Astrology, and Popular Medicine, 1550–1700*. Manchester, UK: Manchester University Press, 2007.

Daidoji, Keiko. "The Adaptation of the *Treatise on Cold Damage* in Eighteenth-Century Japan: Text, Society, and Readers." *Asian Medicine* 8 (2013): 361–93.

DasGupta, Sayantani. "Medicalization." In *Keywords for Disability Studies*, edited by Rachel Adams, Benjamin Reiss, and David Serlin, 120–21. New York: New York University Press, 2015.

de Ferranti, Hugh. "The Kyushu *Biwa* Traditions." In *The Ashgate Research Companion to Japanese Music*, edited by Alison McQueen Tokita and David W. Hughes, 105–26. Burlington, VT: Ashgate, 2008.

de Ferranti, Hugh. *The Last Biwa Singer: A Blind Musician in History, Imagination and Performance*. Ithaca, NY: Cornell East Asia Series, Cornell University, 2009.

de Ferranti, Hugh. "Transmission and Textuality in the Narrative Traditions of Blind Biwa Players." *Yearbook for Traditional Music* 35 (2003): 131–52.

Deshpande, Vijaya. "Indian Influences on Early Chinese Ophthalmology: Glaucoma as a Case Study." *Bulletin of the School of Oriental and African Studies* 62, no. 2 (1999): 306–22.

Deshpande, Vijaya. "Ophthalmic Surgery: A Chapter in the History of Sino-Indian Medical Contacts." *Bulletin of the School of Oriental and African Studies* 63, no. 3 (2000): 370–88.

Ding Lei. "Iyaku iryō to Nichū rentai: Kishida Ginkō no shokatsudō o chūshin ni." *Nihon kenkyū: Kokusai Nihon Bunka Kenkyū Sentā kiyō* 31 (2005): 209–33.

Dormandy, Thomas. *Opium: Reality's Dark Dream*. New Haven: Yale University Press, 2012.

Ehlers, Maren. "Benevolence, Charity, and Duty: Urban Relief and Domain Society during the Tenmei Famine." *Monumenta Nipponica* 69, no. 1 (2014): 55–101.

Ehlers, Maren. *Give and Take: Poverty and the Status Order in Early Modern Japan*. Cambridge, MA: Harvard University Asia Center, Harvard University Press, 2018.

Elman, Benjamin. "Rethinking the Sino-Japanese Medical Classics: Antiquarianism, Languages, and Medical Philology." In *Antiquarianism, Language, and Medical Philology: From Early Modern to Modern Sino-Japanese Medical Discourses*, edited by Benjamin Elman, 1–18. Leiden: Brill, 2015.

Elman, Benjamin. "Sinophiles and Sinophobes in Tokugawa Japan: Politics, Classicism, and Medicine during the Eighteenth Century." *East Asian Science, Technology, and Society: An International Journal* 2, no. 1 (2008): 93–121.

Endō Shōji. "Iinuma-juku to sono monjin no dōkō." In *Zaison rangaku no tenkai*, edited by Tazaki Tetsurō, 77–140. Kyoto: Shibunkaku Shuppan, 1992.

Ericson, Mark David. "The Tokugawa Bakufu and Léon Roches." PhD diss., University of Hawaii, 1978.

Figal, Gerald. *Civilization and Monsters: Spirits of Modernity in Meiji Japan*. Durham: Duke University Press, 1999.

Flavin, Philip. Review of *The Koto: A Traditional Instrument in Contemporary Japan*, by Henry Mabley Johnson. *Asian Music* 37, no. 1 (2006): 127–34.

Flavin, Philip. "Sōkyoku-jiuta: Edo-Period Chamber Music." In *The Ashgate Research*

Companion to Japanese Music, edited by Alison McQueen Tokita and David W. Hughes, 169–96. Burlington, VT: Ashgate, 2008.

Fleming, William D. "Restaging the Forty-Seven Rōnin: Performance and Print in Late Eighteenth-Century Japan." *Eighteenth-Century Studies* 48, no. 4 (2015): 391–415.

Freeberg, Ernest. *The Education of Laura Bridgman: First Deaf and Blind Person to Learn Language.* Cambridge, MA: Harvard University Press, 2001.

Fritsch, Ingrid. *Japans blinde Sänger: Im Schutz der Gottheit Myōon-Benzaiten.* München: Ludicium Verlag, 1996.

"From Segregation to Civil Rights: Americans with Disabilities Act of 1990." In *Gale Encyclopedia of American Law,* 3rd edition, edited by Donna Batten, 13:396–433. Detroit: Gale, 2011.

Frumer, Yulia. *Making Time: Astronomical Time Measurement in Tokugawa Japan.* Chicago: University of Chicago Press, 2018.

Früstück, Sabine. *Colonizing Sex: Sexology and Social Control in Modern Japan.* Berkeley: University of California Press, 2003.

Fukase Yasuaki. *Tennentō konzetsushi: kindai igaku bokkōki no hitobito.* Kyoto: Shibunkaku Shuppan, 2002.

Fukuoka, Maki. *The Premise of Fidelity: Science, Visuality, and Representing the Real in Nineteenth-Century Japan.* Stanford: Stanford University Press, 2012.

Gordon, Andrew. *A Modern History of Japan: From Tokugawa Times to the Present.* New York: Oxford University Press, 2009.

Groemer, Gerald. "The Creation of the Edo Outcaste Order." *Journal of Japanese Studies* 27, no. 2 (2001): 263–93.

Groemer, Gerald. "Edo's 'Tin Pan Alley': Authors and Publishers of Japanese Popular Song during the Tokugawa Period." *Asian Music* 27, no. 1 (1995–96): 1–36.

Groemer, Gerald. "Female Shamans in Eastern Japan during the Edo Period." *Asian Folklore Studies* 66 (2007): 27–53.

Groemer, Gerald. *Goze: Women, Musical Performance, and Visual Disability in Traditional Japan.* New York: Oxford University Press, 2016.

Groemer, Gerald. *Goze to goze uta no kenkyū: shiryō-hen.* Nagoya-shi: Nagoya Daigaku Shuppankai, 2007.

Groemer, Gerald. "The Guild of the Blind in Tokugawa Japan." *Monumenta Nipponica* 56, no. 3 (2001): 349–80.

Groemer, Gerald. *The Spirit of Tsugaru: Blind Musicians, Tsugaru-jamisen, and the Folk Music of Northern Japan, with the Autobiography of Takahashi Chikuzan.* Warren, MI: Harmonie Park Press, 1999.

Groemer, Gerald. *Street Performers and Society in Urban Japan, 1600–1900.* New York: Routledge, 2016.

Groemer, Gerald. "Who Benefits? Religious Practice, Blind Women (*Goze*), Harugoma, and Manzai." *Japanese Journal of Religious Studies* 41, no. 2 (2014): 347–86.

Hall, John Whitney. "The *Bakuhan* System." In *The Cambridge History of Japan,* edited by John Whitney Hall and James L. McClain. Vol. 4, *Early Modern Japan,* 128–82. New York: Cambridge University Press, 1991.

Hardacre, Helen. *Religion and Society in Nineteenth-Century Japan: A Study of the Southern Kantō Region, Using Late Edo and Early Meiji Gazetteers.* Ann Arbor: Center for Japanese Studies, University of Michigan, 2002.

Hardacre, Helen. *Shintō and the State, 1868–1988.* Princeton: Princeton University Press, 1989.

Harris, William V. "Popular Medicine in the Classical World." In *Popular Medicine in*

Graeco-Roman Antiquity: Explorations, edited by William V. Harris, 1–64. Leiden: Brill, 2016.

Hasegawa Haruo, ed. *Rikugun senpei iji seiki.* Tokyo: Hasegawa Haruo, 1892. National Diet Library Digital Collections. http://dl.ndl.go.jp/info:ndljp/pid/798086

Hasegawa Naoya. "Edo fūzoku ni anmashi no waza o egaita Katsushika Hokusai: Hokusai no byōsha ni yoru Edoki no anma." *Idō no Nihon,* no. 795 (December 2009): 135–43.

Hayashi Kazutoshi. "Heike mabushi shoshi." In *DVD-ban Ozaki-ke bon Heike mabushi kaisetsu,* edited by Ogino Kengyō Kenshōkai, 3–4. Nagoya: Sōkō Eshikkusu, 2011.

Heyer, Katharina. *Rights Enabled: The Disability Revolution, from the U.S., to Germany and Japan, to the United Nations.* Ann Arbor: University of Michigan Press, 2015.

Hibi Kayoko. "Kurume-han ni okeru Kansei yonen zaikata showappu no shuhōgawari to ōjōya." In *Kinsei no chiiki to chūkan kenryoku,* edited by Shimura Hiroshi and Yoshida Nobuyuki, 83–122. Tokyo: Yamagata Shuppansha, 2011.

Honma Ritsuko. *Mōjin no shokugyōteki jiritsu e no ayumi: Iwahashi Takeo o chūshin ni.* Hyōgo-ken Nishinomiya-shi: Kansei Gakuin Daigaku Shuppankai, 2017.

Horn, Klaus-Peter, and Bianca Frohne. "On the Fluidity of 'Disability' in Medieval and Early Modern Societies: Opportunities and Strategies in a New Field of Research." In *The Imperfect Historian: Disability Histories in Europe,* edited by Sebastian Barsch, Anne Klein, and Pieter Verstraete, 17–40. Frankfurt am Main: Peter Lang, 2013.

Hoshino Kazuyuki. "Mōsō no shoji kyōten: jishinkyō o megutte." *Komazawa Daigaku bukkyō bungaku kenkyū* 18 (2015): 69–84.

Howell, David. *Geographies of Identity in Nineteenth-Century Japan.* Berkeley: University of California Press, 2005.

Howell, David. "Hard Times in the Kantō: Economic Change and Village Life in Late Tokugawa Japan." *Modern Asian Studies* 23, no. 2 (1989): 349–71.

Hughes, Bill, and Kevin Paterson. "Disability Studies and Phenomenology: The Carnal Politics of Everyday Life." *Disability & Society* 14, no. 5 (1999): 597–610.

Hughes, Bill, and Kevin Paterson. "The Social Model of Disability and the Disappearing Body: Towards a Sociology of Impairment." *Disability & Society* 12, no. 3 (1997): 325–40.

Hur, Nam-lin. *Death and Social Order in Tokugawa Japan: Buddhism, Anti-Christianity, and the Danka System.* Cambridge, MA: Harvard University Asia Center, Harvard University Press, 2007.

Hur, Nam-lin. *Prayer and Play in Late Tokugawa Japan: Asakusa Sensōji and Edo Society.* Cambridge, MA: Harvard University Asia Center, Harvard University Press, 2000.

Husson, Thérèse-Adèle. *Reflections: The Life and Writings of a Young Blind Woman in Post-Revolutionary France.* Translated by Catherine J. Kudlick and Zina Weygand. New York: New York University Press, 2001.

Hyōdō Hiromi. *Heike monogatari no rekishi to geinō.* Tokyo: Yoshikawa Kōbunkan, 2000.

Ichiko Teiji, ed. *Heike monogatari kenkyū jiten.* Tokyo: Meiji Shoin, 1978.

Igarashi Tomio. *Goze: ryogeinin no kiroku.* Tokyo: Ōfūsha, 1987.

Inoue Tatsushichirō. *Ganka eiseigaku.* Tokyo: Handaya Iseki Shōten, 1894. National Diet Library Digital Collections. http://dl.ndl.go.jp/info:ndljp/pid/836224

Inoue Toyotarō. *Ganbyō torahōmu ron.* Edited by Inoue Seiki. Tokyo: Tōkyō Ganka Byōin, 1904. National Diet Library Digital Collections. http://dl.ndl.go.jp/info: ndljp/pid/836303

Inoue Toyotarō. *Kingan torahōmu ryōyōhō.* Edited by Katei Eiseikai. Tokyo: Daigakkan, 1904. National Diet Library Digital Collections. http://dl.ndl.go.jp/info:ndljp /pid/836309

Ishii, Nobuko. "Sekkyō-bushi." *Monumenta Nipponica* 44, no. 3 (1989): 283–307.
Itasaka, Noriko. "The Woman Reader as Symbol: Changes in Images of the Woman Reader in Ukiyo-e." In *The Female as Subject: Reading and Writing in Early Modern Japan*, edited by Peter F. Kornicki, Mara Patessio, and G. G. Rowley, 87–108. Ann Arbor: University of Michigan Center for Japanese Studies, University of Michigan Press, 2010.
Itō Risa. *Ningyō jōruri no doramatsurugī: Chikamatsu ikō no jōruri sakusha to Heike monogatari. Waseda Daigaku gakujutsu sōsho*, no. 19. Tokyo: Waseda Daigaku Shuppanbu, 2011.
Jackson, Terrence. *Network of Knowledge: Western Science and the Tokugawa Information Revolution.* Honolulu: University of Hawai'i Press, 2016.
Jannetta, Ann. "Diseases of the Early Modern Period in Japan." In *The Cambridge World History of Human Disease*, edited by Kenneth F. Kiple, 385–89. New York: Cambridge University Press, 2008.
Jannetta, Ann. *The Vaccinators: Smallpox, Medical Knowledge, and the "Opening" of Japan.* Stanford: Stanford University Press, 2007.
Jansen, Marius B. *The Making of Modern Japan.* Cambridge, MA: Belknap Press of Harvard University Press, 2002.
Jansen, Marius B. "Rangaku and Westernization." *Modern Asian Studies* 18, no. 4 (1984): 541–53.
Johnson, Hiroko. *Western Influences on Japanese Art: The Akita Ranga Art School and Foreign Books.* Amsterdam: Hotei Publishing, 2005.
Josephson, Jason Ānanda. "An Empowered World: Buddhist Medicine and the Potency of Prayer in Japan." In *Deus in Machina: Religion, Technology, and the Things in Between*, edited by Jeremy Stolow, 117–41. New York: Fordham University Press, 2013.
Katafuchi Mihoko. "Edo yōjōron e no michiyuki: jūroku seiki kara jūshichi seiki zenhan ni okeru shintai e no hairyo." *Supōtsushi kenkyū*, no. 16 (2003): 79–85.
Katō Yasuaki. *Nihon mōjin shakaishi kenkyū.* Tokyo: Miraisha, 1974.
Katori Toshimitsu. "Edoki no shinkyū anma to shikaku shōgaisha: Sugiyama-ryū shinjutsu no Edo kara Meiji no tenkai o chūshin ni." *Shakai shinkyūgaku kenkyū* 11 (2016): 7–24.
Katori Toshimitsu. "Mishima sōkengyō Yasu'ichi no shiryō to Tsuchiura no densetsu." *Idō no Nihon*, no. 793 (2009): 100–109.
Katori Toshimitsu. "Sugiyama kengyō Wa'ichi no deshitachi." In *Kinsei ni okeru chiiki shihai to bunka*, edited by Kitahara Susumu, 299–331. Tokyo: Taiga Shobō, 2003.
Kawamura, Kunimitsu. "A Female Shaman's Mind and Body, and Possession." *Asian Folklore Studies* 62 (2003): 255–87.
Kim, Eunjung. *Curative Violence: Rehabilitating Disability, Gender, and Sexuality in Modern Korea.* Durham: Duke University Press, 2017.
Kim, Hoi-eun. *Doctors of Empire: Medical and Cultural Encounters between Imperial Germany and Meiji Japan.* Toronto: University of Toronto Press, 2014.
Kinda'ichi Haruhiko. *Heikyoku kō.* Tokyo: Sanseidō, 1997.
Knecht, Peter. "Japanese Shamanism." In *Shamanism: An Encyclopedia of World Beliefs, Practices, and Culture*, edited by Mariko Nambo Walter and Eva Jane Neumann Fridman, 1:674–80. Santa Barbara: ABC-CLIO, 2004.
Kogawa Kenzaburō. *Kōhon Nihon ganka gakushi.* Tokyo: Tohōdō Shoten, 1904.
Koida Tomoko. *Hotoke to onna no Muromachi: Monogatari sōshi ron.* Tokyo: Kasama Shoin, 2008.

Komoda Haruko. "Heike mabushi no Edo denpa ni tsuite." *Heikyoku shinpojiumu, Aichi Kenritsu Daigaku Bungaku Bunkazai Kenkyūjo nenpō* 5 (2012): 99–109.
Komoda Haruko. *Heike no ongaku: tōdō no dentō.* Tokyo: Daiichi Shobō, 2003.
Komoda Haruko. "Kyōto Daigaku-zō *Heikyoku mabushi*: sono seiritsu jijō to shutten chūki ni tsuite." *Tōyō ongaku kenkyū* 55 (1990): 31–90.
Komoda, Haruko. "The Musical Narrative of *The Tale of the Heike.*" Translated by Alison McQueen Tokita. In *The Ashgate Research Companion to Japanese Music,* edited by Alison McQueen Tokita and David W. Hughes, 77–104. Burlington, VT: Ashgate, 2008.
Komoda Haruko. "Nagoya heikyoku no ryūha o megutte: Maeda-ryū ka Hatano-ryū ka." *Tōyō ongaku kenkyū* 62 (1997): 1–20.
Kornicki, Peter. "Manuscript, not Print: Scribal Culture in the Edo Period." *Journal of Japanese Studies* 32, no. 1 (2006): 23–52.
Kornicki, Peter. "Women, Education, and Literacy." In *The Female as Subject: Reading and Writing in Early Modern Japan,* edited by Peter F. Kornicki, Mara Patessio, and G. G. Rowley, 7–38. Ann Arbor: University of Michigan Center for Japanese Studies, University of Michigan Press, 2010.
Kovacs, Jürgen, and Paul Unschuld, trans. *Essential Subtleties on the Silver Sea: The Yin-Hai Jing-Wei: A Chinese Classic on Ophthalmology.* Berkeley: University of California Press, 1998.
Kudlick, Catherine. "Comment: On the Borderland of Medical and Disability History." *Bulletin of the History of Medicine* 87, no. 4 (2013): 540–59.
Kudlick, Catherine. "Social History of Medicine and Disability History." In *The Oxford Handbook of Disability History,* edited by Michael Rembis, Catherine Kudlick, and Kim E. Nielsen, 105–24. New York: Oxford University Press, 2018.
Kurihara Tsuyakichi. *Hikari usure iku toki: Meiji no mōshōnen ga kyōshi ni naru made.* Tokyo: Azusa Shoten, 1993.
Kurihara Tsuyakichi. *Taishō no Tōkyō mōgakkō.* Tokyo: Azusa Shoten, 1986.
Kuriyama, Shigehisa. *The Expressiveness of the Body and the Divergence of Greek and Chinese Medicine.* 3rd printing. New York: Zone Books, 2002.
Kuriyama, Shigehisa. "The Historical Origins of Katakori." *Japan Review,* no. 9 (1997): 127–49.
Linker, Beth. "On the Borderland of Medical and Disability History: A Survey of the Fields." *Bulletin of the History of Medicine* 87, no. 4 (2013): 499–535.
Low, Morris. "Medical Representations of the Body in Japan: Gender, Class, and Discourse in the Eighteenth Century." *Annals of Science* 53, no. 4 (1996): 345–59.
Machi Senjurō. "Igakkan no gakumon keisei (1): Igakkan seiritsu zengo." *Nihon ishigaku zasshi* 45, no. 3 (1999): 339–70.
Marcon, Federico. "Inventorying Nature: Tokugawa Yoshimune and the Sponsorship of *Honzōgaku* in Eighteenth-Century Japan." In *Japan at Nature's Edge: The Environmental Context of a Global Power,* edited by Ian Jared Miller, Julia Adeney Thomas, and Brett L. Walker, 189–206. Honolulu: University of Hawai'i Press, 2013.
Marcon, Federico. *The Knowledge of Nature and the Nature of Knowledge in Early Modern Japan.* Chicago: University of Chicago Press, 2015.
Mass, Jeffrey P. *Yoritomo and the Founding of the First Bakufu: The Origins of Dual Government in Japan.* Stanford: Stanford University Press, 1999.
Matisoff, Susan. *The Legend of Semimaru: Blind Musician of Japan.* New York: Columbia University Press, 1978.

Matisoff, Susan. "Nō as Transformed by Chikamatsu." *Journal of the Association of Teachers of Japanese* 11, no. 2/3 (1976): 201–16.

Matisoff, Susan, trans. "Semimaru." In *Twenty Plays of the Nō Theatre*, edited by Donald Keene with Royall Tyler, 99–114. New York: Columbia University Press, 1970.

Matsuda Michio, ed. *Yōjōkun.* Tokyo: Chūō Kōronsha, 1973.

McClain, James L. "Failed Expectations: Kaga Domain on the Eve of the Meiji Restoration." *Journal of Japanese Studies* 14, no. 2 (1988): 403–47.

Metzler, Irina. *A Social History of Disability in the Middle Ages: Cultural Considerations of Physical Impairment.* New York: Routledge, 2013.

Mishima, Saiichi. *The History of Ophthalmology in Japan.* Oostende, Belgium: J. P. Wayenborgh, 2004.

Mitchell, David T., and Sharon L. Snyder. *Narrative Prosthesis: Disability and the Dependencies of Discourse.* Ann Arbor: University of Michigan Press, 2000.

Miyachi Takehiko. "Hizen mōsō kō." *Ningen bunka kenkyū* (Nagasaki Junshin Daigaku) 1 (March 2003): 17–31.

Miyano Hiroki. "Kinsei kōki Shōren'in ni yoru mōsō shihai jittai." *Nanakuma shigaku* 9 (2008): 17–40.

Miyazaki Masao. "Shīboruto no sandō tengan'yaku." *Yakushigaku zasshi* 29, no. 3 (1994): 469–83.

Muroki Yatarō. "Jōrurihime monogatari." In *Jōruri no tanjō to kojōruri*, edited by Muroki Yatarō et al. Vol. 7, *Iwanami kōza* (*kabuki bunraku*), 3–26. Tokyo: Iwanami Shoten, 1998.

Murota Yasuo. "Iwahashi Takeo kenkyū oboegaki: sono ayumi to gyōseki o chūshin ni." *Kwansei Gakuin Daigaku jinken kenkyū* 13 (March 2009): 27–46.

Nagai Akiko. "Chikuzen Chikugo no mōsō shūdan to sono shūhen." In *Mibunteki shūen*, edited by Tsukada Takashi, Yoshida Nobuyuki, and Wakita Osamu, 255–93. Kyoto: Buraku Mondai Kenkyūjo, 1994.

Nagai Akiko. *Nikkan mōsō no shakaishi.* Fukuoka-shi: Ashi Shobō, 2002.

Nagao Eiichi Kyōju Taikan Kinen Ronbunshū Kankōkai, ed. *Shinkyū anmashi ronkō: Nagao Eiichi kyōju taikan kinen ronbunshū.* Tokyo: Ōunkai, 2004.

Nagata Naoko. "Kinsei kōki ni okeru kanja no ishi sentaku: Suzuki Heikurō Kōshi nikki o chūshin ni." *Bulletin of the National Museum of Japanese History* 116 (February 2004): 317–42.

Nakamura, Karen. *Deaf in Japan: Signing and the Politics of Identity.* Ithaca: Cornell University Press, 2006.

Nakano Hatayoshi. "Mōsō to biwagaku." *Ōita Kenritsu Geijutsu Bunka Tanki Daigaku kenkyū kiyō* 6 (1967): 11–16.

Nakayama, Izumi. "Posturing for Modernity: Mishima Michiyoshi and School Hygiene in Meiji Japan." *East Asian Science, Technology, and Society: An International Journal* 6, no. 3 (2012): 355–78.

Narita Mamoru. *Mōsō no denshō: Kyūshū chihō no biwa hōshi.* Tokyo: Miyai Shoten, 1985.

Nenzi, Laura. *Excursions of Identity: Travel and the Intersection of Place, Gender, and Status in Edo Japan.* Honolulu: University of Hawai'i Press, 2008.

Nenzi, Laura. "To Ise at All Costs: Religious and Economic Implications of Early Modern Nukemairi." *Japanese Journal of Religious Studies* 33, no. 1 (2006): 75–114.

Nielsen, Kim E. *A Disability History of the United States.* Boston: Beacon Press, 2012.

Nielsen, Kim E. *The Life of Anna Ott: Money, Marriage, and Madness.* Springfield: University of Illinois Press, 2020.

Nielsen, Kim E. *The Radical Lives of Helen Keller.* New York: New York University Press, 2004.

Nishioka Yōko. "Jishin mōsō no shakumon." In *Kōtō denshō "yomi, katari, hanashi" no sekai,* edited by Fukuda Akira, Iwase Hiroshi, and Hanabe Hideo. Vol. 10, *Kōza Nihon no denshō bungaku,* 157–70. Tokyo: Miyai Shoten, 2004.

Nomura Zuiten. *Sōhen-ryū: rekishi to keifu.* Kyoto: Mitsumura Suiko Shoin, 1987.

Ogasawara Yoshiaki. "Shichōkaku shōgaiji kyōiku no akebono ni okeru kigyōka fuiransoropī: Ōsaka Mōain to Godai Gohē o chūshin ni." *Kyōto Kōka Joshi Daigaku kenkyū kiyō* 50:162–72.

Ogata Akiko. "Bakumatsu Higo ni okeru tōdōza." Presentation, December 6, 2008, 1–18. Kumamoto University repository. http://hdl.handle.net/2298/10310

Ogata Akiko. "Kinsei Higo ni okeru tōdōza no kakuritsu." *Kumamoto Daigaku shakai bunka kenkyū* 9 (March 2011): 121–40.

Ogata Akiko. "Zamoto kikiyaku senshutsu kara miru Kumamoto-han no tōdōza." *Kumamoto Daigaku shakai bunka kenkyū* 10 (March 2012): 79–97.

Okumura Mitsuo. *Heikyoku fuhon no kenkyū.* Tokyo: Ōfūsha, 1981.

Ōmachi Keigetsu, ed. *Ekiken jikkun: ge.* Tokyo: Shiseidō, 1911. National Diet Library Digital Collections. http://dl.ndl.go.jp/info:ndljp/pid/754686

Ono Bunkei. *Kaisetsu Shinkyū chōhōki.* Tokyo: Idō no Nipponsha, 1973.

Otake, Tomoko. "New Law Bans Bias against People with Disabilities, but Shortcomings Exist, Say Experts." *Japan Times,* May 2, 2016. https://www.japantimes.co.jp/news/2016/05/02/reference/new-law-bans-bias-against-people-with-disabilities-but-shortcomings-exist-say-experts/

Ott, Katherine. "Disability Things: Material Culture and American Disability History, 1700–2010." In *Disability Histories,* edited by Susan Burch and Michael Rembis, 119–35. Springfield: University of Illinois Press, 2014.

Ōura Hiromasa. "Ashihara kengyō no ashiato." *Nihon ishigaku zasshi* 51, no. 1 (2005): 51–81.

Ōura Hiromasa, Hanawa Toshihiko, and Ishino Shōgo. "Sugiyama Shinden-ryū no keishōsha tachi." *Nihon ishigaku zasshi* 50, no. 1 (2004): 70–71.

Ōura Hiromasa, and Ichikawa Yūri. "Wada Masanaga no nokoshita *Sugiyama shinden-ryū* zenkan no kenshō." *Nihon ishigaku zasshi* 55, no. 3 (2009): 329–45.

Ōura Hiromasa, and Kosoto Hiroshi. "Sugiyama Kengyō Itoku Kenshōkaisho zō no *Sugiyama shinden-ryū.*" *Nihon ishigaku zasshi* 50, no. 2 (2004): 223–41.

Ōura Jikan. *Sugiyama Shinden-ryū rinshō shinan.* Tokyo: Rikuzensha, 2007.

Oyler, Elizabeth. *Swords, Oaths, and Prophetic Visions: Authoring Warrior Rule in Medieval Japan.* Honolulu: University of Hawai'i Press, 2006.

Ozaki Masatada. *Heike chūkō no so: Ogino kengyō.* Nagoya: Aichi-ken Kyōdo Shiryō Kankōkai, 1976.

Ozaki Masatada. "Ogino kengyō to Heike mabushi no kōkeisha." In *DVD-ban Ozaki-ke bon Heike mabushi kaisetsu,* edited by Ogino Kengyō Kenshōkai, 49–64. Nagoya: Sōkō Eshikkusu, 2011.

Paulson, William R. *Enlightenment, Romanticism, and the Blind in France.* Princeton: Princeton University Press, 1987.

Pennington, Lee K. *Casualties of History: Wounded Japanese Servicemen and the Second World War.* Ithaca: Cornell University Press, 2015.

Platt, Brian. *Burning and Building: Schooling and State Formation in Japan, 1750–1890.* Cambridge, MA: Harvard University Asia Center, Harvard University Press, 2004.

Platt, Brian. "Japanese Childhood, Modern Childhood: The Nation-State, the School, and 19th-Century Globalization." *Journal of Social History* 38, no. 4 (2005): 965–85.

Plutschow, Herbert. "The Placatory Nature of *The Tale of the Heike*: Additional Documents and Thoughts." In *Currents in Japanese Culture: Translations and Transformations*, edited by Amy Vladeck Heinrich, 71–80. New York: Columbia University Press, 1997.

Rapp, Rayna, and Faye Ginsburg. "Enabling Disability: Rewriting Kinship, Reimagining Citizenship." *Public Culture* 13, no. 3 (2001): 533–56.

Roberts, Luke S. *Mercantilism in a Japanese Domain: The Merchant Origins of Economic Nationalism in 18th-Century Tosa.* New York: Cambridge University Press, 2002.

Roberts, Luke S. "Shipwrecks and Flotsam: The Foreign World in Edo-Period Tosa." *Monumenta Nipponica* 70, no. 1 (2015): 83–122.

Rogaski, Ruth. *Hygienic Modernity: Meanings of Health and Disease in Treaty-Port China.* Berkeley: University of California Press, 2004.

Rotermund, Hartmut O. "Demonic Affliction or Contagious Disease? Changing Perceptions of Smallpox in the Late Edo Period." *Japanese Journal of Religious Studies* 28, nos. 3–4 (2001): 373–98.

Rotermund, Hartmut O. "Illness Illustrated. Social Historical Dimensions of Late Edo Measles Pictures (Hashika-e)." In *Written Texts–Visual Texts: Woodblock-Printed Media in Early Modern Japan*, edited by Susanne Formanek and Sepp Linhart, 251–82. Amsterdam: Hotei Publishing, 2005.

Rowden, Terry. *The Songs of Blind Folk: African American Musicians and the Cultures of Blindness.* Ann Arbor: University of Michigan Press, 2009.

Rowley, G. G. *An Imperial Concubine's Tale: Scandal, Shipwreck, and Salvation in Seventeenth-Century Japan.* New York: Columbia University Press, 2013.

Rubinger, Richard. *Private Academies of the Tokugawa Period.* Princeton: Princeton University Press, 1982.

Saiki Kazuma. *Kokiroku no kenkyū (ge).* Tokyo: Yoshikawa Kōbunkan, 1989.

Saitō Masao. "Onkodō Hanawa sensei den ni tsuite." In *Hanawa Hokinoichi ronsan (gekan)*, edited by Onko Gakkai, 111–38. Tokyo: Kinseisha, 1976.

Sakuma Jun'ichi. *Goze no minzoku.* Vol. 91, *Minzoku mingei sōsho.* Tokyo: Iwasaki Bijutsusha, 1983.

Saya Makito. *Heike monogatari kara jōruri e: Atsumori setsuwa no hen'yō.* Tokyo: Keiō Gijuku Daigaku Shuppankai, 2002.

Scalenghe, Sara. *Disability in the Ottoman Arab World, 1500–1800.* New York: Cambridge University Press, 2014.

Screech, Timon. *The Lens within the Heart: The Western Scientific Gaze and Popular Imagery in Later Edo Japan.* Honolulu: University of Hawai'i Press, 2002.

Shakespeare, Tom. "The Social Model of Disability." In *The Disability Studies Reader*, edited by Lennard Davis, 214–21. New York: Routledge, 2013.

Shinmura Taku. *Kodai iryō kanninsei no kenkyū.* Tokyo: Hōsei Daigaku Shuppankyoku, 1983.

Shinmura Taku. *Nihon iryōshi.* Tokyo: Yoshikawa Kōbunkan, 2006/2009.

Siebers, Tobin. "Returning the Social to the Social Model." In *The Matter of Disability: Materiality, Biopolitics, Crip Affect*, edited by David T. Mitchell, Susan Antebi, and Sharon L. Snyder, 39–47. Ann Arbor: University of Michigan Press, 2019.

Smits, Gregory. "Shaking Up Japan: Edo Society and the 1855 Catfish Picture Prints." *Journal of Social History* 39, no. 4 (2006): 1045–78.

Snyder, Sharon L., and David T. Mitchell. *Cultural Locations of Disability*. Chicago: University of Chicago Press, 2006.

Spafford, David. *A Sense of Place: The Political Landscape in Late Medieval Japan*. Cambridge, MA: Harvard University Asia Center, Harvard University Press, 2013.

Stanley-Baker, Michael. "'Indian Massage' from Sun Simiao's Prescriptions Worth a Thousand in Gold." In *Buddhism and Medicine: An Anthology of Premodern Sources*, edited by C. Pierce Salguero, 533–37. New York: Columbia University Press, 2017.

Stevens, Carolyn. *Disability in Japan*. New York: Routledge, 2013.

Sugano Noriko. *Edo jidai no kōkōsha: Kōgiroku no sekai*. Tokyo: Yoshikawa Kōbunkan, 1999.

Sugano, Noriko. "State Indoctrination of Filial Piety in Tokugawa Japan." Translated by Sherri Bayouth. Edited by Anne Walthall. In *Women and Confucian Cultures in Premodern China, Korea, and Japan*, edited by Dorothy Ko, JaHyun Kim Haboush, and Joan R. Piggott, 170–92. Berkeley: University of California Press, 2003.

Suzuki Eiichi. "Mito-han no igaku to iryō." *Nihon ishigaku zasshi* 56, no. 2 (2010): 160–62.

Suzuki Noriko. "Edo jidai no igakusho ni miru baidokukan ni tsuite." In *Nihon baidokushi no kenkyū: iryō, shakai, kokka*, edited by Fukuda Mahito and Suzuki Noriko, 37–66. Kyoto: Shibunkaku Shuppan, 2005.

Suzuki Noriko. "Kinsei raibyōkan no keisei to tenkai." In *Rekishi no naka no raisha*, edited by Fujino Yutaka, 83–140. Tokyo: Yumiru Shuppan, 1996.

Suzuki Takatsune. "Heikyoku fuhon toshite no tokushoku." In *DVD-ban Ozaki-ke bon Heike mabushi kaisetsu*, edited by Ogino Kengyō Kenshōkai, 5–12. Nagoya: Sōkō Eshikkusu, 2011.

Suzuki Takatsune. *Heikyoku to Heike monogatari*. Tokyo: Chisen Shokan, 2007.

Suzuki Takatsune. "Koe no denshō, koe no kigōka: Heike ginpu kara Heike mabushi e." *Jinbun kagaku kenkyū* (Niigata Daigaku) 128 (2011): 1–19.

Suzuki Takatsune. "Shiryō shōkai Tōdō ryakki." *Jinbun kagaku kenkyū* (Niigata Daigaku) 110 (2002): 35–101.

Suzuki Takatsune. "Tōdō no koshikimoku: kaidai to honkoku." In *Fugeki mōsō no denshō sekai*, edited by Fukuda Akira and Yamashita Kin'ichi, 3:246–79. Tokyo: Miyai Shoten, 2006.

Suzuki Toshio. "Edo jidai ni okeru yōjōsho no kenkyū: shintai undō no yōjōteki kachi o megutte." *Hokkaidō Daigaku Kyōiku Gakubu kiyō*, no. 22 (1973): 411–24.

Suzuki, Yui. *Medicine Master Buddha: The Iconic Worship of Yakushi in Heian Japan*. Leiden: Brill, 2012.

Takahashi Sada'ichi. *Heike monogatari Kaku'ichi-bon shinkō: Yasakaryū-bon no seiritsu ruden*. Kyoto: Shibunkaku Shuppan, 1993.

Takizawa Toshiyuki. "Jūkyū seiki zenki yōjōron ni okeru ningen keiseikan no kōsatsu." *Kyōikugaku kenkyū* (Nihon Kyōiku Gakkai) 57, no. 2 (1990): 159–68.

Tan, Wei Yu Wayne. "The Brain in Text and in Image: Reconfiguring Medical Knowledge in Late Eighteenth-Century Japan." In *Visualizing the Body in Art, Anatomy, and Medicine since 1800: Models and Modeling*, edited by Andrew Graciano, 87–104. New York: Routledge, 2019.

Tanihara Hidenobu. "Hosokawa Tadaoki to Edo jidai shoki no ganka." *Nihon Ganka Gakkai zasshi* 122, no. 9 (2018): 675–84.

Tanihara Hidenobu. "Hyōshi no kaisetsu: Nihon de saisho no ganka senmon'i: Majima Seigan to Majima-ryū ni tsuite." *Ganka* 55, no. 9 (2013): 977–83.

Tateyama Zennoshin. *Heike ongakushi*. Tokyo: Kimura Yasushige, 1910.

Terao Kōji. "Kinsei jiin no kashitsuke ni tsuite: Shōren'in myōmokukin no kenkyū josetsu." *Sangyō keizai ronsō* (Kyōto Sangyō Daigaku) 2, no. 3 (1967): 107–32.

Thomas, Roger. "Approaches to Oneiric Texts and Imagery in Early Modern Japan." *Journal of Japanese Studies* 45, no. 1 (2019): 57–90.

Thompson, C. Michele. *Vietnamese Traditional Medicine: A Social History.* Singapore: National University of Singapore Press, 2015.

Tokita, Alison McQueen. *Japanese Singers of Tales: Ten Centuries of Performed Narrative.* New York: Routledge, 2015.

Tōkyō Mōgakkō, ed. *Tōkyō mōgakkō ichiran.* Tokyo: Tōkyō Mōgakkō, 1926. National Diet Library Digital Collections. https://dl.ndl.go.jp/info:ndljp/pid/941237

Tomikura Tokujirō. *Heike monogatari kenkyū.* Tokyo: Kadokawa Shoten, 1964.

Toyama baiyaku gyōshi (jōkan). Edited by Takaoka Kōtō Shōgyō Gakkō. Takaoka: Takaoka Kōtō Shōgyō Gakkō, 1935. National Diet Library Digital Collections. https://dl.ndl.go.jp/info:ndljp/pid/1050431

Trambaiolo, Daniel. "Ancient Texts and New Medical Ideas in Eighteenth-Century Japan." In *Antiquarianism, Language, and Medical Philology: From Early Modern to Modern Sino-Japanese Medical Discourses,* edited by Benjamin Elman, 81–104. Leiden: Brill, 2015.

Trambaiolo, Daniel. "Antisyphilitic Mercury Drugs in Early Modern China and Japan." *Asiatische Studien: Zeitschrift der Schweizerischen Asiengesellschaft (Études Asiatiques: Revue de la Société Suisse-Asie)* 69, nos. 3–4 (2015): 997–1016.

Trambaiolo, Daniel. "Epidemics and Epistemology in Early Modern Japan: Japanese Responses to Chinese Writings on Warm Epidemics and Sand-Rashes." In *Translation at Work: Chinese Medicine in the First Global Age,* edited by Harold Cook, 157–75. Leiden: Brill, 2020.

Trambaiolo, Daniel. "Native and Foreign in Tokugawa Medicine." *Journal of Japanese Studies* 39, no. 2 (2013): 299–324.

Trambaiolo, Daniel. "Vaccination and the Politics of Medical Knowledge in Nineteenth-Century Japan." *Bulletin of the History of Medicine* 88, no. 3 (2014): 431–56.

Trambaiolo, Daniel. "Writing, Authority and Practice in Tokugawa Japan, 1650–1850." PhD diss., Princeton University, 2014.

Triplett, Katja. "Using the Golden Needle: Nāgārjuna Boddhisattva's Ophthalmological Treatise and Other Sources in the Essentials of Medical Treatment." In *Buddhism and Medicine: An Anthology of Premodern Sources,* edited by C. Pierce Salguero, 543–48. New York: Columbia University Press, 2017.

Tsukuba Daigaku Fuzoku Mōgakkō Dōsōkai Kōenkai, ed. *Mōa kyōiku bunrigo hyakunen, Nazureba yubi ni akirakeshi: Tsukuba Daigaku Fuzoku Mōgakkō kinen bunshū.* Tokyo: Ōunkai, 2011.

Ubukata Takashige. "Okumura-ke monjo kaisetsu." In *Tōdōza heike biwa shiryō: Okumura-ke zō,* edited by Atsumi Kaoru, Maeda Mineko, and Ubukata Takashige, 399–408. Kyoto: Daigakudō Shoten, 1984.

Ueda Kenji. "Hanawa Hokinoichi to kokugaku." In *Hanawa Hokinoichi ronsan (jōkan),* edited by Onko Gakkai, 29–55. Tokyo: Kinseisha, 1976.

Umeda Chihiro. "Kinsei Nara no mōsō soshiki." In *Kinsei no shūkyō to shakai: chiiki no hirogari to shūkyō,* vol. 1, edited by Aoyagi Shūichi, Takano Toshihiko, and Nishida Kahoru, 92–115. Tokyo: Yoshikawa Kōbunkan, 2008.

Umihara Ryō. *Edo jidai no ishi shūgyō: gakumon, gakutō, yūgaku.* Tokyo: Yoshikawa Kōbunkan, 2014.

Umihara Ryō. "Edo no rangakusha: Bunseiki 'Ika jinmeiroku' no bunseki kara." *Bulletin of the National Museum of Japanese History* 116 (February 2004): 91–108.

Umihara Ryō. "Kinsei ganka'i no mibun sonritsu to gakutō." *Rekishi kagaku* (Ōsaka Rekishi Kagaku Kyōgikai) 199 (2009–11): 19–32.

Umihara Ryō. *Kinsei iryō no shakaishi: chishiki, gijutsu, jōhō.* Tokyo: Yoshikawa Kōbunkan, 2007.

Vaporis, Constantine. *Breaking Barriers: Travel and the State in Early Modern Japan.* Cambridge, MA: Harvard University Asia Center, Harvard University Press, 1994.

Vaporis, Constantine. *Tour of Duty: Samurai, Military Service in Edo, and the Culture of Early Modern Japan.* Honolulu: University of Hawai'i Press, 2008.

Vigouroux, Mathias. "Edo jidai ni okeru shinkyū igaku: sono shisō no enkaku." *Nihon ishigaku zasshi* 54, no. 1 (2008): 74–76.

Vigouroux, Mathias. "The Reception of the Circulation Channels Theory in Japan (1500–1800)." In *Antiquarianism, Language, and Medical Philology: From Early Modern to Modern Sino-Japanese Medical Discourses,* edited by Benjamin A. Elman, 105–32. Leiden: Brill, 2015.

Wakita Osamu. *Kawara makimono no sekai.* Tokyo: Tōkyō Daigaku Shuppankai, 1991.

Wakuda Tetsuji. "Edoki no anma jutsu." *Idō no Nihon,* no. 813 (2011): 41–45.

Waldschmidt, Anne. "Disability Goes Cultural: The Cultural Model of Disability as an Analytical Tool." In *Culture—Theory—Disability: Encounters between Disability Studies and Cultural Studies,* edited by Anne Waldschmidt, Hanjo Berressem, and Moritz Ingwersen, 19–28. Bielefeld: Transcript Verlag, 2017.

Watanabe, Takeshi. *Flowering Tales: Women Exorcising History in Heian Japan.* Cambridge, MA: Harvard University Asia Center, Harvard University Press, 2020.

Weygand, Zina. *The Blind in French Society from the Middle Ages to the Century of Louis Braille.* Translated by Emily-Jane Cohen. Stanford: Stanford University Press, 2009.

Weygand, Zina. "Blind Love: A Love under Constraints." Translated by Tammy Berberi. *Journal of Literary and Cultural Disability Studies* 10, no. 2 (2016): 223–37.

Wheatley, Edward. *Stumbling Blocks before the Blind: Medieval Constructions of a Disability.* Ann Arbor: University of Michigan Press, 2010.

Williams, Duncan Ryūken. *The Other Side of Zen: A Social History of Sōtō Zen Buddhism in Tokugawa Japan.* Princeton: Princeton University Press, 2005.

Wortley, Kathryn. "Yellow Brick Roads: How Japan's Tactile Paving Aids Solo Travel." *Japan Times,* August 22, 2020. https://www.japantimes.co.jp/news/2020/08/22/national/social-issues/tactile-paving-visually-impaired/

Yamada Akira. *Tsūshi: Nihon no shōgaisha—Meiji, Taishō, Shōwa.* Tokyo: Akashi Shoten, 2013.

Yamada, Keisuke. "Rethinking *Iemoto*: Theorizing Individual Agency in the *Tsugaru Shamisen* Oyama-ryū." *Asian Music* 48, no. 1 (2017): 28–57.

Yamada Kōta. "Matsushiro hanryō no mōjin: Kōka san umadoshi Tōjio-mura ameya Heisuke joshi ikken." In *Han chiiki no kōzō to hen'yō: Shinano no kuni Matsushiro-han chiiki no kenkyū,* edited by Watanabe Takashi, 179–240. Tokyo: Iwata Shoin, 2005.

Yamada Tomoko. "Hōraiji to Mikawa Owari no Yakushi shinkō." In *Yakushi shinkō,* edited by Gorai Shigeru, 79–96. Vol. 12, *Minshū shūkyō shisōsho.* Tokyo: Yūzankaku Shuppan, 1986.

Yamashita Hiroaki. *Heike monogatari no seisei.* Tokyo: Meiji Shoin, 1984.

Yamashita Takeshi. *Edo jidai shomin kyōka seisaku no kenkyū.* Tokyo: Azekura Shobō, 1969.

Yokota Noriko. "Monoyoshi kō: kinsei Kyōto no raisha ni tsuite." *Nihonshi kenkyū* 352 (1991): 1–29.

Yonemoto, Marcia. *The Problem of Women in Early Modern Japan.* Berkeley: University of California Press, 2016.

Young, William Evan. "Family Matters: Managing Illness in Late Tokugawa Japan, 1750–1868." PhD diss., Princeton University, 2015.

Zhang, Zhibin, and Paul Unschuld. *Dictionary of the Ben Cao Gang Mu.* Vol. 1, *Chinese Historical Illness Terminology.* Berkeley: University of California Press, 2015.

Bibliography · 260

Index

242 · Index

Printed and bound by CPI Group (UK) Ltd, Croydon, CR0 4YY

09/06/2025

14686136-0001